Colorectal Cancer

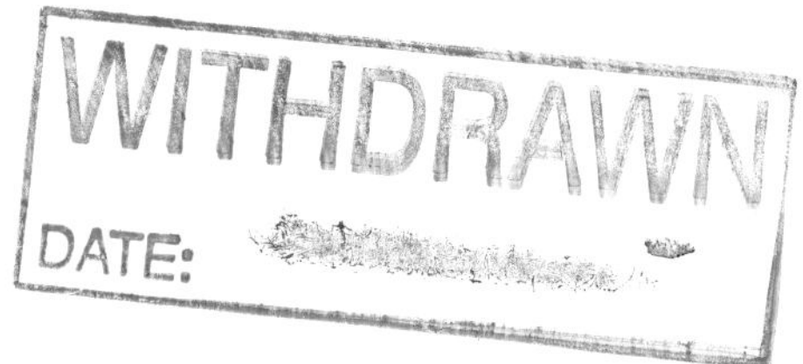

Colorectal Cancer

Edited by

Colin S. McArdle MD FRCS
Professor of Surgery, University of Edinburgh, Royal Infirmary, UK

David J. Kerr MD DSc FRCP
Professor of Clinical Oncology, CRC Institute for Cancer Studies, University of Birmingham, UK

Peter Boyle PhD
Director, Division of Epidemiology and Biostatistics, European Institute of Oncology, Milan, Italy and Professor, The Medical School, University of Birmingham, UK

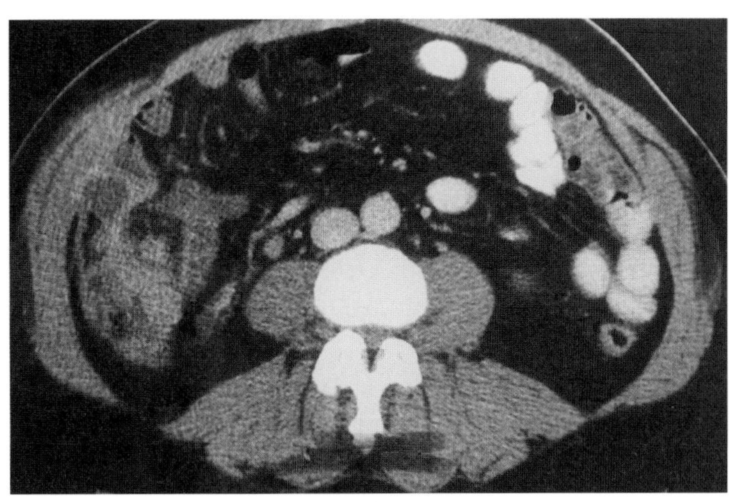

59 St. Aldates
Oxford OX1 1ST, UK

First published 2000

British Library Cataloguing in Publication Data.
A catalogue record for this title is available from the British Library.

ISBN 1 899066 72 1

McArdle, C. (Colin)
Colorectal Cancer
Colin S. McArdle, David J. Kerr and Peter Boyle (eds)

Always refer to the manufacturer's Prescribing Information before prescribing drugs cited in this book.

Design
Ellen Moorcraft

Medical Artwork
Adrian and Gudrun Cornford,
Reinheim, Germany

Page layout
J&L Composition Ltd, UK

Image reproduction
Pixel Tech PTE Ltd, Singapore

Isis Medical Media staff
Commissioning Editor: John Harrison
Editorial Controllers: Sarah Carlson, Fiona Cornell
Production and Editorial Manager: Julia Savory
Production Manager: Sarah Sodhi

Printed and bound by
Craft Print International Ltd, Singapore

Distributed in the USA by
Books International Inc., P.O. Box 605,
Herndon, VA 20172, USA

Distributed in the rest of the world by
Plymbridge Distributors Ltd., Estover Road,
Plymouth, PL6 7PY, UK

CONTENTS

LIST OF CONTRIBUTORS

John H. Anderson MD FRCS
Consultant Surgeon, Department of Surgery, Royal Infirmary, Glasgow, UK

Riccardo A. Audisio MD
Consultant Surgeon, Surgical Oncologist and Honorary Senior Lecturer, University of Liverpool, Department of General Surgery, Whiston Hospital, Prescot, Merseyside, UK

Philippe Autier
Division of Epidemiology and Biostatistics, European Institute of Oncology, Milan, Italy

Dennis M. Balfe
Professor, Mallinckrodt Institute of Radiology, Washington University School of Medicine, St Louis, MO, USA

Jorge Luiz A. Bastos MD
Visiting Fellow, The Liver and Hepatobiliary Unit, Queen Elizabeth Hospital, Edgbaston, Birmingham, UK

D. Timothy Bishop PhD
Professor, ICRF Genetic Epidemiology Laboratory, St James's University Hospital, Leeds, UK

Peter Boyle PhD
Director, Division of Epidemiology and Biostatistics, European Institute of Oncology, Milan, Italy, and The Medical School, University of Birmingham, UK

Simon Bramhall MD FRCS(Gen Surg)
Lecturer in Surgery, The Liver and Hepatobiliary Unit, Queen Elizabeth Hospital, Edgbaston, Birmingham, UK

Steven R. Brown FRCS BMedSci
Research Fellow, ICRF Genetic Epidemiology Laboratory, St James's University Hospital, Leeds, UK

Harry J.G. Burns FRCS MPH
Director of Public Health, Greater Glasgow Health Board, Glasgow, UK

Jack Cuzick PhD
Head of Department of Mathematics, Statistics and Epidemiology, Imperial Cancer Research Fund, London, UK

Sina Dorudi BSc PhD FRCS FRCS(Gen)
Senior Lecturer and Consultant Colorectal Surgeon, St Bartholomew's and the Royal London School of Medicine and Dentistry,The Royal London Hospital, Whitechapel, London, UK

David R. Ferry FRCP PhD
Senior Lecturer in Oncology, CRC Institute for Cancer Studies, University of Birmingham, Edgbaston, Birmingham, UK

Nigel Gray
Division of Epidemiology and Biostatistics, European Institute of Oncology, Milan, Italy

Paul J. Hermanek MD, MDhc
Emeritus Professor of Surgical Pathology, Department of Surgery, Friedrich–Alexander-Universität, Erlangen, Germany

Roger D. James MRCP FRCR
Director, Cancer Services for Kent, The Kent Cancer Centre, Mid Kent Healthcare Trust, Maidstone Hospital, Barming, Kent, UK

David J. Kerr FRCP MD DSc
Professor of Clinical Oncology, CRC Institute for Cancer Studies, University of Birmingham, Edgbaston, Birmingham, UK

Michael J.S. Langman MD FRCP FMedSci
Professor of Medicine, University of Birmingham and Honorary Senior Research Fellow, Division of Epidemiology and Biostatistics, European Institute of Oncology, Milan, Italy

Walter E. Longo MD FACS FASCRS
Associate Professor of Sugery, Division of Colon and Rectal Surgery, St Louis University School of Medicine, St Louis, MO, USA

Colin McArdle MD FRCS
Professor, Department of Surgery, The University of Edinburgh, Royal Infirmary, Edinburgh, UK

Paul McMaster MA, MB, ChM, FRCS
Hepatobiliary and Transplant Surgeon/Professor, Department of Surgery, University of Birmingham, and The Liver and Hepatobiliary Unit, Edgbaston, Birmingham, UK

Patrick Maisonneuve
Division of Epidemiology and Biostatistics, European Institute of Oncology, Milan, Italy

Rachel S. Midgley BSc(Hons) MRCP
MRC Clinical Research Fellow, CRC Institute for Cancer Studies, University of Birmingham, Edgbaston, Birmingham, UK

Josef Rüschoff HMD
Department of Pathology, Klinikum Kassel, Kassel, Germany

Michelle D. Semin
Instructor, Mallinckrodt Institute of Radiology, Washington University School of Medicine, St Louis, MO, USA

Gianluca Severi
Division of Epidemiology and Biostatistics, European Institute of Oncology, Milan, Italy

Franco Uggeri MD
Professor of Surgery, Milan University, School of Medicine, Clinica Chirurgica Generale, Ospedale San Gerardo, Monza, Italy

Norman S. Williams MS FRCS
Professor of Surgery, St. Bartholomew's and the Royal London School of Medicine and Dentistry, The Royal London Hospital, Whitechapel, London, UK

Annie M. Young SRN BSc(Hons)
Research Fellow, Department of Nursing Studies, University of Birmingham, Edgbaston, Birmingham, UK

Chapter 1

EPIDEMIOLOGY OF COLORECTAL CANCER CONTROL

P. Boyle, H.J.G. Burns, N. Gray, P. Maisonneuve, G. Severi, P. Autier and M.J.S. Langman

Introduction

Over two-thirds of a million men and women are newly affected by colorectal cancer each year and nearly 400,000 deaths are caused by this condition annually. A strategy whose adoption and implementation could lead towards colorectal cancer control is presented with supporting evidence.

The usual paradigm of following axes of primary, secondary and tertiary prevention is broken and replaced by apportioning responsibility between various groups within society – the general public, individuals with a genetic risk of colorectal cancer, primary care doctors, health care purchasers and those responsible for specialist medical training. Colorectal cancer is one of the forms of cancer most strongly linked to aspects of lifestyle that may be prevented or detected early by individual action. The association with aspects of dietary practices and physical activity is too strong to ignore and needs implementation despite our ignorance of the time lag between implementation and prevention. A powerful logic suggests that an endoscopic intervention should be available to each individual, probably in the sixth decade, possibly repeated later but quite possibly not. There are two powerful drugs or drug combinations [aspirin and other non-steroidal anti-inflammatory drugs (NSAIDS); hormone replacement therapy (HRT)] which have a beneficial effect on the incidence of colorectal cancer. Again, the lag period has not been fully elucidated, and the drugs have a broad spectrum of effects; nevertheless, the existence of effect appears to be clear. The new cyclo-oxygenase (COX-2) inhibitors could have great potential for the prevention of colorectal cancer without the worrying side effect of bleeding peptic ulcer. The existence of a genetic factor for colorectal cancer is definite and careful history taking can define low-and high-risk groups in advance of the availability of mass genetic testing. Specialist treatment facilities should be provided by health care providers and those responsible for continual specialist training should introduce continuing medical education on a regular basis for consultant, surgeons, radiotherapists and physicians to keep them abreast of developments in their field.

To achieve the goal of colorectal cancer control it is necessary to make decisions regarding public health; part of this decision process involves deciding at which point enough epidemiological evidence is available to allow a confident change of focus from information generation to health actions. The challenge for those responsible for public health programmes is the urgent need to build this knowledge into preventive programmes which fit the health scheme of their country and the cultural background within which people, physicians and funding agencies operate. To achieve colorectal cancer control it is necessary at some point to abandon a neutral stance and face up to collective responsibilities. This may well be the time to do so for colorectal cancer: adoption of the guidelines presented here could reduce colorectal cancer mortality rates by well over half and perhaps three-quarters.

Colorectal cancer is estimated to be the third most common type of cancer worldwide.[1] It affects men and women almost equally, with approximately one-third of a million new cases diagnosed in each gender group each year.[1] In advanced colorectal cancer in which curative resection is possible, 5-year survival in patients with Dukes' B tumours is 45% which falls to 30% for those with Dukes' C tumours.[2] Five-year survival in those with resected Dukes' A tumours is around 80% and survival following simple resection of an adenomatous pedunculated polyp containing carcinoma in situ (or severe dysplasia) or intramucosal carcinoma is generally close to 100%. Nevertheless, it is estimated that there are 394,000 deaths from colorectal cancer worldwide annually.[3]

The aetiology of colorectal cancer is increasingly well understood,[4] and there is a strong body of evidence to support the potential of chemoprevention of colorectal cancer.[5] The published results of three trials have reported the effectiveness of annual haemocult testing in reducing mortality from colorectal cancer,[6–8] and retrospective studies of sigmoidoscopy confirm that this approach may greatly reduce mortality rates.[9–12] Treatment advances continue to be made gradually;[13] major differences in outcome have been demonstrated according to the nature of the treatment centre,[14] the ability of the surgeon[15] and between countries.[16]

The ultimate goal of all cancer research and cancer treatment is to prevent people dying from the disease in question. Knowledge has been accruing rapidly regarding actions and interventions which could lead to a reduction in death from colorectal cancer, by either reducing the risk of developing the disease, identifying the disease at a stage when it is more curable, or improving the outcome of therapy. Such a package of actions is aimed at colorectal cancer control, where progress will eventually come through contributions from the various elements of a control and prevention strategy.

There has always been the tendency inadvertently to blame individuals for their own cancers ('how many cigarettes did you smoke; why did you eat so much fat?') but there are groups other than the individual who should accept their responsibility and take a role in prevention. A smoker cannot alone to be held guilty of his habit if society allows cigarettes to be sold and smoked: society, through pricing policy, bans on advertising and restrictions on smokers' behaviour could affect smoking rates. The performance of doctors could be improved through their own efforts and health care providers and purchasers could improve health outcomes by introducing better facilities and standards of care. As regards colorectal cancer control, the general population, those members of the population with special risk profiles, primary care doctors, health care purchasers and those responsible for specialist higher medical training each have their own contribution to make.

Ten actions, the adoption and implementation of which could assist the control of colorectal cancer are outlined and discussed in this chapter. Prospects for preventing death from colorectal cancer are now brighter than they were as few as 10 years ago.[17] As stated above, to achieve this goal it is nec-

essary to make public health decisions from an informal stance guided by sufficient epidemiological evidence. This is a major point, as it is too easy for well-oiled, smooth-running data-collection 'machinery' to run on in a quasi-automatic mode without generating health actions.

Turning research findings into public health actions for colorectal cancer control requires a profound change of mentality of the epidemiological community. It is too easy to say that more studies are needed, when they are unlikely to alter existing conclusions. It is also essential to consider the implementation of cancer control activities in a manner different to that of cancer control research. Basically, although everyone is involved in cancer control activities, prime responsibility for the implementation of certain changes is vested in certain groups within a society.

The magnitude of the problem

DESCRIPTIVE EPIDEMIOLOGY OF COLORECTAL CANCER

The diseases of colon and rectal cancer appear to be distinct; however, unfortunately, there are recognized difficulties in distinguishing colon and rectal cancer in mortality statistics for a variety of reasons.[18] Wherever possible, the distinction between colon and rectum will be maintained in this chapter. In general terms, colon cancer is a disease of economically 'developed' countries. Before 60 years of age, the disease is slightly more common in women, whereas thereafter it is more frequent in men [18]

In men, seven of the ten highest rates of incidence of colon cancer are recorded in population groups in the United States with other high rates in Newfoundland (Canada), Hiroshima (Japan) and non-Maori in New Zealand (Table 1.1). It is potentially of considerable significance that these high rates are to be found in a variety of African-American population groups such as in Detroit [35.0/100,000 per annum (p.a.)], Los Angeles (34.8), San Francisco (33.8), Atlanta (32.4) and New Orleans (31.4). In men, the lowest rates of incidence are found in a variety of population groups in developing countries, with the lowest rate reported in Setif (Algeria) (0.5/100,000). In women, the highest rates of incidence again include African-American population groups in North America, with the lowest rates recorded in a similar group of populations as in men (Table 1.1). In each gender group, a number of low-rate regions are found in India.

The pattern is somewhat different for cancer of the rectum. In men and women, it is difficult to ignore the high rates in each gender in the Czech Republic and the high rates in Japanese population groups in Japan and in the United States (Table 1.2). Again, low annual rates per 100,000 are to be found in a variety of population groups in the developing countries with the lowest rates around 2 in men and 1 in women (Table 1.2).

When statistics for colon and rectum (colorectum), are combined the highest rate in men is recorded in the Japanese community in Hawaii (53.5/100,000). The high rates of incidence in men resident in the neighbouring French *départements* of Bas-Rhin and Haut-Rhin merit further study (Table 1.3). Again, the lowest rates are from less developed countries and the low rates consistently recorded in India are of considerable interest (Table 1.3).

Ethnic and racial differences in the incidence of colon cancer, as well as studies on migrants, suggest that environmental factors have a major role in the aetiology of the disease. In Israel, male Jews born in Europe or America are at higher risk for colon cancer than those born in Africa or Asia. Furthermore, the change in risk for the offspring of those Japanese who have migrated to the United States that was predicted by Haenszel and Kurihara[19] has now taken place, the incidence rates approaching or surpassing those in Caucasians in the same population and being three or four times higher than among Japanese in Japan.

In a long-term perspective, rates of incidence of colon cancer are rising slowly, in particular in areas formerly at low risk, with left-sided tumours having shown greater increases.[20] In Australia between 1973 and 1993, colorectal cancer occurred most frequently in

Table 1.1. *Ten highest and ten lowest average, annual, all-ages, age-standardized rates per 100,000 population for colon cancer in men and women worldwide (mid-1990s)*

Colon, Male ICD9 153 Registry	No. of cases	Rate	Colon, Female ICD9 153 Registry	No. of cases	Rate
US, Detroit: Black	806	35.0	New Zealand: non-Maori	3650	29.6
US, Los Angeles: Black	771	34.8	Canada, Newfoundland	503	28.1
US, Hawaii: Japanese	462	34.4	US, San Francisco: Black	408	27.9
US, San Francisco: Black	353	33.8	US, Detroit: Black	899	27.9
US, Hawaii: White	293	32.7	US, San Francisco: Japanese	57	27.0
US, Atlanta: Black	300	32.4	US, Los Angeles: Black	860	26.5
Japan, Hiroshima	939	31.6	US, Atlanta: Black	400	26.2
Canada, Newfoundland	504	31.4	US, New Orleans: Black	314	25.8
US, New Orleans: Black	247	31.4	Canada, Nova Scotia	1028	25.2
New Zealand: non-Maori	3045	31.2	US, Connecticut: Black	188	25.2
Kuwait: Kuwaitis	22	3.5	Korea, Kangwha	7	2.3
Uganda, Kyadondo	16	3.2	Kuwait: non-Kuwaitis	13	2.2
Mall, Bamako	22	3.1	India, Bangalore	128	2.0
India, Bangalore	162	2.4	China, Qidong	79	2.0
India, Trivandrum	17	2.4	Mali, Bamako	13	1.4
China, Qidong	64	2.1	India, Madras	84	1.3
India, Madras	122	1.8	India, Karunagappally	5	1.3
India, Karunagappally	5	1.5	India, Trivandrum	8	1.0
India, Barshi, Paranda, Bhum	6	0.7	Algeria, Setif	7	0.6
Algeria, Setif	4	0.5	India, Barshi, Paranda, Bhum	4	0.4

Data abstracted from ref. 137.

the sigmoid colon and the rectum; in the right colon, cancer occurred most commonly in the caecum. From 1973 to 1993, incidence rates increased in the right colon (by 2.8% p.a. in men and 2.0% p.a. in women) and in the left colon (1.6% in men and 0.7% in women). The incidence rate of cancer of the rectum also increased, by 2.0% p.a. in men and by 0.7% p.a. in women.[21] More complex patterns are seen in high-risk countries.

Although mortality rates are increasing in US Blacks for both sexes, in Whites the increase is confined to older men and rates are decreasing in women. In the United States, rates of

Table 1.2. *Ten highest and ten lowest average, annual, all-ages, age-standardized rates per 100,000 population for rectal cancer in men and women worldwide (mid-1990s)*

Rectum, Male ICD9 154 Registry	No. of cases	Rate	Rectum, Female ICD9 154 Registry	No. of cases	Rate
Canada, Yukon	25	33.7	Canada, Yukon	12	14.4
Czech Republic	7970	24.2	Israel: born in America or Europe	1053	12.8
Zimbabwe, Harare: European	23	22.4	Czech Republic	5602	11.6
France, Haut-Rhin	446	21.5	South Australia	673	11.5
Slovakia	2984	20.6	Israel: All Jews	1533	11.4
New Zealand: non-Maori	1955	20.1	France, Haut-Rhin	343	11.2
Japan, Hiroshima	576	19.4	New Zealand: Non-Maori	1362	11.2
US, San Francisco: Japanese	28	19.3	Australia, Victoria	1876	11.0
Australia, Victoria	2610	19.2	Australian Capital Territory	74	11.0
US, Hawaii: Japanese	235	19.0	Germany, Saarland	691	10.9
India, Bangalore	212	3.1	Viet Nam, Hanoi	70	2.5
Israel: non-Jews	31	3.1	Algeria, Setif	27	2.3
Thailand, Chiang Mai	101	3.1	India, Trivandrum	18	2.3
India, Trivandrum	21	3.1	Kuwait: non-Kuwaitis	13	2.3
Thailand, Khon Kaen	63	3.0	Thailand, Khon Kaen	48	1.9
Mali, Bamako	26	2.9	Kuwait: Kuwaitis	11	1.9
Brazil, Belem	30	2.8	Uganda, Kyadondo	11	1.8
Algeria, Setif	24	2.7	India, Barshi, Paranda, Bhum	10	1.1
India, Barshi, Paranda, Bhum	23	2.6	Mali, Bamako	8	0.7
India, Karunagappally	6	1.6	India, Karunagappally	1	0.3

Data abstracted from ref. 137.

incidence are rising slowly in women. Increasing rates are observed in the Nordic countries whereas, in England and Wales, mortality rates are declining in all age groups in both sexes.

The most recent incidence and mortality data from Europe have been assembled into a single compendium.[22] The highest incidence rates for colon cancer in men (between 27 and 31/100,000 p.a.) are found in four regions of northern Italy (Trieste, Ferrara, Varese and Genoa) and in the *départements* of Haut-Rhin and Bas-Rhin in France (Figure 1.1). The lowest rates (between 8 and 13/100,000) were found

Table 1.3. *Ten highest and ten lowest average, annual, all-ages, age-standardized rates per 100,000 population for colon and rectal cancer combined in men and women worldwide (mid-1990s)*

Colorectum, Male ICD9 153–154 Registry	No. of cases	Rate	Colorectum, Female ICD9 153–154 Registry	No. of cases	Rate
US, Hawaii: Japanese	697	53.5	New Zealand: non-Maori	5012	40.8
New Zealand: non-Maori	5000	51.3	Canada, Newfoundland	678	38.3
Japan, Hiroshima	1515	51.0	US, Detroit: Black	1172	36.6
France, Haut-Rhin	1041	49.9	US, Los Angeles: Black	1182	36.6
Italy, Trieste	547	49.4	US, San Francisco: Black	527	36.4
France, Bas-Rhin	1445	49.2	Israel: born in America or Europe	3034	35.8
Canada, Yukon	39	49.0	US, San Francisco: Japanese	76	35.4
US, Detroit: Black	1100	48.3	US, Atlanta: Black	529	35.0
Czech Republic	15906	48.2	Canada, Nova Scotia	1400	35.0
US, Los Angeles: Black	1061	47.9	South Australia	2047	34.2
Brazil, Belem	73	7.3	Thailand, Khon Kaen	129	5.2
Ecuador, Quito	123	7.3	Uganda, Kyadondo	26	5.1
Thailand, Chiang Mai	240	7.2	India, Bangalore	300	4.8
Mali, Bamako	48	6.0	Kuwait: non-Kuwaitis	26	4.5
India, Madras	367	5.6	India, Madras	258	4.2
India, Bangalore	374	5.5	India, Trivandrum	26	3.3
India, Trivandrum	38	5.4	Algeria, Setif	34	2.9
India, Barshi, Paranda, Bhum	29	3.3	Mali, Bamako	21	2.1
Algeria, Setif	28	3.1	India, Karunagappally	6	1.7
India, Karunagappally	11	3.1	India, Barshi, Paranda, Bhum	14	1.5

Data abstracted from ref. 137.

in areas of Poland, Belarus, Southern Italy, Spain and Finland. Rates tended to be high in Germany and Switzerland, intermediate in the United Kingdom and relatively low in Sweden and areas of central and eastern Europe. Among women, the highest rates were around 20/100,000 in Germany, Ireland, Central Italy, Denmark and Scotland and the lowest rates (around 5–10/100,000) in Poland, Belarus, Croatia, Latvia and Spain) (Figure 1.2).

There is an overall tendency for rates of incidence of rectal cancer to be high and low in areas similar to those for colon cancer, although there are some notable (and interesting) exceptions. The highest rate of incidence of rectal cancer in both sexes has been reported from the population of the former Czechoslovakia: the highest rates were 24.2/100,000 in Czech men and 11.2/100,000 among Slovakian women (Figures 1.3, 1.4). The rates of incidence of colon cancer were intermediate in both Czech and Slovakian men and women.

There is a considerable variation in the mortality rates of colorectal cancer within Europe. Among men, the highest mortality rate per 100,000 was 37.2 in the Czech Republic and the lowest rates were in Albania and Greece (9.1) (Figure 1.5). Among women, the highest mortality rate was 20.7 in the Czech Republic and the lowest again in Albania and Greece (7.4). Ignoring the obvious outliers, there is a clear fourfold variation in colorectal cancer mortality rates between the countries of Europe (Figures 1.5, 1.6).

Temporal trends in colorectal cancer mortality (ICD9 153 and ICD9 154)

The major problem when comparing rates of mortality from colon and rectal cancer separately between populations is the problem of attribution of 'vaguely' defined cancers on the death certificate. The root of the problem was the habit of ascribing any death described by the certifying physician as 'cancer of the large intestine' to the three-digit code for colon: this, of course, could have been a rectal cancer. For this and several other reasons, it is preferable to investigate rates of mortality from colon and rectal cancer together as a single entity. However, there is a recognized loss of information that could be available if mortality data were of a higher quality.

In Canada, the truncated and overall age-adjusted mortality rates remained relatively stable in men until the early 1970s, and have been decreasing ever since. In women, both the truncated and overall age-adjusted mortality rates have been decreasing since 1955. Examination of birth cohorts shows that the rates have been stable or decreasing in successive birth cohorts in men and women for the age groups examined, although the decrease in rates has been more pronounced in women. Canada is one of the few countries outside the Nordic countries where national incidence and mortality data are available.[23] The incidence and mortality rates of colorectal cancer are higher by about 50% in men than in women. In each gender group, the incidence and mortality rates increased to a peak in the mid-1980 and the 'all ages' rates have subsequently declined (Figure 1.7).

In Japan, both the truncated and overall age-adjusted mortality rates have been increasing in both men and women since 1955. Examination of rate by birth cohorts suggests a consistent increase in rates in successive birth cohorts born before 1940 in both sexes. For cohorts born after that date, the rates seem to have levelled off and may even have declined in either gender.[24]

In Czechoslovakia, both the truncated and the overall age-adjusted mortality rates have been increasing in both men and women since 1955. Birth cohort examination indicates an increase in rates in successive birth cohorts in both gender groups, although the rates in younger age groups seem to be levelling off. Thus, it could be that the rapidly rising rates in both men and women will start to level off and fall in the medium term.

In Poland, both the truncated and overall age-adjusted mortality rates have been increasing since 1959 in both men and women. Examination by birth cohorts suggests an increase in rates in successive birth cohorts for almost all age groups examined, and in both sexes.

In Germany, both the truncated and overall age-adjusted mortality rates increased between 1955 and 1979. Thereafter, the rates in women have been decreasing more so in the truncated rates. In men, after a brief and slight decrease between 1980 and 1983, the rates seem to have increased again in the last few years. Birth cohort examination shows an increase in rates for earlier birth cohort and a decrease in recent birth cohorts at all age groups examined, and in both men and women.

In the United Kingdom, the overall age-adjusted mortality rates have shown a slight decrease in men since 1955, although the truncated rates remain relatively unchanged. In women, both the truncated and overall age-adjusted mortality rates have been decreasing

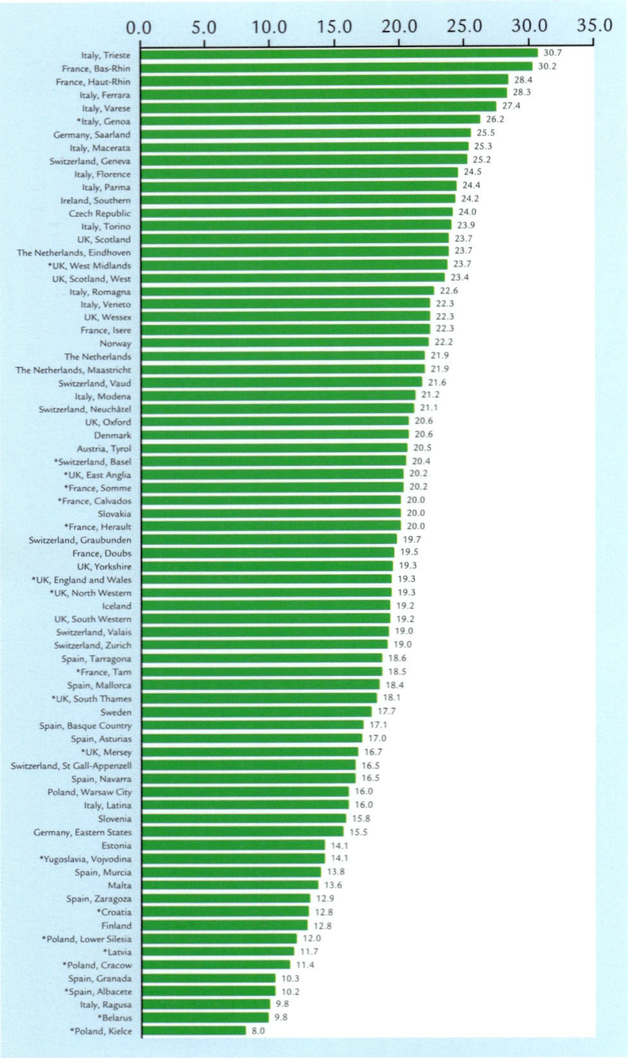

Figure 1.1. *Average, annual, age-standardized incidence rates per 100,000 of colon cancer in men in European cancer registry regions, c.1990. (From ref. 137.)*

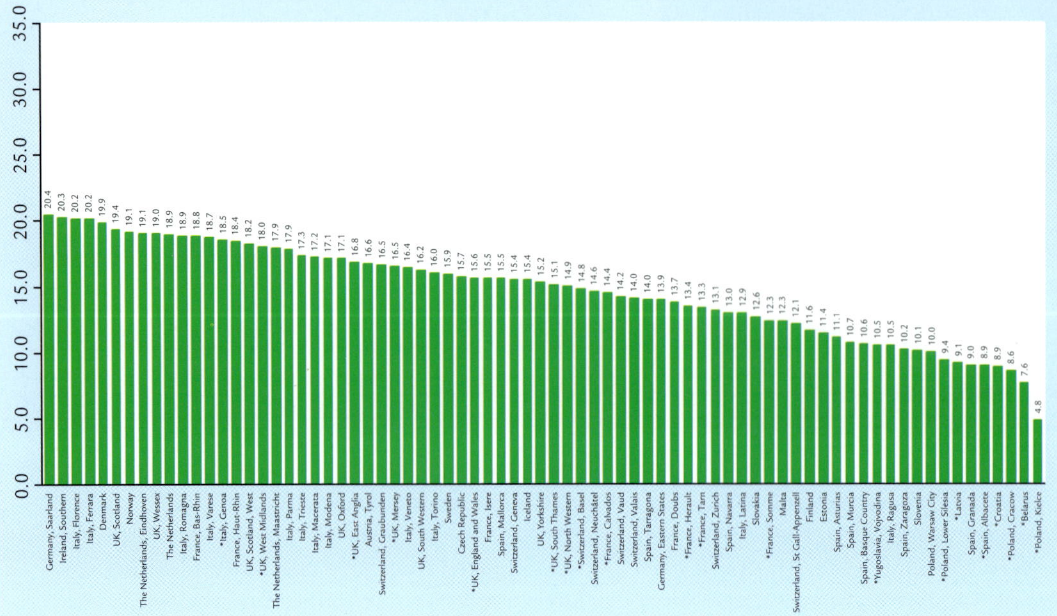

Figure 1.2. *Average, annual, age-standardized incidence rates per 100,000 of colon cancer in women in European cancer registry regions, c.1990. (From ref. 137.)*

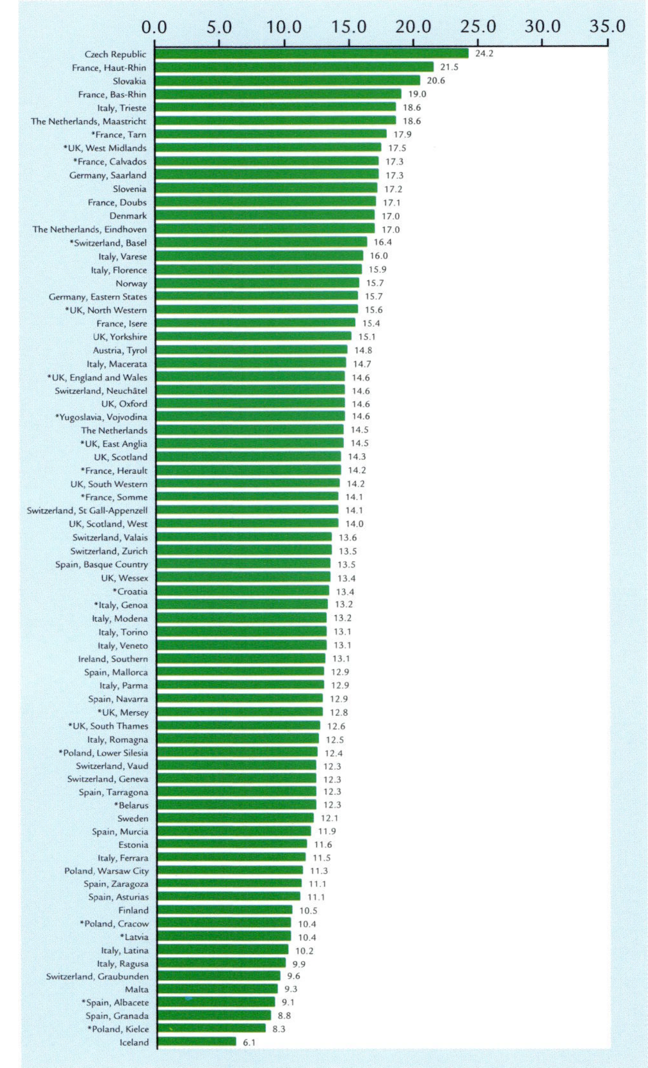

Figure 1.3. *Average, annual, age-standardized incidence rates per 100,000 of rectal cancer in men in European cancer registry regions, c.1990. (From ref. 137.)*

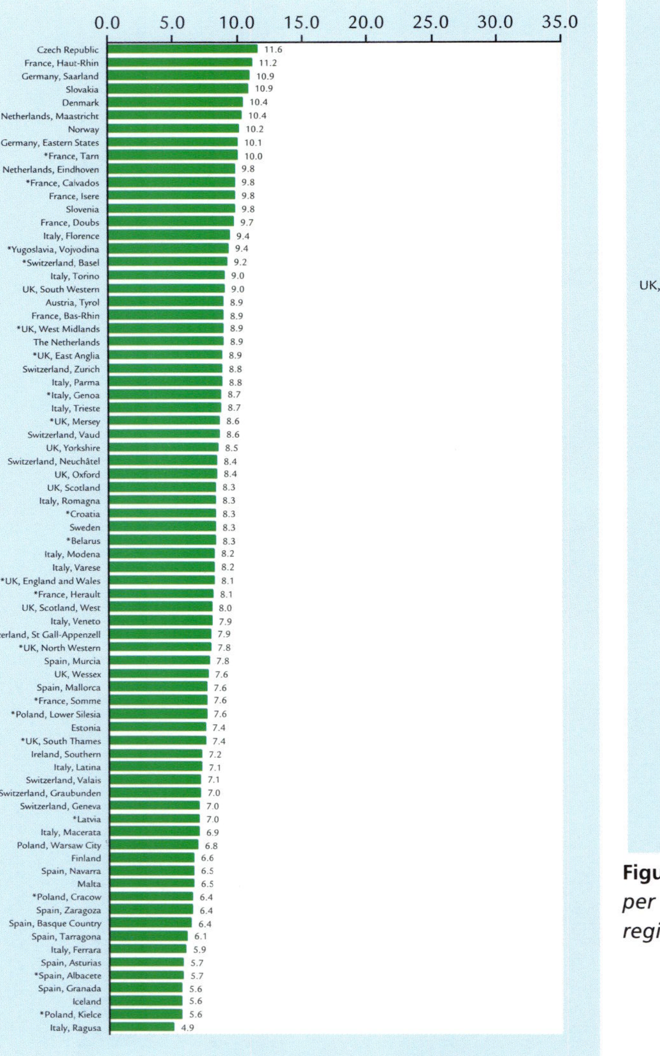

Figure 1.4. *Average, annual, age-standardized incidence rates per 100,000 of rectal cancer in women in European cancer registry regions, c.1990. (From ref. 137.)*

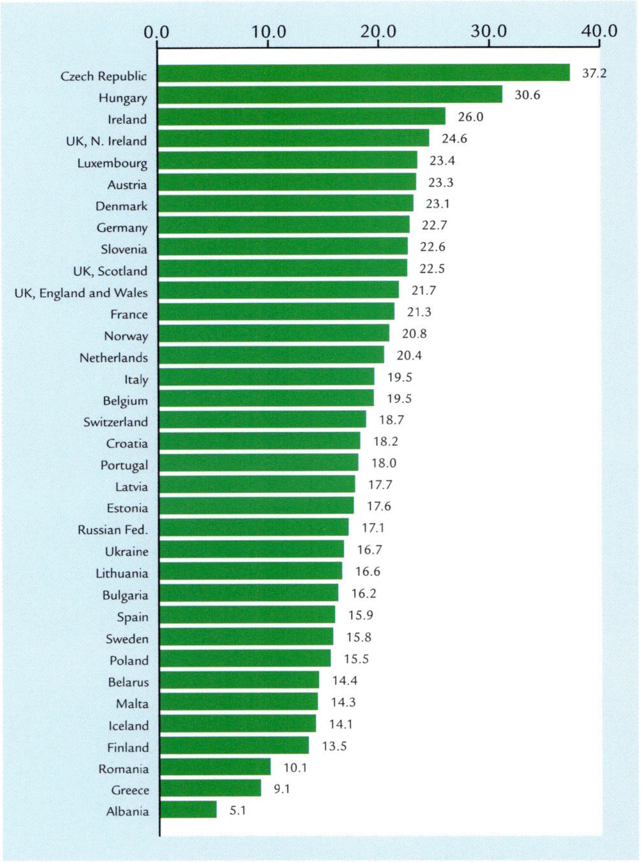

Figure 1.5. *Average, annual, age-standardized mortality rates per 100,000 of colorectal cancer in men in European cancer registry regions, c.1990. (From ref. 137.)*

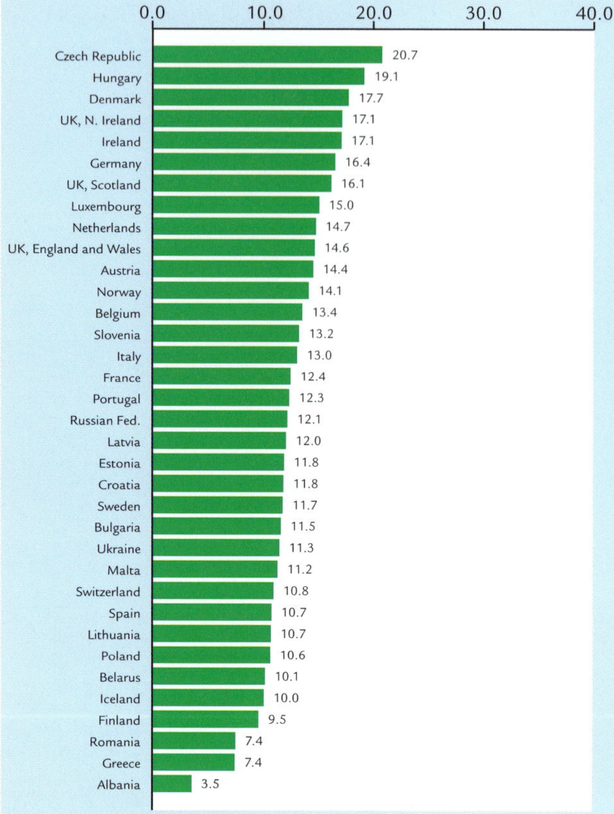

Figure 1.6. *Average, annual, age-standardized mortality rates per 100,000 of colorectal cancer in women in European cancer registry regions, c.1990. (From ref. 137.)*

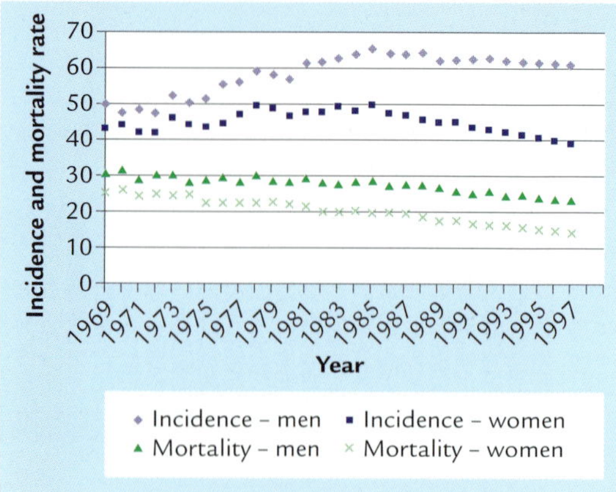

Figure 1.7. *Average, annual age-standardized incidence and mortality rates from colorectal cancer in men and women in Canada, 1965–1997.*

during the entire study period. Examination by birth cohorts shows similar rates in successive birth cohorts born before 1930 and a slight decrease in those born subsequently after. In women, the rates have been decreasing in successive birth cohorts for all the age groups examined.

In Denmark, there is no clear overall time trend for either truncated or overall age-adjusted mortality rates in men since 1955. In women, however, a slight decrease has been observed for both truncated and overall age-adjusted mortality rates during the entire study period. Birth cohort examination suggests that the rates are similar in men and are decreasing in women in successive birth cohorts.

In Italy, the rates of mortality from colorectal cancer in both men and women have been increasing steadily since 1955. After 1980, there has been a levelling-off in rates in women, particularly in the truncated age range.

In Australia, both the truncated and overall age-adjusted mortality rates have been increasing in men since 1955, although the increase in the overall age-adjusted mortality rates seems to have slowed down over the last few years. In women, a slight decrease has been observed for both truncated and overall age-adjusted mortality rates since the early 1970s. Birth cohort examination shows an increase in rates in men in successive birth cohorts born before 1935 and a decrease in rates born subsequently. In women, the rates are similar or have decreased in successive birth cohorts for most of the age groups examined – except for the age groups between 40 and 49 where a slight increase in rates in successive birth cohorts was observed. Interesting data have been published recently regarding a comprehensive analysis of the descriptive epidemiology of colorectal cancer in New South Wales.[21]

Colorectal cancer was the second most common cancer reported in men and women in New South Wales in 1993.[21] The age-standardized incidence rates in men and women in 1993 were 46.1 and 31.0 respectively: this is considerably lower than the incidence rates in Canada (Figure 1.7). From 1973 to 1993, the incidence rates rose by an average of 1.9% p.a. in men and 0.9% in women, whereas mortality rates were steady in men and fell by 0.9% in women. These increases in incidence in men occurred over the age of 45 and in women between the ages of 45 and 74. The overall mortality rate in men remained stable, despite a fall in rates in younger men. In women, the fall in mortality of 0.9% p.a. could be attributed to falls in the very youngest and oldest age groups.[21]

Boyle *et al.* reported that, worldwide, the rates of colorectal cancer were approaching each other: since 1950, in areas where the rate was initially high, rates were now falling and, in areas where the rates were initially low, rates were increasing. The one glaring exception to this rule is in Czechoslovakia where mortality rates are high and rising in both men and women, in both the 'all-ages' group and in the restricted 35–69 age range.

Actions towards colorectal cancer control

GENERAL PUBLIC

One consequence of epidemiological research on cancer to investigate the contribution of lifestyle factors to cancer risk has been to focus blame on the individual who gets cancer. Smoking, alcohol drinking, dietary imprudence, sunlight exposure and even vital agents tend to direct responsibility towards the individual.[25] It is frequently not the case that the individual is principally responsible for decisions regarding factors which influence his or her risk of cancer, and it should be recognized that society, including government and industry, could have a more active role in lifestyle carcinogenesis: government legislation, including taxation policy and other actions, could have profound effects on smoking habits, for example.

It is more than a rhetorical question to ask if governments around the world truly wish to have tobacco controlled. Industry, too, has a positive role in many areas of prevention. There is continual advice to reduce intake of saturated fat in the Western diet to reduce the risk of several important diseases, but this is thwarted to a large extent by the high saturated-fat content of many common foods; could, for example, vegetable-based margarine be used routinely in many bakery products and could fries and hamburgers be prepared routinely in vegetable oil?

The responsibility for cancer control should be shared; nevertheless, each individual in our society has lifestyle choices to make and should be made more aware of the actions that could lead to a reduction in cancer risk of colorectal cancer, as well as of other forms of cancer and serious diseases. These actions are outlined below.

1. Increase intake of vegetables and fruits. Eat five servings of fruit and vegetables each day, whenever possible; systematically replace snacks such as chocolate bars, biscuits and crisps with an apple, orange or other piece of fruit or vegetable

The original hypothesis of the protective effect of dietary fibre against colorectal cancer was based on a clinical/pathological observation and a hypothetical mechanism whereby increasing intake of dietary fibre increases faecal bulk and reduces transit time; more-recent thinking suggests that this mechanism may not be as relevant to colorectal carcinogenesis as previously thought.[26] The term 'fibre' encompasses many components, each of which has specific physiological functions. The most common classification is into insoluble, non-degradable constituents (mainly present in cereal fibre) and soluble, degradable constituents such as pectin and plant gums, which are present mainly in fruit and vegetables. Epidemiological studies have reported differences in the effect of these components. For example, Tuyns *et al.*[27] and Kune *et al.*[28] found a protective effect for total dietary fibre intake in case–control studies, and the same effect was found in one prospective study;[29] however, in many studies no such protective effect was found (see Willett[30] for review).

Most studies in humans have found no protective effect of fibre from cereals but have found a protective effect of fibre from vegetable and, perhaps, fruit sources.[30] This could conceivably reflect an association with other components of fruits and vegetables, with 'fibre' intake acting merely as an indicator of consumption. A potential pathway for this association was recently investigated in a novel epidemiological study design.[31] Cruciferous vegetable intake exhibited a significant inverse association with colorectal cancer risk (odds ratio [OR] = 0.59; 95% confidence interval [CI] = 0.34, 1.02). When tumours were characterized by *p53* overexpression (*p53* positive) aetiological heterogeneity was suggested for family history of colorectal cancer (OR = 0.39; 95% CI = 0.16, 0.93), intake of cruciferous vegetables (test for trend, $P = 0.12$) and beef consumption (test for trend, $P = 0.08$). Cruciferous-vegetable consumption exhibited a significant association when *p53*-positive cases were compared with controls (OR = 0.37; 95% CI = 0.17, 0.82). When *p53*-negative cases were compared with controls, a significant increase in risk was observed for family history of cancer (OR = 4.46; 95% CI = 2.36, 8.43) and beef consumption (OR = 3.17; 95% CI = 1.83, 11.28). The *p53* (positive) dependent pathway appears to be characterized by an inverse association with cruciferous vegetable intake, and that of *p53*-independent tumours characterized by a family history of colorectal cancer and of beef consumption.[31]

Although calcium has been proposed as potentially having a modifying role in colorectal carcinogenesis,[32] little supporting evidence has been forthcoming from epidemiological studies.[33] These studies in humans are of limited value because of questionable study design or the inadequacy of the estimation of diet. A number of studies have reported positive associations with alcohol consumption,[34] but it remains to be proved whether the putative association is with alcohol *per se* and not with the energy contribution of alcohol. There is some experimental evidence that vitamin E and selenium may be protective against tumours of the colon[35] and there is support for the hypothesis that vitamin A or its precursor β-carotene (or both) are also protective.[24] Lactobacilli, found in some dairy products, may have a beneficial effect on the intestine.[36] Of 12 case–control studies of sufficient quality that have addressed the issue of coffee consumption and the risk of colorectal cancer, 11 have indicated inverse (protective) associations.[37] No association has been found with tea drinking or caffeine intake from any sources considered.[37]

Dietary factors are the most important lifestyle determinants of colorectal cancer risk. Methodological problems in nutritional epidemiology preclude a completely unequivocal interpretation of the available data, although the situation is becoming very much clearer. The authors' interpretation is that an effect of saturated fat appears to exist independently of energy intake and that vegetable fibre, directly or indirectly, appears to be protective, as does coffee consumption. Meat intake may also increase risk but whether this is independent of its fat content or its contribution to energy is currently unclear; if independent, the risk could be related to mutagenic products formed in the cooking process. Intake of cereal fibre appears to be protective against the formation of colorectal polyps, although it does not appear to have a role in the later stages of the carcinogenic process involving transformation of the adenomatous polyp into the carcinoma.

The best message to the general public at present is to increase the intake of vegetables and fruits. To be more precise, it is recommended to eat five servings of fruit and vegetables each day, whenever possible, defining a serving as (for example) vegetables with a main dish, a salad before or with a meal, a glass of orange juice, and an apple or orange as a snack. The maximum effect could be attained by systematically replacing snacks such as chocolate bars, biscuits and crisps with an apple, orange or another piece of fruit or vegetable.

2. Reduce intake of calories, and of animal fats in particular. Frequently substitute fish and poultry for beef, lamb and pork as a main course

It has been a fairly consistent finding in those studies that have examined the issue, that energy intake is higher in patients with colorectal cancer than it is in comparison groups: however, the mechanism is complex.[30] Physically active individuals are likely to consume more energy but physical activity reduces the risk of colorectal cancer,[38–41] and also the risk of adenomas.[42–43] The available data, however, show no consistent association between obesity and colorectal cancer risk (although analysis and interpretation of this factor is difficult in retrospective studies where weight loss may be a sign of the disease). This positive effect of energy does not therefore appear to be merely the result of overeating, and may reflect differences in metabolic efficiency. (If the possibility that the association with energy intake is a methodological artefact is excluded, as it seems unlikely that such a consistent finding would emerge from such a variety of study designs in a diversity of population groups, it would imply that individuals who utilize energy more efficiently may be at a lower risk of colorectal cancer.)

There is conflicting evidence from epidemiological studies regarding the role of intake of dietary fat and its association with colorectal cancer risk: this evidence is obtained from ecological studies, animal experiments, and case–control and cohort studies, although there have been few methodologically sound analytical studies performed in humans. Many of these studies have failed to demonstrate that the observed association with fat intake is independent of energy intake: for example, a recent meta-analysis carried out to examine the effects of the intake of dietary fat on colorectal cancer risk,[44] included 13 case–control studies that had previously been conducted and in which 5287 cases and 10,470 controls were analysed simultaneously, positive associations with energy intake were observed with 11 of the 13 studies. There was little evidence of energy-independent effect of either total fat (with ORs of 1.00, 0.95, 1.01, 1.02 and 0.92 for the quintiles of residuals of total fat intake [*P* for trend 0.67]) or for saturated fat, where the ORs in quintiles were 1.00, 1.08, 1.06, 1.21 and 1.06 (*P* for trend 0.39).[44]

There is, however, conflicting evidence from prospective studies. Willett *et al.*[45] published results obtained from the United States Nurses Health study (a prospective design) involving follow-up of 88,751 women aged 34–59 who were without cancer or inflammatory bowel diseases at recruitment. After adjustment for total energy intake, consumption of animal fat was found to be associated with increased colon cancer risk. The trend in risk was highly significant ($P = 0.01$) with the relative risk in the highest compared with the lowest quintile being 1.89 (95% CI = 1.13, 3.15). No association was found with vegetable fat; two other prospective studies did not replicate these findings, however.[46–47]

The issue of the role of fat as opposed to calories being a major risk factor for colorectal cancer is not merely academic. Whether the substitution of fat by other sources of calories is likely or unlikely to reduce meaningfully the risk of colorectal cancer is a major, open question, the answer to which is of direct consequence to public health recommendations.

The Nurses' Health Study[45] examined the independent role of different types of meat. The relative risk of colon cancer in women who ate beef, pork or lamb as a main dish every day was 2.49 (95% CI = 1.24, 5.03), compared with those women reporting consumption less than once a month. The authors interpreted their data as providing evidence for the hypothesis that a high intake of animal fat increases the risk of colon cancer, and they support existing recommendations to substitute fish and chicken for meats high in fat.[45]

The Nurses' Health Study[45] provides the best epidemiological evidence to date identifying increased meat consumption as a risk factor for colon cancer independently of its contribution to fat intake and total energy intake. Risk of colorectal cancer appears to be increased by increasing consumption of fat, protein and meat, and to be reduced by increased consumption of fruit and vegetables.[48] It has been hypothesized that alterations to serum triglycerides and/or plasma glucose could be one possible vehicle for the effects of various aetiological factors.[49] Laboratory evidence strongly suggests that cooked meats may be carcinogenic, particularly with regard to aminoimidazoazerenes (AIAs), which are produced when meats are cooked.[50–51] There is now evidence that AIAs, as well as being highly mutagenic in bacterial assays, are mammalian carcinogens: feeding experiments in mice have produced tumours in various anatomical sites.[52] The situation is not, however, entirely straightforward for example, it has been shown that anticarcinogenic compounds are produced in fried ground beef[53] thus, in the same food there is the potential for mixtures of potentially carcinogenic and anticarcinogenic substances.

The specific fatty acids in the diet may also be important: animal experiments suggest that linoleic acid (an n-6 polyunsaturated fatty acid) promotes colorectal carcinogenesis,35,54 and that a low fat diet rich in eicopentaenoic acid (an n-3 polyunsaturated fatty acid) has an inhibitory effect on colon cancer;55 however, there have been no epidemiological studies conducted to date regarding n-3 and n-6 fatty acids and colorectal cancer risk.

It seems clear that everyone should eat a little less and, particularly, to curb intake of saturated fat. However, humans do not look upon food in terms of macro- or micronutrients but they eat certain foodstuffs. In addition to the advice to eat more fruit and vegetables, it is recommended to reduce the intake of fatty foods and, in particular, frequently to substitute fish and poultry for beef, lamb and pork as a main course. Thus, there are prospects for primary prevention although it is difficult to know how successfully to bring about such large-scale alterations to the diets of large proportions of populations.

3. Increase physical activity levels

There appears to be strong evidence from epidemiological studies that males with high levels of occupational or recreational physical activity appear to be at a lower risk of colon cancer.[56] Such evidence comes from follow-up studies of cohorts who are physically active or who have physically demanding jobs, as well as from case–control studies that have assessed physical activity by, for example, measurement of resting heart rate, or by questionnaire; the association remains, even after control for potentially confounding factors such as diet and body mass index (BMI). The risk of colorectal cancer and self-reported occupational and recreational physical activity was investigated recently in a population-based cohort in Norway.[41] Physical activity at a level equivalent to walking 4 h/week was associated with a decreased risk of colon cancer among women when compared with the (referent) sedentary group (RR = 0.62; 95% CI = 0.40, 0.97): this was particularly marked in the proximal colon (RR = 0.51; 95% CI = (0.28, 0.93). The trend in reducing risk with increased physical activity was similar in women and in men aged over 45.[41]

A case–control study of new adenoma cases and adenoma-free controls demonstrated that physical activity in leisure protected women against colorectal adenomas. There was no evidence of a protective effect of work activity among either women or men, although men who did not participate in any sport were at an increased risk for adenomas (OR = 1.68; 95% CI = 0.93, 3.20).[42] Giovannucci *et al.*[43] took the opportunity to examine the role of physical activity, BMI and the pattern of adipose distribution with the risk of colorectal adenomas. Within the Nurses' Health study, 13,057 female nurses, aged 40–65 years in 1986, had an endoscopy between 1986 and 1992. During this period, 439 were newly diagnosed with adenomas of the distal colorectum. After controlling for age, prior endoscopy, parental history of colorectal cancer, smoking, aspirin use and dietary intake, physical activity was associated inversely with the risk of large adenomas (greater or equal to 1cm) in the distal colon (RR = 0.57, 95% CI = 0.310, 1.08) comparing high and low quintiles of average weekly energy expenditure from leisure activities. Much of this benefit came from activities of moderate intensity, such as brisk walking.

Additionally, BMI was associated directly with risk of large adenomas in the distal colon (RR = 2.21; 95% CI = 1.18, 4.16), for BMI of 29 kg/m^2 or over compared with BMI values of less than 21 kg/m^2. The relationships between BMI or physical activity were considerably weaker for rectal adenomas.[43] This study indicates a similar association between physical activity and occurrence of adenomas in many respects similar to that for colorectal cancer. Exercise appears to protect against adenomas and colorectal cancer, as increasing BMI serves to increase the risk of both.

The reason for such an inverse association has not been identified but has been postulated as being the effect of exercise on bowel transit time,[57] on the immune system,[58] or on serum cholesterol and bile acid metabolism.[59] The same consistent results have not been reported on studies in women, but one possible explanation is that the smaller variation in, for example, occupational activity among women may make such an association more difficult to detect.

Whittemore *et al.*[40] performed a case–control study of Chinese in North America and China, thus ingeniously utilizing the major difference in risk of colorectal cancer that exists between the two continents. Colorectal cancer risk in both continents was increased with increasing intake of total energy – specifically saturated fat; however, no relationship was found with other sources of energy in the diet. Colon cancer risk was elevated among men employed in sedentary occupations and, in both continents and in both sexes, the risks for cancer of the colon and rectum increased with increased time spent seated: the association between colorectal cancer risk and saturated fat was stronger among the sedentary than the active. Risk among sedentary Chinese Americans of either sex increased more than fourfold from the lowest to the highest category of saturated fat intake. Among migrants to North America, risk increased with increasing years spent in North America. Attributable risk calculations suggest that, if these associations are causal, saturated fat intakes exceeding 10 g/day, particularly in combination with physical inactivity, could account for 60% of colorectal cancer incidence among Chinese American men and 40% among Chinese American women.[40]

4. Participate in organized population-screening programmes. In their absence, give strong consideration to having a sigmoidoscopy (or colonoscopy) with polyp removal once between the ages of 50 and 59

When surgical resection is possible, survival is largely dependent on disease stage: the 5-year survival rate is 82% in patients with Dukes' A tumours, and 64, 37 and 4% in patients with Dukes' B, C and D tumours, respectively.[60] As previously mentioned, 5-year survival in patients with resected Dukes' A tumours is around 80% and survival following simple resection of an adenomatous polyp containing carcinoma *in situ* (or severe dysplasia) or intramucosal carcinoma is generally close to 100%; however, there are still nearly 400,000 deaths from colorectal cancer worldwide annually,[3] and this is an important public health issue.

The major differences in survival between early-and late-stage disease clearly indicate the advantage in detecting colorectal cancer at an early stage. Knowledge of the natural history of colorectal cancer, the great majority of which develop through the polyp–carcinoma sequence is being augmented by a deeper understanding of the molecular genetics involved,[61,62] and the genetic events involved in colorectal cancer susceptibility are being uncovered with increasing frequency.[63,64] It has been postulated elsewhere[17] that colorectal cancer may emerge as the first major neoplasm to be preventable, allying successful treatment with successful prevention strategies[5] and using prescription rather than proscription. Inherent in a successful colorectal cancer control programme should be the role of population screening.

The simplest advice to the public is to ensure that any change in bowel habits or unexpected presence of blood in the stool should be investigated, although the impact of this strategy on colorectal cancer incidence and mortality is unknown.[25] Faecal occult blood testing (FOBT) is aimed at the detection of early asymptomatic cancer and is based on the assumption that such cancers will bleed and that small quantities of blood lost in the stool may be detected chemically or immunologically. FOBT has been reported, from case–control studies to reduce colorectal cancer mortality rates by 31%[65] and 57% in women.[66] There are now three randomized trials of FOBT each demonstrating a reduction in colorectal cancer mortality.[6–8] Mandel *et al.*[6] reported a reduction of 33% in colorectal cancer mortality after 13 years in subjects who were offered annual screening with FOBT, but a non-significant reduction (of 6%) in those who were offered biennial screening. In the two more recent studies, the colorectal cancer mortality rates in the group offered biennial FOBT were respectively 0.85[14] and 0.82[15] the rates in the control population. An (approximate) combined analysis of these latter studies produces a relative risk of colorectal cancer death of 0.84 (95% CI = 0.75–0.94).[67] However, in these latter trials, part of the reduction in colorectal cancer mortality was probably attributable to better medical attention and better symptom awareness to screened subjects, rather than to FOBT test itself.[68] In these trials, physicians were directly involved in the clinical study; they knew to which arm patients were randomized, and were aware that many colorectal cancers would arise as interval cancers. As a matter of fact, in the two trials, interval colorectal cancers were more numerous than screen-detected colorectal cancer in subjects who accepted at least one FOBT. It is, therefore, highly probable that in subjects who were put forward to use FOBT, more attention was paid to early symptoms of the eventual presence of interval colorectal cancer, leading to earlier diagnosis of malignant lesions. This hypothesis is supported by the observation that, in both studies, interval colorectal cancers were detected at an earlier stage than was colorectal cancer diagnosed in the control group.[6–8] This is surprising, as one would expect interval cancers not to be detected earlier than in the absence of a screening test.

There are both advantages and disadvantages to FOBT. On the one hand it is low cost, although the investigation of false positives (around 1–3% per test) certainly increases the cost of a screening programme, and it 'examines' the entire colon and rectum. However, FOBT is currently characterized by a low sensitivity (with around 40% of cancers and 80% of adenomas missed by the test)[69,70] and by detection of colorectal cancers at the later stages in the natural history at which lesions bleed which leads to a short lead time and the requirement for frequent testing. Rehydration of the slides results in increased positivity, but also in an increased number of colonoscopies and a decreased specificity of the test. The costs must be weighed against the benefits before public health policy on this topic is formulated; however, it is apparent that a better test (higher sensitivity and specificity) is required.

Until a randomized controlled trial is undertaken and reported, the efficacy of flexible sigmoidoscopy as a screening test for preventing death from colorectal cancer will remain technically unproved: it has recently been demonstrated, under certain assumptions, to be less effective than other potential screening strategies for colorectal cancer.[71] Nevertheless, impressive reductions in rectal cancer and cancer of the distal colon have been reported from observational and demonstration studies: 85% reduction in 21,000 subjects undergoing 'clearing' proctosigmoidoscopy followed by annual proctosigmoidoscopy with removal of all lesions detected;[9] 70% reduction in risk of colorectal cancer for 10 years following sigmoidoscopy;[72] 80% reduction in incidence following examination mostly performed by flexible sigmoidoscopy,[12] and an 85% reduction of rectal cancers achieved by the removal of adenomas.[11] Although the initial examination may be expensive, there is an advantage that polyps may be removed at the time of the initial procedure and no follow-up visits will be required thereby leading to a potential reduction in the incidence of colorectal cancer which has not been demonstrated by FOBT. It may well be that colonoscopy turns out to be the most effective proposition.

There are now some extremely important issues to address in the area of colorectal cancer screening, as follows:

1. Should FOB testing now be recommended as a population screening method? This decision depends on many factors, including the value placed on the magnitude of the mortality reduction, the false-positive rate associated with haemoccult testing which is the subject of intense debate at present,[73–76] the acceptance of the test by the general population and the economic costs involved.[77–78] Given the small gains in mortality reduction to be expected from FOBT, and no alteration to the underlying incidence of the disease, the public health relevance of recommending screening programmes based on the use of currently available technology is still questionable.
2. Should consideration be given to other screening modalities for colorectal cancer? Screening with sigmoidoscopy has been demonstrated in case–control and non-randomized studies to reduce the incidence and mortality from colorectal cancer by over 50%[17,79] FOBT does not appear to reduce the incidence of colorectal cancer. It will be important to develop more sensitive screening methods, able to detect the majority of cancerous lesions at an early stage or lesions before they have evolved in cancer, that enable substantial reductions in mortality from colorectal cancer to be obtained. In this scenario, there is considerable hope in the potential from endoscopic techniques. These methods would be able to detect more than 90% of cancers and large polyps within reach of the endoscope. Since polyps can be removed during an endoscopy, these methods allow both prevention and detection of colorectal cancer. Although one must be cautious with results from observational studies aiming at assessing efficacy of screening technologies,[80] data available so far indicate a 60–80% decrease in colorectal cancer mortality among those subjects who underwent a sigmoidoscopy,[12,72] and a 76–96% decrease in colorectal cancer incidence achieved by the removal of colonic polyps.[81] According to these results, an endoscopic examination of the bowel once every 5–10 years would be sufficient. Colonoscopy could yield better results than sigmoidoscopy, as the entire colon would be explored.
3. Since a large proportion of individuals undergoing FOBT have positive tests and are referred for colonoscopy, could it

prove effective to bypass FOBT testing and go directly to a screening colonoscopy or flexible sigmoidoscopy? This latter strategy is currently being assessed in a large, randomized trial, and is a clear reflection of the tremendous potential for early detection of colorectal cancer by screening.[82] This should continue to be a priority research activity. 1

While awaiting the results of haemoccult testing on colorectal cancer mortality, advances in technology have overtaken events, and developments in the technology of flexible sigmoidoscopy have made this an attractive proposition for assessment. The effects estimated from retrospective studies of infrequent sigmoidoscopy are most impressive; it is almost impossible to consider bias, confounding or chance as alternative explanations of the differences observed. Infrequent sigmoidoscopy will almost certainly lead to a reduction in the incidence and mortality from colorectal cancer.[81,82] It would be extremely unlikely that the results available would be overturned by those of randomized trials, although recent experience tells that the preventive effect may be less than that found in retrospective studies.[80] Developments in the technology of colonoscopy – both scientific and medical – now make this in turn an interesting intervention to assess and, with the advantage that it covers the entire bowel, it could be more effective in reducing the incidence of colorectal cancer: it is impossible to believe that it would be less efficient than sigmoidoscopy.

Colorectal endoscopy is often presented as an expensive technique, not without risk. However, technologies constantly evolve and, in the near future, flexible sigmoidoscopy or colonoscopy could become easier to perform with great safety and at low cost.[83,84] Furthermore, it is not impossible that cost-effectiveness of colonoscopic screening would compare favourably with cost-effectiveness of FOBT screening since, first, reductions in colorectal cancer mortality would most probably be much higher and secondly, costs of colonoscopies would be offset by savings from having to treat fewer patients with colorectal cancer, or treating patients with early-stage colorectal cancer.[85] Finally, endoscopic screening could be proposed as a priority for subsets of the population at higher risk of developing colorectal cancer. Regular endoscopic examinations are already part of the follow-up of subjects with inherited predisposition to colorectal cancer (e.g. subjects with familial polyposis or hereditary non-polyposis colorectal cancer), and there is much research aimed at better identification of subjects or families at higher risk for colorectal cancer.[86]

Decreasing trends in mortality from colorectal cancer have already been noted in many parts of the world.[23,87,88] The reasons for the decline in colorectal cancer mortality are multiple – changes in diet patterns, occasional removal of polyps, earlier diagnosis, and improved management of colorectal cancer. Earlier diagnosis encompasses various methods, from physicians and patients giving more attention to early symptoms of eventual presence of colorectal cancer to sporadic screening tests in asymptomatic subjects, using one or a combination of the proposed screening methods. Given available trial results, widespread adoption of haemoccult testing in the general population will have a modest influence on mortality and no impact on incidence. The current dilemma is whether to wait for 10 years for the results of randomized trials of sigmoidoscopy or colonoscopy screening or whether this classical step could be omitted, as the supporting evidence at present is so strong. A population-based randomized trial should be conducted to test the magnitude of mortality reduction to be expected and the cost-effectiveness obtained from a single full colonoscopic examination of the large bowel. At present, opportunistic colorectal endoscopic examination is offered to a steadily larger proportion of asymptomatic subjects. Hence, if such a trial is not performed very soon, it is probable that an appropriate control group (i.e. subjects without colonoscopic examination or other screening for colorectal cancer) will be difficult to obtain.

The costs of a colonoscopy continue to fall and the economic argument could be strengthened if better control was made of the large number of arguably unnecessary colonoscopies performed on survivors of colorectal cancer at frequent intervals and other susceptible groups.89 Of course, it must be recognised that technology continues to advance and in a short period it is conceivable that some robotic device will be available to replace the colonoscope – and at a reduced price and with fewer potential hazards for the patient.

So what should be recommended to the general public about colorectal cancer screening? Doing nothing is no longer an option, as it has been shown that annual FOB testing reduces the mortality of colorectal cancer, although not by a very impressive amount. One can reflect on the need for a trial of colonoscopy, but the main goal of such a large-scale trial will be to try to evaluate the policy of colorectal cancer screening by colonoscopy by careful evaluation of the side effects, and of the costs and issues such as the acceptance rate of initial screens and subsequent screens. It will be some time before colonoscopy can be recommended to the general public and governments for population screening. However, for the motivated individual, there are strong circumstantial and theoretical grounds for believing that colonoscopy would lead to a reduction in risk of developing colorectal cancer, as well as reducing the risk of dying from the disease. It is predictable that the reduction of risk of colorectal cancer associated with sigmoidoscopy will be less than that for colonoscopy since the sigmoidoscope reaches a smaller proportion of the entire bowel than the colonoscope.

5. Consult a doctor as soon as possible if you have a noticeable and unexplained change in bowel habits, notice blood in the stool, have colicky pain in the abdomen or have recurrent sensation of incomplete evacuation after defaecation

Ensuring that any change in bowel habits, unexpected presence of blood in the stool, chronic colicky pain in the abdomen or the recurrent sensation of incomplete evacuation after defaecation is investigated is potentially useful as secondary prevention and serves as a reminder about the signs or symptoms that could easily be observed by anyone and that are possibly related to colorectal cancer. It is unequivocally established that cancer survival is better for early, localized disease than for the later-stage, advanced form of the disease; thus, the earlier in the process that a cancer can be diagnosed and treated then the better this is for the patient. Potential symptoms of colorectal cancer should not be ignored but should serve as a clear warning for the individual to consult his or her doctor for advice. The signs and symptoms described are not specific for cancer; when any symptom is present, the individual should see a doctor.

It has generally been accepted that this is good advice and that such actions ameliorate health outcomes although proof of benefit has tended to be qualitative. According to data from Glasgow (United Kingdom) for two time periods (1974–1979 and 1980–1984) around three out of ten cases of colorectal cancer present as surgical emergencies.[90] In both time periods, curative resection rates were lower in emergency (45 and 35% in 1974–1979 and 1980–1984, respectively) than in elective cases (58 and 60%); operative mortality rates were higher in emergency admissions (19 and 29%) compared with elective admissions (9 and 10%) and 5-year survival rates were considerably higher in elective (30.6 and 24.5%) than in emergency admissions (11.8 and 11.3%).[90] Paying attention to symptoms which frequently refer to invasive colorectal cancer, thereby avoiding an emergency admission, could lead to improved rates of survival.

INDIVIDUALS WITH A GENETIC RISK OF COLORECTAL CANCER

6. By reason of a strong family history of colorectal cancer in relatives, or the presence of a disease such as familial adenomatous polyposis, there are individuals who are at an increased risk of colorectal cancer. Such people should be carefully followed and should participate in whatever screening programme is indicated

The natural history and the role of several risk factors in the aetiology of colorectal cancer are becoming more clearly understood[61–62] and the genetic events involved in colorectal cancer susceptibility are being uncovered with increasing frequency:[64,91] the recent rate of progress in our understanding of the genetics of colorectal cancer is impressive.[92,93] Arguably more is known about the genetics of colorectal cancer than any other common form of the disease.[94] There are a number of clinical syndromes that predispose to colorectal cancer: the majority are inherited as autosomal dominant genes (on average, a carrier of this mutation passes on the mutation to half of the offspring). Offspring have a high chance of developing colorectal cancer. These syndromes include those which predispose to large numbers of polyps [for example, familial adenomatous polyposis (FAP)], those which predispose to adenomatous polyps with high malignant potential [for example, hereditary non-polyposis colorectal cancer (HNPCC)], and those syndromes associated non-adenomatous polyps with an increased risk less than that associated with adenomatous polyps (for example, Peutz–Jeghers syndrome). Apart from these syndromes, epidemiological studies provide evidence that other, weaker, genetic factors are also involved in the pathogenesis of colorectal cancer.[93] Virtually all studies conducted indicate that families of patients with colorectal cancer are more likely to have a history of colorectal cancer than families of 'controls': the increased risk of cancer in relatives is between 2 and 4 when compared with the general population.[92]

Several specialist clinics and screening protocols have been established for patients belonging to families with these symptoms. Increasingly, intense surveillance protocols are being made available and these should be brought to the attention of patients with these diseases and their primary care physicians. Where high-risk patients can be identified, they should be informed of the importance of participating in surveillance/screening protocols and should endeavour to do so.

PRIMARY CARE DOCTORS

7. Patients who consult with possible symptoms of bowel cancer should have an adequate physical examination, including a careful digital rectal examination whenever indicated

Having sensitized the general population and members of families who are at high risk of colorectal cancer to early symptoms of the disease, it is vitally important to alert the primary care physician to the current possibilities with regard to colorectal cancer. Individuals who present to their primary care physician with potential symptoms of colorectal cancer should have a careful history taken and an appropriate physical examination. Of those who present with rectal bleeding, the great majority will not have colorectal cancer but will generally have a banal complaint such as haemorrhoids. Whenever colon or rectal cancer is among the differential diagnoses, a careful digital rectal examination should be performed and the primary care physician should not hesitate to refer the patient for a specialist opinion if colorectal cancer is suspected.

8. Doctors should advise their healthy patients appropriately about the possible benefits of aspirin (and other NSAIDS) and of hormone replacement therapy in the possible prevention of colorectal cancer

There is currently insufficient evidence, on the basis of randomized clinical trials for the chemoprevention of colorectal cancer; on these classical grounds of evidence-based medicine it is not possible to advocate use of any compound for chemoprevention in a general population study. The molecule(s) responsible for the effect of fruits and vegetables are not yet clearly identified. Taken overall, there are suggestions of benefit from vitamin A or β-carotene, vitamin C, vitamin D, vitamin E, calcium supplements, folate and anti-inflammatory drugs and H_2 antagonists: the study of relatively novel chemical entities such as protease inhibitors is at an earlier stage. Prolonged treatment is too speculative a possibility for all of the above compounds, in reducing the risk of developing colorectal cancer, and/or in preventing polyp occurrence.[5]

It is difficult to overlook the abundant evidence that the use of NSAIDs is associated with reduced risks of colorectal cancer and adenomatous polyps.[95–99] Effects have been demonstrated consistently, although not completely uniformly, in case–control and cohort studies, and appear to be related to dose and duration of treatment (reviewed in ref. 5). Effects are biologically plausible because NSAID use appears to prevent or reduce the frequency of carcinogen-induced animal colonic tumours,[100–101] because NSAIDs appear to reduce growth rates in colon cancer cell lines and because polyp formation in familial adenomatous polyposis coli appears to be retarded.[102–103]

Use of these drugs is attractive because they are licensed for human treatment and their effects, outside the issue of cancer prevention, are well understood. Little evidence exists in the basis of trials to prevent cancer recurrence. Use of indomethacin or other cyclo-oxygenase antagonists has been suggested to improve natural killer cell activity, and to enhance non-specific immunotherapy of experimental lung tumour metastases.[104–106] In a randomized study in cervical cancer in 160 patients, use of indomethacin enhanced survival of those given radiation treatment by 27% at 5 years and 41% at 10 years.[107] NSAIDs have classic adverse effects on the kidney (interstitial nephritis), skin (rash and photosensitivity), lung (predisposition to asthma) and liver (hepatitis – particularly with diclofenac). However, none of these, individually or collectively, is as frequent as gastrointestinal bleeding from peptic ulcers and, to a lesser extent, from the colon.[108] Risks vary up to 20-fold between agents and by up to 10-fold by dose.[109] For continued aspirin use, ORs appear to be 2.3 (75 mg daily) and 3.2 (150 mg daily), with higher risks at higher doses.[108,109] Risks can almost certainly be reduced by using the enteric-coated drug, but available evidence has generally been obtained with standard preparations. Whether it would be wise to alter deliberately the delivery pattern in treating large intestinal disease is unclear. Enteric-coated preparations are probably completely absorbed in the small bowel and the non-enteric in the stomach and small bowel, so differences may be immaterial. Since, in the US Physicians' Health Study, low-dose aspirin (325 mg on alternate days) appeared to be relatively ineffective in preventing colon cancer,[110] doses of at least 325 mg daily may be required. It is unclear, however, whether, in that study, follow-up was sufficiently prolonged; risk reduction in US nurses became apparent only after 20 years of continuous use.[111] Consequently, the US Physicians Trial may also have had a less than optimal intervention period.

There is currently much interest surrounding the development of COX-2 inhibitors.[112] Traditional NSAIDS such as aspirin inhibit both COX-1 and COX-2 enzyme activity. These enzymes are both involved in prostaglandin synthesis, although COX-1 is constitutively expressed and is important in maintaining the integrity of the gut and the kidney whereas COX-2 is inducible by inflammation such as is found in rheumatoid arthritis. It is the blocking of COX-1 activity that causes the gastrointestinal and renal toxicity associated with prolonged aspirin use. The development of specific COX-2 inhibitors should, in theory, be associated with fewer side effects and should also retain a potential chemotherapeutic effect against colorectal carcinogenesis.[103,113,114]

There are a variety of reasons for believing that COX-2 is involved in the development of colorectal cancer: there is an increase in COX-2 expression in adenomatous polyps in humans and in malignant tumours of the large bowel; intestinal polyps from Min+ mice (which have a germline mutation in the *Apc* gene and are a model for human FAP) and carcinogen-induced rat colon tumours also show increased levels of COX-2.[115] Chemoprevention by selective COX-2 inhibitors has been demonstrated in cell culture,[116] in the azoxymethane-treated rat model of colon cancer[117] and in ApcD716 mice.[115] It has been demonstrated that one molecule which exhibits only COX-2 (O-[acetoxyphenyl] hept-2–ynyl sulphide [APHS]) is 60 times more effective in blocking COX-2 activity than aspirin and that it irreversibly inhibits enzyme activity in macrophages and colon cancer cells.[118] Development of molecules such as this for clinical use will have profound effects on patients with both rheumatoid and osteo-arthritis and may well have a significant role in future programmes of colorectal cancer prevention.

More recently, the issue of HRT and the reduced risk of colorectal cancer risk has come to the fore: it remains one of the outstanding clinical research issues at present.[119] A Medline search was used to identify observational studies published between January 1974 and December 1993 for a meta-analysis of HRT and colorectal cancer risk.[120] The overall risk for colorectal cancer and oestrogen replacement therapy was 0.92 (95% CI = 0.74, 1.5). There was not a separate effect when colon and rectal cancer were considered as separate entities.[120] Subsequent to this report, further studies have been published.

A case–control study from Seattle, USA among 193 women aged 30–62 years with colon cancer and an equal number of controls was conducted to examine the relationship between colon cancer and female hormone use.[121] Use of non-contraceptive hormones after age 40 was associated with a reduced risk of colon cancer (OR=0.60; 95% CI = 0.35, 1.01). The risk among women with 5 or more years of use was 0.47 (0.24, 0.91).[121]

Colorectal cancer mortality was examined in some detail in the American Cancer Society

Prospective Study. With the risk set to 1.0 among women reported never to be users of HRT (the referent group), the risk associated with 'ever' use was 0.69 (95% CI = 0.60,0.79).[122] Relative to the risk in never users, the risk associated with less than 1 year of use was 0.81 (0.63,1.03), with between 2 and 5 years of use 0.76 (0.61,0.95); and for between 6 and 10 years of use 0.55 (0.39, 0.77). For 11 or more years of use of HRT the risk was 0.54 (0.39,0.76).

Kampman *et al.*[123] recently reported a large case–control study throughout the United States. The use of HRT was significantly related inversely to risk with the effect limited to women who were recent users (OR = 0.71; 95% CI = 0.56, 0.89). There was no trend with duration of use of HRT and there was no difference in the effect at different sites of the colon. An analysis of the records of women in the Breast Cancer Detection Demonstration Project revealed 313 cases of colorectal cancer and a small reduction in risk among recent HRT users (RR = 0.78; 95% CI = 0.55, 1.11).[124]

Of 21 published studies of HRT and colorectal cancer risk, 14 support an inverse association, of which seven show a statistically significant reduction in risk.[125] The risk seems lowest among the most recent users. Although there are still some contradictions in the available literature, it appears likely that use of HRT reduces the risk of colorectal cancer in women. The risk appears to be halved with 5–10 years of such use. The role of unopposed oestrogens, compared with combination HRT, is an open issue for colorectal cancer.

HEALTH CARE PROVIDERS

From time to time there can appear to be some confusion about the role of health care purchasers: they should not exist to find the cheapest health care available for the population but to find the health care that provides the best outcomes and then to deliver it in the most cost-effective manner available to the population covered. This should involve identifying sources of variation in the outcome of therapy over and above the characteristics of the individual cancer, and bringing about their alteration in the community in the most cost-effective manner to maximize the outcome of treatment in patients in their area. Recently, a number of important sources of variation have been identified in the outcome of colorectal cancer.

9. Specialist clinics should be established within geographical regions, with multidisciplinary management protocols utilized for patients discovered to have colorectal cancer

For a long time it has been thought that there is a variation in the outcome of treatment of cancer. Thirty cancer registries throughout Europe have participated in the EUROCARE project, which was designed to investigate variations in survival between these registry regions. Approximately 800,000 patients with cancer were included in this database and the regions were assembled into 12 countries for presentation of the results.[16] For colon cancer, the relative 5-year survival in men ranged from highest values in Switzerland (51%), the Netherlands (50%) and France (45%) to the lowest values in Estonia (40%), England (35%) and Poland (21%). There was also considerable variation reported in rectal cancer in men with the highest survival rates reported from Switzerland (50%), Finland (43%) and the Netherlands (41%) and the lowest survival rates in Scotland (31%), Estonia (30%) and Poland (15%).

This is a remarkable dataset, but the findings must be treated with some caution as there are limitations to the information that constrain the straightforward interpretation of these results: for example, criteria for admission of cases to the study were not standardized in the participating registries (the problem of Death Certificate Only registrations was not consistently dealt with); the date of diagnosis varied (some registries use date of registration, some use date treatment commenced and some use date of first symptoms); completeness of follow-up varied between regional registries (in France the death certificate is a private document, making linkage between *département* of death and *département* of diagnosis extremely difficult) and national registries (follow-up in Denmark and the United Kingdom is virtually complete as a result of national cause-of-death registries); furthermore, no allowance was made for the case-mix of the patients. Notwithstanding these sources of potential bias, it is unlikely that biases explain all the variation noted and it could be concluded that there is variation in the outcome of colorectal cancer treatment in Europe, although it may be exaggerated in the data presented in the EUROCARE study.[16]

Rectification of this situation could be of important benefit to colorectal cancer patients throughout Europe: indeed, such variation is unlikely to be restricted to this single continent. Rectification depends on prior identification of the factors contributing to this situation. Stiller,[14] in a detailed review of all cancer sites, has demonstrated convincingly that centralized referral or entry to clinical trials has frequently been associated with a higher survival rate and has never been shown to be associated with a reduced survival rate.[14] Studies that have specifically investigated colorectal cancer have been consistent with this overall observation.[126–130] Determinants of success in the outcome of colorectal cancer are not straightforward to identify: for example, the simplest definition of specialization is volume, and this is not associated with outcome.[15]

McArdle and Hole[15] have published a very influential article on variations in the outcome of colorectal cancer according to a number of factors including the individual surgeon. Employing data on all patients diagnosed in one large teaching hospital in Glasgow between 1974 and 1979, they noted that management of these patients was divided between 13 consultant surgeons, none of whom had a specific interest in colorectal surgery. They found wide variations in the aggressiveness of the surgeons (an overall 52% curative resection rate ranged from 40 to 76% according to individual surgeons), the quality of surgical technique (wound dehiscence rate overall was 5% ranging from 0 to 11%) and the postoperative mortality rate (which was overall 16% but varied between 8 and 30% according to surgeon). After adjusting for case-mix and important prognostic variables, the relative hazard ratio (fixed overall as 1.0) varied from 0.59 to 1.61 according to surgeon.[15] In other words, 10-year survival varied almost threefold between surgeons.

There are undoubted sources of variation in the outcome of treatment of colorectal cancer unrelated to the cancer itself. Treatment in specialist centres or according to a treatment protocol is associated with an increased survival rate. It is also evident that surgical technique may be more relevant to the outcome of treatment of colorectal cancer care than for most other sites of cancer, where the surgery is less technically demanding. The case for the establishment of specialist clinics within geographical regions employing multidisciplinary management protocols is convincing. The role of the health care provider or purchaser is to ensure that this quality of care is available to patients at the minimum price that can be achieved.

SPECIALIST TRAINING

10. Continual specialist training should be introduced on a regular basis for consultant surgeons, radiotherapists and physicians to keep them abreast of developments in their field

The optimum treatment for most cancers is evolving gradually and higher medical training is a never-ending process. This may be more important for colorectal cancer, where surgical technique is an important element of outcome, radiotherapy has an increasingly important role and medical management is evolving fairly rapidly. The need for a system of continuing medical education in Europe is now overdue and it is good that strides are currently being taken in this direction.

Discussion

For hundreds of years, epidemiology has had as its basis astute clinical observations such as those of the excess of breast cancer in nuns,[131] puerperal fever and the hygiene of the obstetrician[132] and cancer of the lip and pipe smoking.[133] These, and other observations have been reviewed by Clemmesen:[134] undoubtedly other associations noted have not stood the test of time.

The scientific basis of epidemiology really emerged only in the second half of this century although there were at least two prototype case–control studies were previously conducted.[135–136] The statistical under-pinning of the subject emerged from the major United States Schools of Public Health (Harvard and Johns Hopkins) and from London, Oxford and Paris as the twentieth century progressed. As the theoretical basis of epidemiology was developed, terminology was introduced to help create a unifying theory, satisfactory for understanding the conceptual basis of the subject.

Cancer control, a term used to cover all steps leading to reduction or prevention of cancer mortality, has always been considered under the three headings of primary, secondary and tertiary prevention. Although this is a very appropriate distinction to classify the various types of actions that could prevent cancer deaths, it may not be the most appropriate paradigm for a major initiative to move epidemiology through its theoretical and information-gathering phase to its next phase involving public health implementation of these findings. Without this progression, information may wither on the vine and significant numbers of preventable deaths may occur.

One consequence of all the aetiological research on lifestyle factors and (particularly chronic) diseases has been, however inadvertently, to blame the patient for the development of the disease. The furthest this has been taken has been the well-publicized refusal in parts of England to perform cardiac bypass surgery, when indicated on clinical grounds, because an individual happens to smoke cigarettes. Society, of which we are part, has given its members cheap and easy access to what has become the most widely used dependency-inducing drug: the blame for addiction should not be completely shouldered by the addict in such circumstances. Prevention guidelines, for example the European Code Against Cancer,[18] implicitly place the blame and responsibility for prevention at the door of each individual.

Consideration of the example of colorectal cancer reveals that there are true prospects for greatly reducing the mortality from this condition. However, achievement of colorectal cancer control can be achieved only by realizing that there are other groups within our Society who have responsibility for this, apart from the individual, and that the theoretical model of primary, secondary and tertiary prevention is not the basis of practical control strategies. Deaths, theoretically preventable, will continue to occur unless individual groups are identified who are given responsibility for particular actions. Primary care physicians, health care purchasers, those responsible for specialist medical training, each have defined contributions to reducing colorectal cancer mortality (Appendix 1.1). Of course, the individual within our society should be aware that he/she has lifestyle choices to make and that some of these could lead to reductions in the risk of colorectal cancer as well as of other serious diseases.

The major reductions in the incidence and mortality of colorectal cancer reported from retrospective assessment of sigmoidoscopy are frequently around 80% and are difficult to ignore.[9–12] The ability to use this information logically is not straightforward. Given the usual requirements of evidence-based medicine – the need for a meta-analysis or at least findings from randomized trials, it seems priority to embark on large, long-term randomized trials. However, given the biological plausibility, the relative ease and safety of the procedure and the impressive size of the reduction, could this step be passed over? This apparent statistical heresy has precedents in oncology: the two major advances in cancer cure in the modern era – mustine, vincristine, procarbazine and prednisolone (MOPP) and megavoltage radiotherapy for Hodgkin's disease and *cis*-platinum-based chemotherapy for testicular cancer – have not been the consequences of randomized phase III trials: results of treatment were so obvious that such trials were not necessary. Perhaps the same case should be made for colonoscopy in the prevention of colorectal cancer death.

The change in knowledge of colorectal cancer since 1980 has been enormous and this could be the first major neoplasm where control strategies could have major impact on reducing mortality. A number of groups within society have defined responsibilities to contribute to this goal and decisions need to be taken about when data gathering should end and prevention action should begin. There are gambles involved in embarking on coordinated programmes such as outlined herein. However, for colorectal cancer the 'bet' is small and the winnings could be high. If the opportunity is not seized, many deaths may occur that could otherwise have been avoided.

Acknowledgements

This work was conducted within the framework of support by the Italian Association for Cancer

Research (Associazione Italiana per la Ricerca sul Cancro).

References

1. Parkin DM, Pisani P, Ferlay J. Estimates of the worldwide incidence of eighteen major cancers in 1985. *Int J Cancer* 1993; 55: 594–606

2. Morson BC. *Gastrointestinal Pathology*. Oxford: Blackwell Scientific, 1979

3. Pisani P, Parkin DM, Ferlay J. Estimates of the worldwide mortality rate from 18 major cancers in 1985. Implications for prevention and projections of future burden. *Int J Cancer* 1993; 55: 891–903

4. Boyle P, Maisonneuve P, Audisio RA. Epidemiology of gastrointestinal cancer. In: McCulloch P, Kingsnorth A (eds) *Management of Gastrointestinal Cancer*, London: BMJ Publishing Group, pp. 1–36

5. Langman MJS, Boyle P. Chemoprevention of colorectal cancer. *Gut* 1998;43: 578–585

6. Mandel J, Bond J, Church T *et al.* Reducing mortality from colorectal cancer by screening for fecal occult blood. *N Engl J Med* 1993; 328: 1365–1371

7. Hardcastle JD, Chamberlain JO, Robinson MHE *et al.* Randomised controlled trial of faecal-occult-blood screening for colorectal cancer. *Lancet* 1996; 348: 1472–1477

8. Kronberg O, Fenger C, Olsen J *et al.* Randomised study of screening for colorectal cancer with faecal-occult-blood test. *Lancet* 1996; 348: 1467–1471

9. Gilbertson VA, Nelms JM. The prevention of invasive cancer of the rectum. *Cancer* 1978; 41: 1137–1139

10. Selby JV, Friedman GD, Quesenbery CJ, Weiss NS. A case–control study of screening sigmoidoscopy and mortality from colorectal cancer. *N Engl J Med* 1992; 326: 653–657

11. Atkin WS, Morson BC, Cuzick J. Long-term risk of colorectal cancer after excision of rectosigmoid adenomas. *N Engl J Med* 1992; 326: 658–662

12. Newcomb PA, Norfleet RG, Storer BE *et al.* Screening sigmoidoscopy and colorectal cancer mortality. *J Natl Cancer Inst* 1992; 84: 1572–1575

13. Cunningham D, Findlay M. The chemotherapy of colon cancer can no longer be ignored. *Eur J Cancer* 1993; 29: 2077–2079

14. Stiller CA. Centralised treatment, entry to trials and survival. *Br J Cancer* 1994; 70: 352–362

15. McArdle CS, Hole DJ. Impact of variability among surgeons on postoperative morbidity and mortality and ultimate survival. *Br Med J* 1991; 302: 1501–1505

16. Berrino F, Sant M, Verdacchia A *et al.* Survival of cancer patients in Europe: the EUROCARE study. *IARC Scientific Publications*. Lyon: IARC 1995

17. Boyle P. Progress in preventing death from colorectal cancer. *Br J Cancer* 1995; 72: 528–530

18. Boyle P, Smans M, Zaridze D. Descriptive epidemiology of colorectal cancer. *Int J Cancer* 1985; 36: 9–18

19. Haenzel W, Kurihara M. Studies of Japanese migrants. I. Mortality from cancer and other diseases among Japanese in the United States. *J Natl Cancer Inst* 1968; 40: 43–68

20. Haenzel W, Core P. Cancer of the colon and rectum and adenomatous polyps. A review of epidemiologic findings. *Cancer* 1971; 28: 14–24

21. Bell J, Coates M, Day P, Armstrong BK. *Colorectal Cancer in New South Wales in 1972 to 1993*. Sydney: Cancer Council, New South Wales Health Department, 1996

22. Levi F, Lucchini F, Boyle P *et al.* Cancer incidence and mortality in Europe, 1988–92. *J Epidemiol Biostat* 1998; 3: 295–373

23. Canadian Cancer Society. *Canadian Cancer Statistics*, 1997. Toronto: Canadian Cancer Society, 1997

24. Boyle P, La Vecchia C, Maisonneuve P *et al.* Cancer epidemiology and prevention. In: Peckham M, Pinedo H, Veronesi U (eds) *Oxford Textbook of Oncology*. Oxford: Oxford University Press, pp. 199–273

25. Boyle P, Veronesi U, Tubiana M *et al.* European School of Oncology Advisory Report to the European Commission for the 'Europe Against Cancer Programme'. European Code Against Cancer. *Eur J Cancer* 1995; 29: 1395–1405

26. Kritchevsky D. Diet, nutrition and cancer: the role of fibre. *Cancer* 1986; 58: 1830–1836

27. Tuyns AJ, Haeltermann M, Kaaks R. Colorectal cancer and the intake of nutrients: oliogo-saccharides are a risk factor, fats are not. A case–control study in Belgium. *Nutr Cancer* 1987; 10: 181–196

28. Kune S, Kune GA, Watson LF. Case–control study of dietary aetiological factors: the Melbourne colorectal cancer study. *Nutr Cancer* 1987; 9: 21–42

29. Heilbrun LK, Hankin JH, Nomura AMY *et al.* Colon cancer and dietary fat, phosphorus and calcium in Hawaiian-Japanese men. *Am J Clin Nutr* 1986; 43: 306–309

30. Willett WC. The search for the causes of breast and colon cancer. *Nature* 1989; 338: 389–394

31. Freedman AN, Michalek AM, Marshall JR *et al.* Familial and nutritional risk factors for *p53* overexpression in colorectal cancer. *Cancer Epidemiol Biomarkers Prev* 1996; 5: 285–291

32. Newmark HL, Wargovich MJ, Bruce WR. Colon cancer and dietary fat, phosphate and calcium: a hypothesis. *J Natl Cancer Inst* 1984; 72: 1323–1325

33. Sorenson AW, Slattery ML, Ford MH. Calcium and colon cancer: a review. *Nutr Cancer* 1988; 11: 135–145

34. Longnecker MP, Orza MJ, Adams ME *et al.* A meta-analysis of alcoholic beverage consumption in relation to risk of colorectal cancer. *Cancer Causes Contr* 1990; 1: 59–68

35. Zaridze DG. Environmental etiology of large-bowel cancer. *J Natl Cancer Inst* 1983; 70: 389–400

36. Goldin BR, Gorbach SL. The effect of milk and lactobacillus feeding on human intestinal bacterial enzyme activity. *Am J Clin Nutr* 1984; 39: 756–761

37. IARC. *Monographs on the evaluation of the carcinogenic risk of chemicals to man.* Volume 44. *Coffee, tea, mate, methylxanthines (caffeine, theophylline, theobromine) and methylglyoxal.* Lyon: IARC, 1988

38. Vena JE, Graham S, Zielezny M, *et al.* Occupational exercise and risk of cancer. *Am J Clin Nutr* 1987; 45: 318–327

39. Slattery ML, Schumacher ML, Smith M *et al.* Physical activity, diet and role of colon cancer in Utah. *Am J Epidemiol* 1988; 128: 989–999

40. Whittemore AS, Wu-Williams AH, Lee M *et al.* Diet, physical activity and colorectal cancer among Chinese in North America and China. *J Natl Cancer Inst* 1990; 82: 915–926

41. Thune I, Lurid E. Physical activity and risk of colorectal cancer in men and women. *Br J Cancer* 1996; 73: 1134–1140

42. Sandler RS, Pritchard ML, Bangiwala SI. Physical activity and the risk of colorectal adenomas. *Epidemiology* 1995; 6: 602–606

43. Giovannucci E, Colditz GA, Stampfer MJ, Willett WC. Physical activity, obesity and risk of colorectal cancer in women (United States). *Cancer Causes Contr* 1996; 7: 253–263

44. Howe GR, Aronson KJ, Benito E *et al.* The relationship between dietary fat intake and risk of colorectal cancer: evidence from the combined analysis of 13 case–control studies. *Cancer Causes Contr* 1997; 8: 215–228

45. Willett WC, Stampfer MJ, Colditz GA *et al.* Relation of meat, fat, and fiber intake to the risk of colon cancer in a prospective study among women. *N Engl J Med* 1990; 323: 1664–1672

46. Bostick RM, Potter JD, Kushi LH *et al.* Sugar, meat, and fat intake and risk factors for colon cancer incidence in Iowa women (United States). *Cancer Causes Contr* 1994; 5: 1664–1672

47. Goldbohm RA, van den Brandt PA, van't Veer P *et al.* A prospective cohort study on the relation between meat consumption and the risk of colon cancer. *Cancer Res* 1994; 54: 38–52

48. Potter JD, Slattery ML, Bostwick RM, Gapstur SM. Colon cancer: a review of the epidemiology. *Epidemiol Rev* 1993; 15: 499–545

49. McKeown-Eyssen G. Epidemiology of colorectal cancer revisited: are serum triglycerides and/or plasma glucose associated with risk. *Cancer Epidemiol Biomarkers Prev* 1994; 3: 687–695

50. Sugimura T. Past, present and future of mutagens in cooked foods. *Environ Health Perspect* 1986; 67: 5–10

51. Felton JS, Knize MG, Shen NH *et al.* Identification of the mutagens in cooked beef. *Environ Health Perspect* 1986; 67: 17–24

52. Schiffman MH, Felton JS. Fried foods and the risk of colon cancer. *Am J Epidemiol* 1990; 131: 376–378

53. Ha WI, Grim NK, Periza MW. Anticarcinogenics from fried ground beef: heat-altered derivatives of linoleic acid. *Carcinogenesis* 1987; 8: 1881–1887

54. Sakaguchi M, Hiramatsu Y, Takada H *et al.* Effect of dietary unsaturated and saturated fats on azoxymethane-induced colon carcinogenesis in rats. *Cancer Res* 1984; 44: 1472–1477

55. Minoura YT, Takata T, Sakaguchi M *et al.* Effect of dietary eicopentaenoic acid on azoxymethane induced colon carcinogenesis in rats. *Cancer Res* 1988; 46: 4790–4794

56. Shephard RJ. Exercise in the prevention and treatment of cancer – an update. *Sports Med* 1993; 15: 258–280

57. Holdstock DJ, Misiewicz JJ, Smith T *et al.* Propulsion (mass movements) in the human colon and its relationship to meals and somatic activity. *Gut* 1970; 11: 91–99

58. Simon HB The immunology of exercise. *JAMA* 1984; 252: 2735–2738

59. Bartram HP, Wynder EL. Physical activity and colon cancer risk? Physiological consideration. *Am J Gastroenterol* 1989; 84: 109–112

60. Kune GA, Kune S, Fields B *et al.* Survival in patients with large-bowel cancer. *Dis Colon Rectum.* 1990; 33: 938–946

61. Fearon ER, Vogelstein B. A genetic model for colorectal tumorigenesis. *Cell* 1990; 61: 759–767

62. Morotomi M, Guillem J, LoGerfo P, Weinstein IB. Production of diacylglycerol, an activator of protein kinase C, by human intestinal microflora. *Cancer Res* 1990; 50: 3595–3599

63. Bodmer WF, Balley CJ, Bodmer J *et al.* Localization of the gene for familial adenomatous polyposis on chromosome 5. *Nature* 1987; 328: 614–618

64. Hall NR, Murday VA, Chapman P *et al.* Genetic Linkage in Muir–Torre syndrome to the same chromosomal region as cancer family syndrome. *Eur J Cancer* 1994; 30: 180–182

65. Selby JV, Friedman GD, Quesenberry CP, Weiss NS. Effect of fecal occult blood testing on mortality from colorectal cancer: a case–control study. *Ann Intern Med* 1993; 118: 1294–1297

66. Wahrendorf J, Robra BP, Wiebelt H *et al.* Effectiveness of colorectal cancer screening: a population-based case–control study in Saarland, Germany. *Eur J Cancer Prev* 1993; 1: 221–227

67. Hardcastle JD. Screening for colorectal cancer. *Lancet* 1997; 349: 358

68. Faivre J, Tazi MA, Autier P, Bleiberg H. Should there be mass screening using faecal occult blood test for colorectal cancer? *Eur J Cancer* 1998; 34: 773–780

69. Rozen P, Ron E, Fireman Z *et al.* The relative value of fecal occult blood tests and flexible sigmoidoscopy in screening for large bowel neoplasia. *Cancer* 1987; 60: 2553–2558

70. Allison J, Feldman R, Tekawa I. Hemocult screening in detecting colorectal neoplasm. *Ann Intern Med* 1990; 112: 328–333

71. Winawer SJ, Fletcher RH, Miller L *et al.* Colorectal cancer screening: clinical guidelines and rationale. *Gastroenterology* 1997; 112: 594–642

72. Selby JV, Friedman GD, Quesenberry CP, Weiss NS. A case–control study of screening sigmoidoscopy and mortality from colorectal cancer. *New Eng J Med* 1992; 326, 653–657

73. Church TR, Ederer F, Mandel JS. Faecal occult blood screening in Minnesota: sensitivity of the screening test. *J Natl Cancer Inst* 1997; 89: 1440–1448

74. Ederer F, Church TR, Mandel JS. Faecal occult blood screening in Minnesota: role of chance detection of lesions. *J Natl Cancer Inst* 1997; 89: 1423–1428

75. Lang CA, Ranshoff DF. On the sensitivity of faecal occult blood test screening for colorectal cancer. *J Natl Cancer Inst* 1997; 89: 1392–1393

76. Launoy G, Smith TC, Duffy SW, Bouvier V. Colorectal cancer mass screening: estimation of faecal occult blood test sensitivity, taking into account cancer mean sojourn time. *Int J Cancer* 1997; 73: 208–210

77. Simon JB. Should all people over the age of 50 have regular fecal occult-blood tests: postpone population screening until problems are solved. *N Engl J Med* 1998; 338: 1151–1152

78. Fletcher RH. Should all people over the age of 50 have regular fecal occult-blood tests: if it works, why not do it? *N Engl J Med* 1998; 338: 1153–1154

79. Greenberg R, Baron J. Prospects for preventing colorectal cancer death. *J Natl Cancer Inst* 1993; 85, 1182–1184

80. Hosek RS, Flanders WD, Sasco, AJ. Bias in case–control studies of screening effectiveness. *Am J Epidemiol* 1996; 143: 193–201

81. Winawer SJ, Zauber AG, Ho MN *et al.* Prevention of colorectal cancer by colonoscopic polypectomy. *N Eng J Med* 1993; 329: 1977–1981

82. Mandel J. Colon and rectal cancer. In: Reintgen DS, Clark RA (eds) *Cancer Screening.* St Louis: Mosby, 1996 pp. 55–96

83. Bhattacharya I, Sack EM. Screening colonoscopy: the cost of common sense. *Lancet* 1996; 347: 1744–1745

84. Rogge JD, Elmore MF, Mahoney SJ *et al.* Low-cost, office-based, screening colonoscopy. *Am J Gastroenterol* 1994; 89: 1775–1780

85. Atkin WS, Cuzick J, Northover JMA, Whynes DK. Prevention of colorectal cancer by once-only sigmoidoscopy. *Lancet* 1993; 341: 736–740

86. Toribara NW, Sleisenger MH. Screening for colorectal cancer. *N Eng J Med* 1995; 332: 861–867

87. Chu KC, Tarone RE, Chow W, Hankey BF, Reis LAG. Temporal patterns in colorectal cancer incidence, survival and mortality from 1950 through 1990. *J Nat Cancer Inst* 1994; 86: 997–1006

88. Coleman MP, Esteve J, Dameicki P *et al.* Trends in cancer incidence and mortality. *IARC Scientific Publications No.* 121, Lyon: IARC, 1993

89. Northover J. Realism or nihilism in bowel cancer follow-up. *Lancet* 1998; 351: 1074–1075

90. McArdle CS, Wotherspoon H, Hole DJ, Murray GD. Colorectal cancer: a continuing problem. *Gastrointest Cancer* 1996; 1: 171–176

91. Bodmer WF, Balley CJ, Bodmer J *et al.* Localization of the gene for familial adenomatous polyposis on chromosome 5. *Nature* 1987; 328: 614–618

92. Bishop DT, Thomas HJW. The genetics of colorectal cancer. *Cancer Surv* 1990; 9: 585–604

93. Bishop DT, Hall NR. The genetics of colorectal cancer. *Eur J Cancer* 1994; 30: 1946–1956

94. Ponz de Leon M. Familial and hereditary tumours. *Recent Results Cancer Res* 1994; 136: 1–156

95. Peleg I, Maibach HT, Brown SH, Wilcox CM. Aspirin and non-steroidal anti-inflammatory drug use and the risk of subsequent colorectal cancer. *Arch Intern Med* 1994; 154: 394–399

96. Rosenberg L, Palmer JR, Zauber AG *et al.* A hypothesis: non-steroidal anti-inflammatory drugs reduce the incidence of large bowel cancer. *J Natl Cancer Inst* 1991; 83: 355–358

97. Kune GA, Kune S, Watson JF. Colorectal cancer risk, chronic illnesses, operations and medications: case–control results from the Melbourne Colorectal Cancer Study. *Cancer Res* 1988; 48: 4399–4404

98. Giovannucci E, Rimm EB, Stampfer MJ *et al.* Aspirin use and the risk of colorectal cancer and adenoma in male health professionals. *Ann Intern Med* 1994; 121: 241–246

99. Logan RF, Little J, Hawtin PG, Hardcastle JD. Effect of aspirin and nonsteroidal anti-inflammatory drugs on colorectal adenomas: case–control study of subjects participating in the Nottingham faecal occult blood screening programme. *Br Med J* 1993; 307: 285–289

100. Narisawa T, Sato M, Tani M, Takahashi I. Inhibition of development of methyl-nitrosourea induced colonic tumours by peroral administration of indomethacin. *Jpn J Cancer Res* 1982; 73; 377–381

101. Reddy BS, Rao CV, Rivenson A, Kelloff G. Inhibitory effect of aspirin on azoxymethane-induced colon carcinogenesis in F 344 rats. *Carcinogenesis* 1993; 14: 1493–1497

102. Labayle D, Fischer D, Vielh P *et al.* Sulindac causes regression of rectal polyps in familial adenomatous polyposis. *Gastroenterology* 1991; 101: 635–639

103. Giardiello FM, Hamilton SR, Krush AJ *et al.* Treatment of colonic and rectal adenomas with sulindac in familial adenomatous polyposis. *N Engl J Med* 1993; 328: 1313–1316

104. Lala PK, Parhar RS, Singh P. Indomethacin therapy abrogates the prostaglandin mediated suppression of natural killer activity in tumorbearing mice and prevents tumor metastasis. *Cell Immunol* 1986; 99: 108–118

105. Narisawa T, Takahashi M, Masuda T *et al.* Prevention of peritoneal carcinomatosis recurrence with a prostaglandin synthesis inhibitor, indomethacin. *Gan To Kagaku Ryoho* 1987; 14: 2496–2501

106. Schultz RM, Altorn MG. Potentiation of non-specific immunotherapy of experimental lung metastases by indomethacin. *J Immuno-pharmacol* 1983; 5: 277–280

107. Weppelmann B, Monkemeier D. The influence of prostaglandin antagonists on radiation therapy of carcinoma of the cervix. *Gynecol Oncol* 1984; 17: 196–199

108. Langman MJS, Weil J, Wainwright P *et al.* Risks of bleeding peptic ulcer associated with individual non-steroidal anti-inflammatory drugs. *Lancet* 1994; 343: 1075–1078

109. Weil J, Colin Jones D, Langman MJS *et al.* Prophylactic aspirin and risk of peptic ulcer bleeding. *Br Med J* 1995; 310: 827–830

110. Gann PH, Manson JE, Glynn RJ, Buring JE, Hennekens CH. Low dose aspirin and incidence of colorectal tumours in a randomised trial. *J Natl Cancer Inst* 1993; 85: 1220–1224

111. Giovannucci E, Egan KM, Hunter DJ *et al.* Aspirin and the risk of colorectal cancer in women. *N Engl J Med* 1995; 333: 609–614

112. Rustgi AK. Cyclooxygenase-2: the future is now. *Nature Medicine* 1998; 4: 773–774

113. Shiff SJ, Rigas B. Nonsteroidal anti-inflammatory drugs and colorectal cancer: evolving concepts of their chemotherapeutic actions. *Gastroenterology* 1998; 113: 1992–1998

114. Piazza GA, Alberts DS, Hixson LJ *et al.* Sulindac sulfone inhibits azoxymethane-induced colon carcinogenesis in rats without reducing prostaglandin levels. *Cancer Res* 1997; 57: 2909–2915

115. Oshima M, Dinchuk JE, Kargman SL *et al.* Suppression of intestinal polyps in *APC* delta 716 knockout mice by inhibition of prostaglandin endoperoxidase-2 (COX-2). *Cell* 1996; 87: 803–809

116. Sheng H, Shao J, Kirkland SC, *et al.* Inhibition of human colon cancer cell growth by selective inhibition of cyclooxygenase-2. *J Clin Invest* 1997; 99: 2254–2259

117. Kalgutar AS, Kozak KR, Crews BC *et al.* Aspirin-like molecules that covalently inactivate cyclooxygenase-2. *Science* 1998; 280: 1268–1270

118. Reddy BS, Rao CV, Seibert K. Evaluation of cyclooxygenase-2 inhibitor for potential chemopreventive properties in colon carcinogenesis. *Cancer Res* 1996; 56: 4566–4569

119. Veronesi U, Maisonneuve P, Costa A *et al.* on behalf of the Italian Tamoxifen Study Group. Prevention of breast cancer with tamoxifen: The Italian Randomised Trial among Hysterectomised Women. *Lancet* 1998; 352: 93–97

120. MacLennan SC, MacLennan AH, Ryan P. Colorectal cancer and oestrogen replacement therapy: a meta-analysis of epidemiological studies. *Med J Austr* 1991; 162: 491–193

121. Jacobs EJ, White E, Weiss NS. Exogenous hormones, reproductive history and colon cancer. *Cancer Causes Contr* 1994; 5: 359–366

122. Calle EE, Miracle-McMahill HL, Thun MJ, Heath CW. Estrogen replacement therapy and risk of fatal colon cancer in a prospective cohort of postmenopausal women. *J Natl Cancer Inst* 1995; 87: 517–523

123. Kampman E, Potter JD, Slattery ML *et al.* Hormone replacement therapy, reproductive history and colon cancer: a multicentre case-control study in the United States. *Cancer Causes Contr* 1997; 8: 146–158

124. Troisi R, Schairer C, Chow WL *et al.* A prospective study of menopausal hormones and risk of colorectal cancer in the United States. *Cancer Causes Contr* 1997; 8: 75–79

125. Calle EE. Editorial: Hormone replacement therapy and colorectal cancer: interpreting the evidence. *Cancer Causes Contr* 1997; 8: 127–129

126. Hakama M, Karjalainen S, Hakulinen T. Outcome-based equity in the treatment of colon cancer patients in Finland. *Int J Technol Assess.Health Care* 1989; 5: 619–630

127. Mohner M, Slislow W. Untersuchung zum Einfluss der regional zentralisierten Behandlung auf die Uberlebenschancen beim Rektumkarzinom in der DDR. *Zentralbl Chir* 1990; 115: 801–812

128. Launoy G, Le Coutour X, Gignloux M *et al.* Influence of rural environment on diagnosis, treatment and prognosis of colorectal cancer. *J Epidemiol Community Health* 1992; 46: 365–367

129. Pickering RM, Chadwell IR and Mounteney L. Importance of district of residence and known primary site for bowel cancer survival: analysis of data from Wessex Cancer registry. *J Epidemiol Community Health* 1992; 46: 266–270

130. Kingston RD, Walsh S, Jeacock J. Colorectal surgeons in district general hospitals produce similar survival outcomes to their teaching hospital colleagues: review of five year survivals in Manchester. *J R Coll Surg Edinb* 1992; 37: 235–237

131. Ramazzini B. De morbis artificum. Diatriba. J Corona, Venezia, 1743

132. Semmelweis IP. The etiology, the concept and the prophylaxis of childbed fever, 1861. Translated and republished in *Med Class* 1941; 5: 350–773

133. Melzer R. Uber den Lippenkrebs und die Ursache seines haufigen Vorkommens in Krain. *Jena Ann Med Physiol* 1850; II: 480–484

134. Clemmesen J. *Statistical Studies in Malignant Neoplasms. I. Review and Results.* Copenhagen: Munksgaard, 1965

135. Lane-Claypon JE. A further report on cancer of the breast, with special reference to its associated antecedent conditions. *Rep Min Health No. 32*, London: Ministry of Health, 1926

136. Muller FH. Tabaksmisbrauch und Lungenkarzinom. *Z Krebsforsch* 1940; 49: 57–85

137. Parkin DM, Whelan SL, Ferlay L *et al.* (eds) Cancer incidence in five continents, Vol. VII. *IARC Scientific Publications No. 143.* Lyon: IARC, 1997

Appendix 1.1: guidelines for colorectal cancer control

The goal of all cancer research and treatment is to prevent people dying from the disease. Knowledge has been accruing rapidly regarding actions and interventions which could lead to a reduction in death from colorectal cancer, either by reducing the risk of developing the disease, by identifying the disease at a stage when it is more curable or by improving the outcome of therapy. Such a package of actions is aimed at colorectal cancer control, which will be achieved by contributions in a number of areas and requiring actions on the part of several separate sections of society, as outlined below.

GENERAL PUBLIC

1. Increase intake of vegetables and fruits. Eat five servings of fruits and vegetables each day whenever possible: systematically replace snacks such as chocolate bars, biscuits and crisps with an apple, orange or another piece of fruit or vegetable.
2. Reduce intake of calories, and of animal fats in particular. Frequently substitute fish and poultry for beef, lamb and pork as a main course.
3. Increase physical activity levels: this can be accomplished by activities of moderate intensity such as brisk walking.
4. Participate in organized population-screening programmes. In their absence, give serious consideration to having a sigmoidoscopy (or colonoscopy) with polyp removal once between the age of 50 and 59 years.
5. Consult a doctor as soon as possible if you have a noticeable and unexplained change in bowel habits, notice blood in the stool, have colicky pain in the abdomen or have a recurrent sensation of incomplete evacuation after defaecation.

INDIVIDUALS WITH A GENETIC RISK OF COLORECTAL CANCER

6. Individuals with a strong family history of colorectal cancer, or the presence of a disease such as familial adenomatous polyposis, are at an increased risk of colorectal cancer. Such people should be carefully followed and should participate in whatever screening programme is indicated.

PRIMARY CARE DOCTORS

7. Patients who consult with possible symtoms of bowel cancer should have an adequate physical examination, including a careful digital rectal examination whenever indicated.
8. Doctors should advise their healthy patients appropriately about the possible benefits of aspirin and hormone replacement therapy in the possible prevention of colorectal cancer

HEALTH CARE PURCHASERS

9. Specialist clinics should be established within geographical regions, with multidisciplinary management protocols available for patients discovered to have colorectal cancer.

SPECIALIST TRAINING

10. Continual specialist training should be introduced on a regular basis for consultant surgeons, radiotherapists and physicians to keep them abreast of developments in their field.

Chapter 2

IMAGING OF COLORECTAL CANCER*

D. Balfe and M. Semin

Introduction

RATIONALE FOR RADIOLOGICAL STAGING AND FOLLOW-UP

Carcinoma of the colorectum is a prevalent and lethal disease; in the United States, an estimated 131,200 cases will be diagnosed in 1997, and about 54,900 deaths will be due to this disease. There have been advances in nearly every field related to the diagnosis and treatment of colorectal cancer, yet the 5-year survival of patients with invasive cancers has improved only slightly. It is generally agreed that improvement in the rate of discovery of adenomatous polyps, the precancerous mucosal lesion, will have the most beneficial effect by reducing the disease prevalence.

Once the disease is detected, staging procedures, of varying cost and complexity, are instituted in all patients. Therapeutic manoeuvres follow, and the patients are entered into a follow-up regimen, in which they participate for a substantial percentage of their remaining lives. All of this represents considerable expense in an increasingly cost-conscious era. Accordingly, it is worthwhile to review the goals and benefits of both staging and follow-up for patients with colorectal carcinoma.

GOALS FOR STAGING

The general goal for staging patients with any cancer is to determine the overall extent of disease prior to institution of therapy. Since, in colon cancer patients, the only clearly effective therapy is surgical removal of the tumour, it can be argued that diagnostic manoeuvres designed to obtain precise local staging information are not useful. As suggested by Cohen, 'preoperative evaluation and staging should focus on techniques that might either preclude surgery entirely, alter the planned operation either

* A version of this chapter first appeared in *Imaging in Oncology*, (Janet Husband and Rodney Reznek, eds) Oxford: Isis Medical Media, 1998.

preoperatively or intraoperatively, or suggest the need for preoperative adjuvant therapy.'[1] With present technology, the only group of colon cancer patients who might profit from preoperative staging are those with unexpectedly advanced systemic disease, who would thus avoid needlessly radical surgery.[2–7]

There are more treatment options available for patients with rectal cancer and, therefore, more reason to obtain staging information. Some well-localized tumours are amenable to simple local resection; more advanced cancers allow a choice among sphincter-sparing low anterior resection, abdominoperineal resection or perioperative adjuvant radio- or chemotherapy.[8,9] For these choices to be made rationally, precise information about the local extent of the tumour must be known. It is particularly important to have reliable information regarding those tumours in which pathological staging is not obtained at the time that therapy is instituted; judgement of the success or failure of preoperative adjuvant therapy relies on knowing exactly what was being treated.

In academic centres, there is some justification for performing expensive staging manoeuvres, even though patients may not directly benefit: as new treatment ideas emerge, more and more patients may receive part of their cancer therapy prior to pathological staging, and the assessment of the efficacy of novel therapies will depend on accurate imaging information.

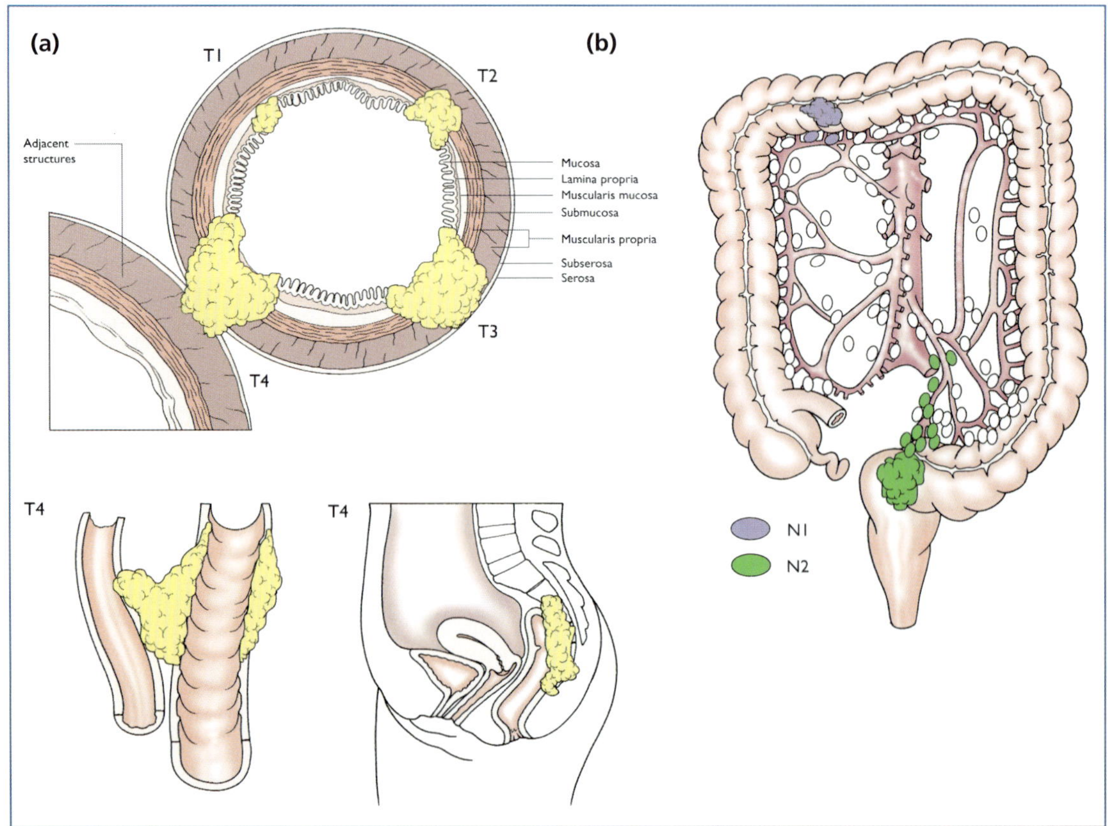

Figure 2.1. *Staging colorectal cancer: (a) primary tumour (T); (b) lymph nodes (N).*

STAGING SYSTEMS

It has been well documented that the biological behaviour of colorectal cancer (and, therefore, the prognosis of the patient with that disease) is strongly linked to the following:

- *The degree of penetration of the cancer through the bowel wall;*
- *The presence or absence of lymphatic dissemination;*
- *The presence or absence of systemic metastases.*

Staging systems in common use reflect this correlation. The original staging system, introduced by Dukes' to apply to rectal cancers, has undergone a number of modifications. This has led to confusion, since not all of the modifications have been universally adopted. A staging system commonly in use in the United Kingdom is given in Table 2.1. Stage D was added by Turnbull, and is more generally used in the United States than in Europe.

A logical system that avoids some of the communication problems experienced by proponents of the modified Dukes' classifications is the TNM system (Table 2.2), which has been recommended for adoption by the American College of Surgeons' Commission on Cancer. This identifies the depth of local tumour invasion (T), the status of regional lymph nodes (N) (Figure 2.1) and the presence or absence

Table 2.1. *Staging system commonly used in the United Kingdom*

Stage	Description
A	Carcinoma limited to the bowel wall
B	Local spread of cancer beyond the bowel wall, but no involvement of lymph nodes
C	Lymph node involvement C1: Local nodes only C2: Apical nodes
D	Distant metastases present

Table 2.2. *The TNM staging system*

T	Description
TX	Primary tumour cannot be assessed
T0	No evidence of primary tumour
Tis	Carcinoma *in situ*
T1	Tumour invades the submucosa
T2	Tumour invades the muscularis propria
T3	Tumour invades through the muscularis propria into the subserosa or into non-peritonealized pericolic or perirectal tissues
T4	Tumour perforates the visceral peritoneum or directly invades other organs or structures
N	**Description**
NX	Regional lymph nodes cannot be assessed
N0	No regional lymph node metastasis
N1	Metastasis found in 1–3 regional lymph nodes
N2	Metastasis found in ≥ 4 regional lymph nodes
M	**Description**
MX	Presence of distant metastases cannot be determined
M0	No distant metastases
M1	Distant metastases

Table 2.3. *Combined tumour stage*

Stage	Description (TNM)			Modified Dukes' classification
0	Tis	N0	M0	
I	T1, T2	N0	M0	A
II	T3,T4	N0	M0	B
III	Any T	N1, N2	M0	C
IV	Any T	Any N	M1	D

of distant metastases (M). These three parameters are then incorporated into the final stage. This system is in use at the authors' institution. The combined tumour stage is as shown in Table 2.3.

One test for the adequacy of any staging system is to determine that patients classified in each specific stage have similar prognostic outcomes. The reported variations in patient survival in stage II (60–80%) and stage III (20–50%) suggest that further modifications, utilizing biological factors, such as tumour grade or gene content, will be necessary.

GOALS FOR FOLLOW-UP

Similar to the controversy surrounding staging procedures, there is reason to question the utility of performing close surveillance of patients after they have undergone primary therapy for colorectal carcinoma.[10–12] It is undeniably expensive to perform repeated imaging tests, and it is relatively rare to find recurrent disease that is amenable to cure. Therefore, aggressive follow-up protocols are most appropriately restricted to programmes that are involved in therapeutic research trials, in which setting it is important to document the precise time and site of the first recurrence. The assumption implicit in all surveillance programmes is that early detection of recurrence translates to improved chance for cure; in colorectal cancer, this assumption has yet to be validated.[10]

However, there are specific instances in which it is valuable to detect recurrent disease in an asymptomatic patient: isolated local recurrence in rectal cancer, and low-volume, well-circumscribed hepatic and pulmonary recurrences are amenable to resection for cure.[10,13–15] As more aggressive and (it is hoped), more successful chemotherapeutic agents become available, this short list may expand. It is, therefore, important to be aware of the strengths and limitations of available imaging methods in the detection of disease recurrence—specifically, the performance of these methods in local, hepatic and pulmonary sites.

It should be mentioned that one of the goals for surveillance in the group of patients previously treated for colorectal cancer is the identification of a metachronous carcinoma. Colonoscopy or barium enema (or some combination of the two methods) should be employed in this group, since they are at higher risk than the general population to develop another cancer.[16] The discussion that follows outlines the relative accuracy of each available imaging method in both staging and follow-up of patients with colorectal cancer.

Imaging in staging

COMPUTED TOMOGRAPHY

Staging at presentation

T-staging

With the introduction of computed tomography (CT) of the whole body in the mid-1970s, radiologists were for the first time able to depict solid organs such as the liver and pancreas, and the mesentery and wall of the hollow structures in the alimentary tract. Considerable enthusiasm accompanied the application of this novel technique to staging gastrointestinal neoplasms. Early studies [17–20] reported staging accuracies in excess of 90%, fuelling the demand for the routine use of this technique. Later studies,[21,22] in which a greater fraction of patients had localized (rather than extensive) primary tumours, showed that CT was considerably more accurate in assessing T4 carcinomas (Figures 2–4) than in differentiating between T2 and T3 lesions, and that its sensitivity for local invasion ranged from 48 to 55%. The major difficulty (as yet not overcome) is that CT findings do not discriminate between direct tumour infiltration of the pericolonic fat and the desmoplasia commonly induced by localized tumour within the same mesenteric fat (Figure 2.5). Additionally, the spatial resolution of CT is insufficient to detect focal tumour spread external to the muscularis propria or serosa. Numerous studies with quite similar results have been published,[23–28] and consistently document this failure. The study by Shank *et al.*[23] is noteworthy in that it assessed inter- and intra-observer variability. The two interpreting investigators agreed with each other's assessment in only 37% of cases; a single observer who evaluated the same dataset on two different occasions reached the same conclusion in only 51% of cases.

The Radiologic Diagnostic Oncology Group (RDOG) reported on the performance of CT in the local staging of 314 patients (111 of whom had rectal cancer).[29] In this study, rectal insufflation of air was performed to ensure adequate luminal distension. The accuracy of CT in predicting perirectal tumour invasion was 74%, while for pericolonic tumour invasion it was 72%.

The use of water as a negative contrast agent has some theoretical advantages over the use of air, since the luminal surface of the wall can be displayed at standard window settings.[30,31] Given adequate preparation and

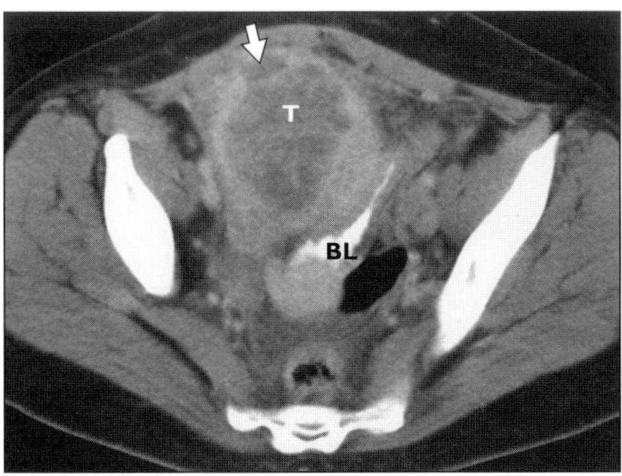

Figure 2.2. *Computed tomography CT scan in a T4 caecal cancer. Section through the true pelvic inlet shows a large mass (T) arising from the caecum (the original of the mass was shown on other images). The anterior surface of the mass has invaded the right rectus muscle (arrow) and its posterior surface invades the anterior wall of the bladder (BL), causing marked distortion of the bladder lumen.*

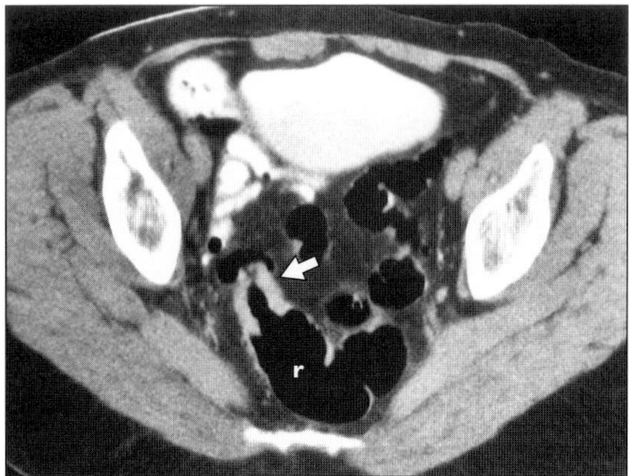

Figure 2.3. *CT scanning after inflation. CT scan obtained in the prone position after air inflation of the rectum (r) shows an annular mass (arrow) arising in the distal sigmoid colon. Small masses and their mesenteric boundaries are much more easily assessed when the lumen is disturbed.*

luminal distension, however, it is not clear how water distension can affect the ability of CT to predict subtle pericolonic invasion and differentiate it from peritumoral fibrosis. However, two recent reports suggested considerably increased T-staging accuracy using water as a contrast medium for both rectal[30] and colonic[31] primary cancers. This method requires further testing before it is possible to assess its performance definitively.

Although CT is not reliable in predicting pericolonic infiltration, it may be useful in predicting those patients at risk for recurrence from primary rectal carcinoma. A pilot study of 51 patients[32] showed that, of the 14 patients in whom CT demonstrated perirectal soft-tissue infiltration to or through the perirectal fascia, four developed local recurrence (as opposed to three of the 37 who lacked that finding).

N-staging

Detection of normal-sized, tumour-bearing nodes has been the Holy Grail of cross-sectional imaging for the last two decades. As Thoeni and Rogalla[33] state in their review of the subject of cross-sectional imaging for colorectal cancer,[33] '... although asymmetry and size can be used to determine lymph node abnormality, the pathological nature of the enlargement cannot be determined by CT ... many metastatic foci are found in lymph nodes measuring less than 1 cm in diameter. Benign or malignant disease can produce lymphadenopathy ...'. The large comparative study reported by the RDOG[29] found a sensitivity for detecting lymph node metastases in 322 patients to be 38% for rectal cancer and 56% for colonic cancer (Figures 2.6 and 2.7); the overall accuracy in all patients studied was only 62%. Lymph node status was not addressed in all papers dealing with the subject of staging, but in those with sufficient data, CT sensitivity ranged between 68 and 79%; in each report, the major difficulty was insensitivity to small, tumour-bearing nodes.[22,24,30] Although CT has relatively high specificity, false-positive assessments, due to hyperplastic nodes attaining diameters in excess of 1.5 cm, are well documented. In summary, the major drawback to using CT to stage colorectal cancer is its inaccuracy in evaluating pericolonic lymph nodes.

Detection of local recurrence

Shortly after the introduction of CT as a practical clinical method, there was considerable interest in its use in patients who had undergone previous abdominoperineal resections for low rectal carcinomas, since this group was difficult to assess by traditional radiological means. Early reports[34–36] suggested that CT might be sensitive to recurrent cancer before

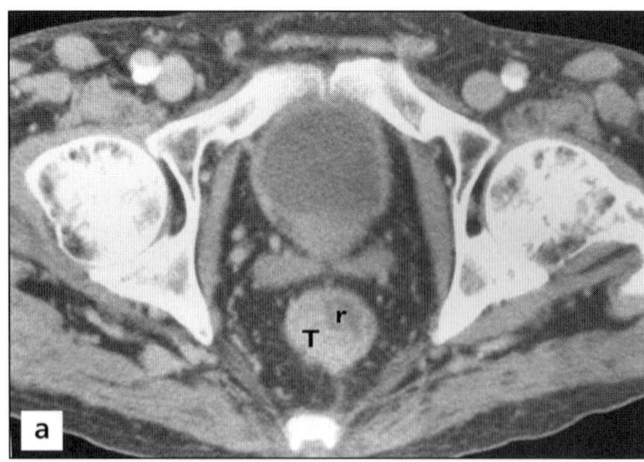

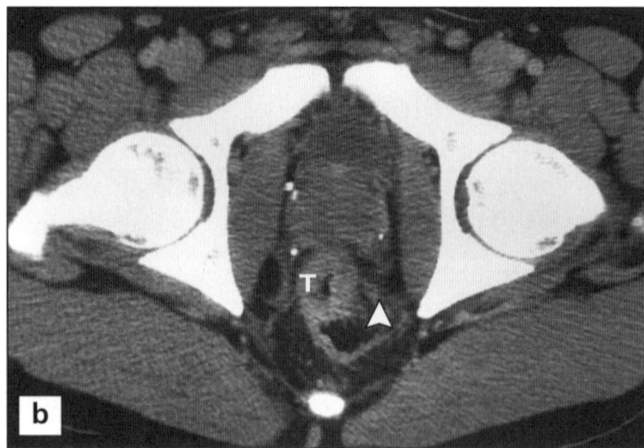

Figure 2.4. *Pitfalls in CT staging of cancers of the colorectum. (a) CT understaging occurred in this patient with a well-circumscribed tumour (T) on the right posterolateral rectal wall, producing marked distortion of the rectal lumen (r). The CT stage was T2 but the pathological specimen showed invasion of the perirectal fat. (b) CT overstaging occurred in this patient with an annular rectal tumour (T). There is asymmetric thickening of the left perirectal fascia (arrowhead) separating the ischiorectal fossa from the perirectal fat; the CT stage was therefore T3. The pathological specimen showed inflammatory changes only.*

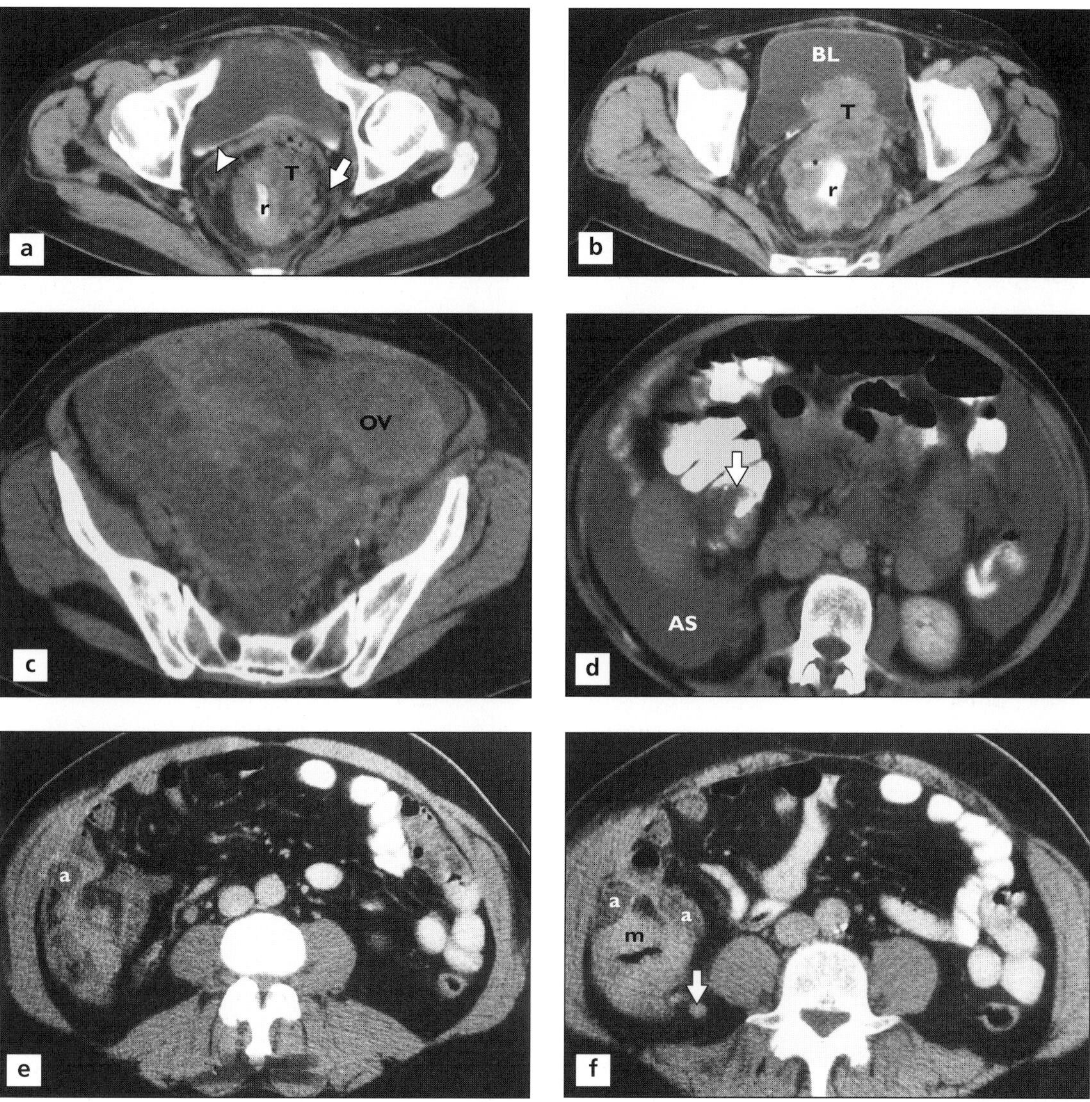

Figure 2.5. *CT staging of local extension in colorectal cancer. (a) CT section through the lower rectum shows a large circumferential tumour (T) causing extensive distortion of the rectal lumen (r). A large perirectal lymph node (arrowhead) is observed. There is extensive thickening of the perirectal fascia (arrow) which was due to inflammation rather than tumour; (b) slightly more cephalic section in the same patient shown in (a) shows direct invasion by the tumour (T) into the posterior wall of the bladder (BL); (c) CT section through the pelvic brim shows enormous tumour replacing the ovaries (OV); (d) CT section in the same patient as (c) shows moderate amount of ascites (AS) and a mass (arrow) distorting the caecal tip. This was interpreted as an ovarian primary cancer with serosal metastasis to the caecum, but was determined at pathological examination to be a caecal carcinoma with peritoneal metastases to both ovaries; (e) CT section through the lower abdomen in a patient clinically suspected of having appendicitis. There is a fluid collection (a) with a surrounding rim of enhancement abutting the transversus abdominis muscle; (f) CT section obtained at a slightly more caudal level in the same patient as (e) shows several other small abscesses (a). The appendix (arrow) is normal, but there is a mass (m) producing circumferential thickening of the caecal wall. The surgical specimen showed perforation of a large caecal carcinoma. Stage for stage, perforated cancers have a far worse prognosis than those uncomplicated by perforation.*

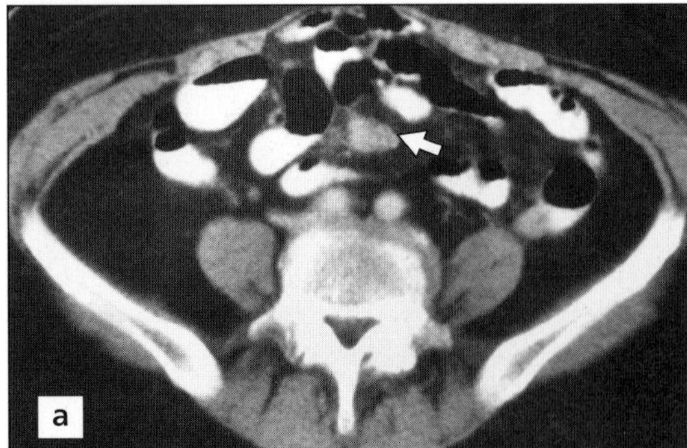

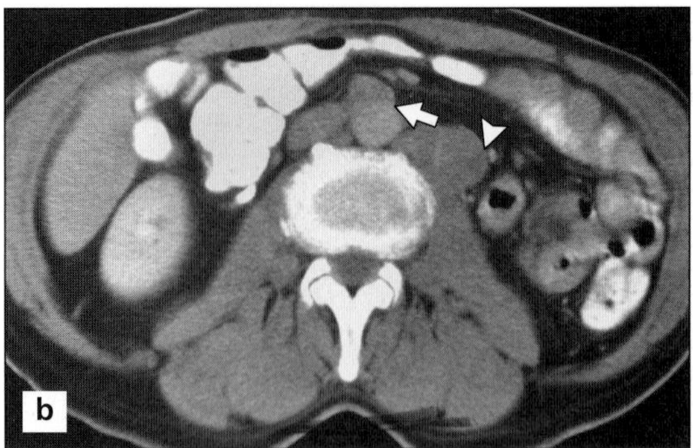

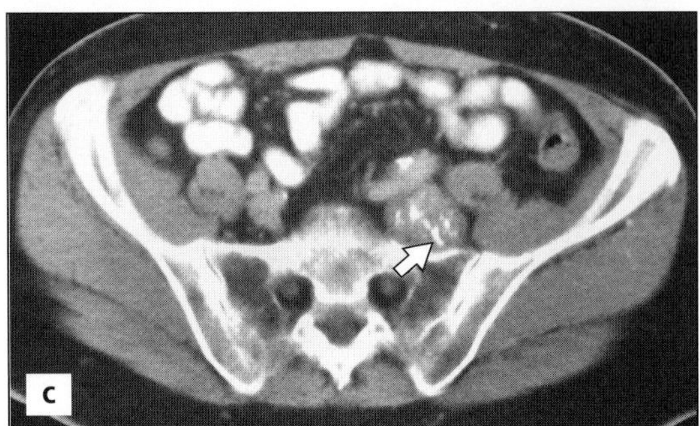

Figure 2.6. *CT of nodal metastases. (a) CT section through the lower abdomen in a patient with a primary adenocarcinoma of the sigmoid colon shows a large nodal metastasis (arrow) in the mesosigmoid; (b) CT section in another patient with a primary adenocarcinoma of the sigmoid colon shows metastases in the retroperitoneum (arrowhead) and anterior to the aorta (arrow) near the origin of the inferior mesenteric artery; (c) CT section through the sacrum in a patient with mucinous adenocarcinoma of the sigmoid colon shows characteristic calcification (arrow) within a parasacral node.*

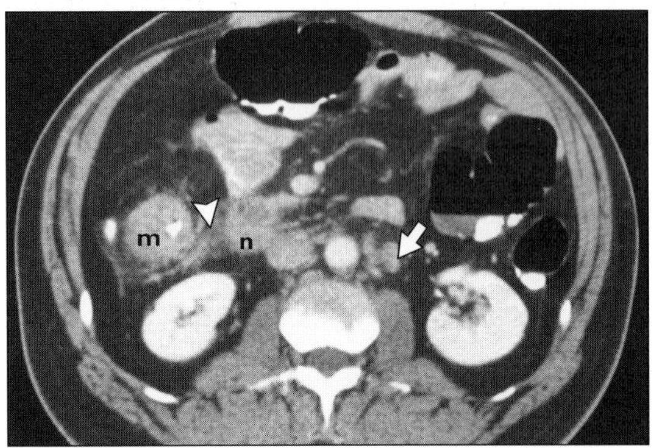

Figure 2.7. *CT section through the mid-abdomen in a patient with a large (T3M2) carcinoma of the ascending colon. The primary mass (m) is producing marked luminal distortion, and there is evidence of direct invasion of the mesenteric fat (arrowhead). A regional mesenteric node (n) is present, and there are multiple matted left para-aortic nodes (arrow), indicating extensive tumour spread.*

clinical symptoms or carcinoembryonic antigen (CEA) elevation prompted a search (Figures 2.8 and 2.9); later reports have disputed this claim. In a study of 66 patients in whom postoperative CT was used as a routine part of the follow-up protocol, 33 patients ultimately developed recurrent disease. Of these, 31 had symptoms or laboratory findings that suggested recurrence before the CT became positive.[37] In a recent report comparing CT with magnetic resonance imaging (MRI) in detecting recurrence after either abdominoperineal resection or low anterior resection, the accuracy of CT (68%) was considerably poorer than that of MRI (95%) in the 18 patients who underwent both examinations.

One recent report,[38] in which 21 cases were detected with local tumour recurrence, noted that CT detected only three of the eight patients with documented recurrence after low anterior resection. Results in patients with abdominoperineal resections were somewhat better than the studies reported above; 12 of 13 documented recurrences were found and, in five of these, the CT was the first diagnostic test to suggest the recurrence.

Overall, the major difficulty with CT in detecting recurrent cancer is its insensitivity to local tumour at the anastomotic site, inability to detect tumour within a fibrotic surgical scar, and inability to differentiate between hyperplastic and tumorous lymph nodes. The role

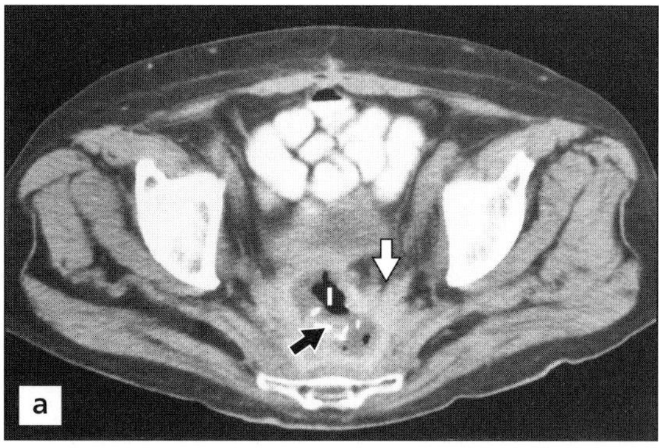

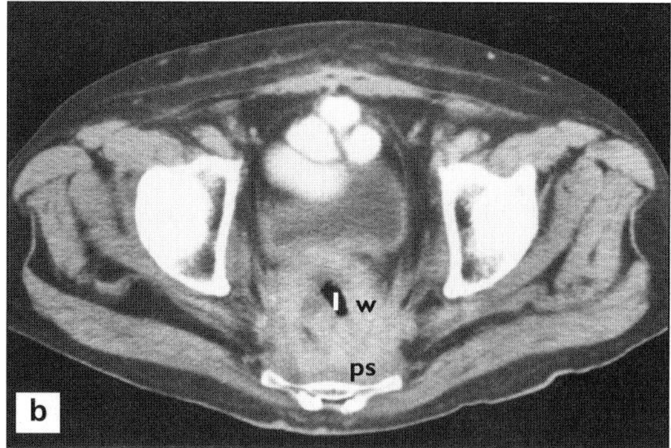

Figure 2.8. *CT depiction of recurrence after low anterior resection. (a) CT section obtained near the anastomotic staple line (black arrow) 11 months after resection of a primary adenocarcinoma of the rectum. There is infiltration of the posterior pelvis by high-attenuation tumour, which extends to the left pelvic sidewall (white arrow). Invasion of the rectal wall produces marked narrowing of the lumen (l); (b) CT section just caudal to (a) shows tumour invasion of the presacral fat (ps) and extensive infiltration of the rectal wall (w).*

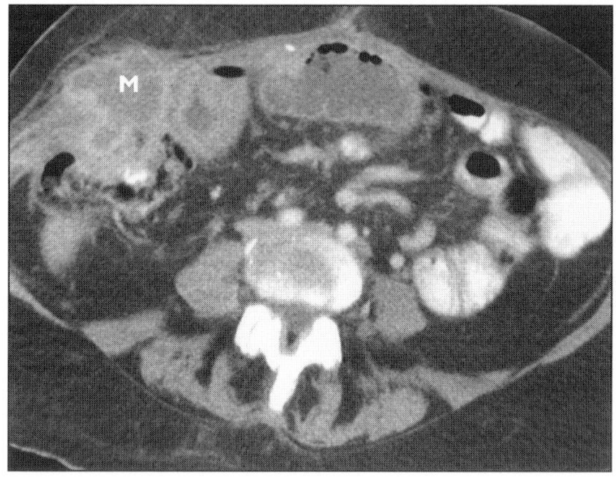

Figure 2.9. *Anterior abdominal wall invasion by recurrent tumour (M) is shown in this patient who had undergone resection of a perforated primary caecal adenocarcinoma 6 months earlier.*

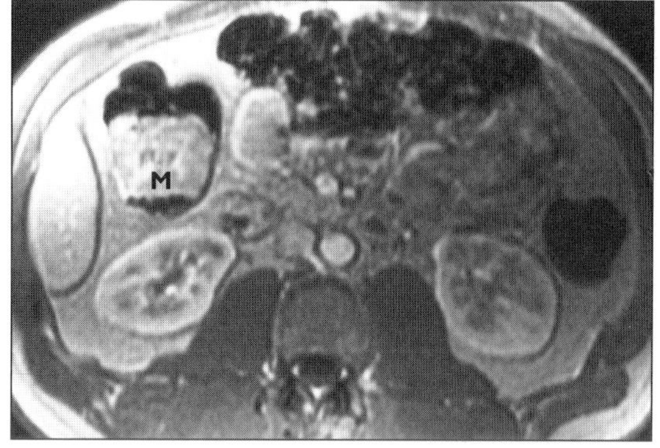

Figure 2.10. *MR image (MRI) through the mid abdomen shows a polypoid mass (M) in the ascending colon, with high intensity after intravenous gadolinium diethylenetriamine-pentaacetic acid (Gd-DTPA) administration. The MRI correctly predicted the absence of invasion into the pericolic fat.*

of CT for a postoperative patient seems limited to confirmation of tumour recurrence by providing a targeting method for percutaneous biopsy.

MAGNETIC RESONANCE IMAGING

Staging at presentation

T-staging

When MRI was introduced into clinical practice in the mid-1980s, there was considerable enthusiasm surrounding its potential for accurate tumour staging and follow-up. There is no question that MRI affords much greater contrast between tissues of different composition than does CT. Early papers[24,25] evaluated CT in comparison to MRI using a standard body coil, without intravenous gadolinium diethylenetriaminepentaacetic acid (Gd-DTPA) enhancement. They noted approximately equal performance of CT compared with MRI for local tumour assessment (Figure 2.10). The largest comparative study[29] published to date compared the accuracy of MRI with that of CT in staging 79 rectal cancers and 149 colon cancers. Using standard 1.0 or 1.5 T-weighted whole-body imaging units, without intravenous Gd-DTPA administration, the sensitivity of MRI to perirectal tumour invasion was 49%, compared with 76% for CT; the two methods had virtually identical specificity. For extrarectal tumours, MRI was only 37% sensitive to pericolic tumour infiltration (compared with CT, 70%), although its high specificity (91%, compared with 68% for CT) afforded the two methods equivalent accuracy.

Somewhat better results have been achieved using similar techniques at single centres: de Lange *et al.*[39] used a Helmholtz coil to attempt staging of 29 patients with rectal cancer, achieving 100% sensitivity to perirectal invasion in the 17 patients in whom it was present, with 75% specificity, overstaging three of the 12 patients in whom the tumour was confined to the wall. Thaler *et al.*[40] compared MRI with endoscopic ultrasound in a series of 37 patients with rectal cancer, reporting 77% sensitivity and 86% specificity to perirectal fat invasion.

A potential advantage (limited to the rectum) of MRI is that endorectal coils may be placed, limiting the field of view, but significantly increasing the spatial resolution. Specifically, it has been established that the use of endorectal coils permits delineation of the layers comprising the rectal wall, in a manner similar to endoluminal ultrasound. Recent results[41–43] confirm that the technique is capable of identifying the muscularis propria, and have reported accuracies ranging from 79 to 92% for evaluation of local tumour invasion. One study[44] compared MRI using an endorectal coil and intraluminal ultrasound; nine of the 15 patients studied had both examinations. In this small group, ultrasound outperformed MRI in three cases, MRI was superior in two cases, and the two studies were equivalent in four patients.

N-staging

MRI is capable of detecting small lymph nodes and differentiating them from adjacent vascular structures, attributes that make it theoretically superior to CT. Unfortunately, there are no clear-cut signal characteristics that allow the interpreter to determine whether a detected node contains metastatic tumour. The report of the RDOG[29] evaluated the nodal status of 260 patients studied with MRI, and determined a sensitivity to malignant perirectal adenopathy of 37% and, to pericolic metastatic nodes of 14%, for a combined sensitivity of 23%. The overall sensitivity for CT imaging in this group was slightly higher (49%) but the accuracy of both examinations was comparable (CT, 62%; MRI, 64%). Other studies using body coils[24,25,39] confirm the relatively unimpressive performance of MRI for nodal staging, reporting sensitivities in the range 43–60%.

Endorectal coils allow much higher spatial resolution of perirectal structures, and are capable of detecting lymph nodes as small as 2 mm.[42] In the group of 36 patients reported, this technique had a sensitivity of 81%; however, the MRI readers interpreted the presence of any non-fat-containing lymph node as evidence of metastatic disease; accordingly, their increased sensitivity was accompanied by reduced specificity (75%), resulting in only modest gain in overall accuracy (78%) compared with previous studies.

Detection of local recurrence

It has been repeatedly documented that CT is relatively insensitive to tumour recurring in a resection site, particularly when radiotherapy has been administered. Early studies using MRI suggested that the signal intensity of viable tumour was much higher on T2-weighted images than that of mature fibrotic tissue from postoperative scarring (Figure 2.11). However, de Lange *et al.*[45] elegantly demonstrated that non-viable tumour, inflammation and oedema can each mimic the signal intensity of recurrent tumour. A recent study of 18 patients [46] compared MRI with CT in evaluating rectosigmoid resection sites. In this selected group (14 of the patients ultimately developed recurrent cancer) MRI was superior to CT in both sensitivity (91% vs 82%) and specificity (100% vs 69%).

Magnetic resonance imaging performance in local staging and follow-up

In summary, there are no data to demonstrate that standard (body-coil) MRI is superior to CT in local staging of colon or rectal cancer, and both methods are decidedly inferior to endorectal ultrasound in determining perirectal

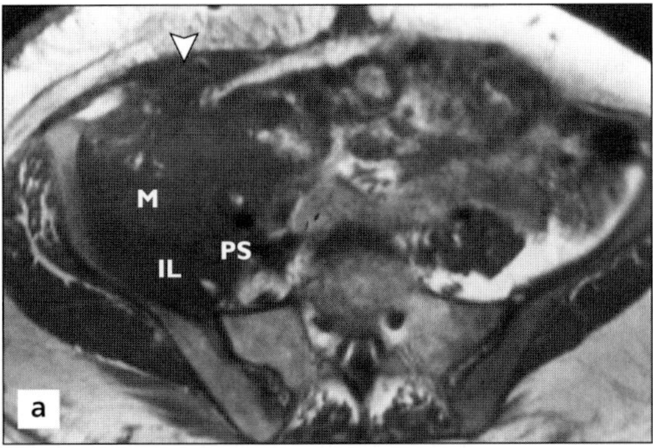

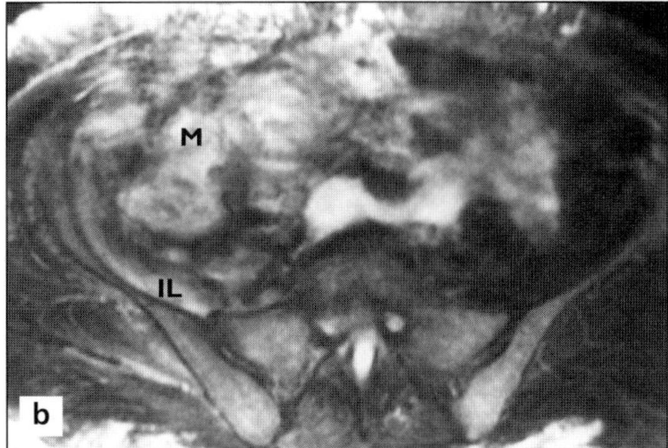

Figure 2.11. *Magnetic resonance imaging (MRI) of recurrent caecal carcinoma. (a) T1-weighted image through the iliac fossa shows a large mass (M) infiltrating the right iliac fossa, obscuring the normal fat planes surrounding the iliacus (IL) and psoas (PS) muscles. The anterior aspect of this mass abuts the anterior abdominal wall (arrowhead); (b) T2-weighted image at the same level shows the increased intensity of the iliacus muscle (IL), presumably a reflection of oedema or inflammation.*

tumour spread. Large, multi-institutional studies will be required before a firm statement can be made regarding the relative performances of endorectal MRI and intraluminal ultrasound. There are technical problems confronting investigators who favour routine use of endorectal MRI: for example, patients with bulky intraluminal tumours present difficulties in adequate tube positioning. Almost all patients are uncomfortable during the MRI period, and motion degradation is a well-documented problem; this is not a major concern in performing intraluminal ultrasound, since it is a 'real-time' method.

As yet, the potential for MRI to detect metastatic lymphadenopathy, using criteria other than size and morphology, has not shown practical value. Body-coil MRI is inferior to CT in detecting lymphadenopathy in local or remote sites. Endorectal coils are effective in increasing spatial resolution for detecting local nodes in rectal cancer patients, but no study to date has demonstrated superiority of MRI to intraluminal ultrasound. Although it remains a fruitful area for research investigation, MRI should not be considered a routine method for local staging of colorectal cancer.

It remains a point for debate whether MRI is superior to CT in evaluating postoperative patients. There is certainly a role for CT in confirming suspicious masses seen when imaging symptomatic patients, but it is not clear whether either cross-sectional imaging method is sufficiently sensitive to detect the rare asymptomatic isolated local recurrence. Alternative methods, such as immunoscintigraphy and positron emission tomography (PET), to be discussed in later sections, appear to be more promising in this regard.

INTRALUMINAL ENDOSCOPIC ULTRASOUND

Staging at presentation

T-staging

Intraluminal (endorectal) ultrasound (EUS) was first introduced in 1983 as a method for staging rectal carcinoma. During the decade that followed, numerous studies[26–28,40,44,47–60] have documented the accuracy of the technique.

Precise results regarding the accuracy of T- and N-staging differ among institutions, but several generalizations can be made with some confidence. Firstly, ultrasound reliably displays the layers of the rectal wall, normally allowing differentiation between the submucosa and the muscularis propria, and between the muscularis propria and the surrounding fat (Figures 2.12, 2.13). Secondly, the overall accuracy of the method in assessing the degree of tumour penetration into the rectal wall is fairly high, averaging between 80 and 85%.[61] The sonographic method makes this determination much more accurately than CT or standard body-coil MRI;[26–28,40,49] endorectal coil MRI[44] requires further evaluation. Thirdly, ultrasound is most reliable for superficial tumours. As

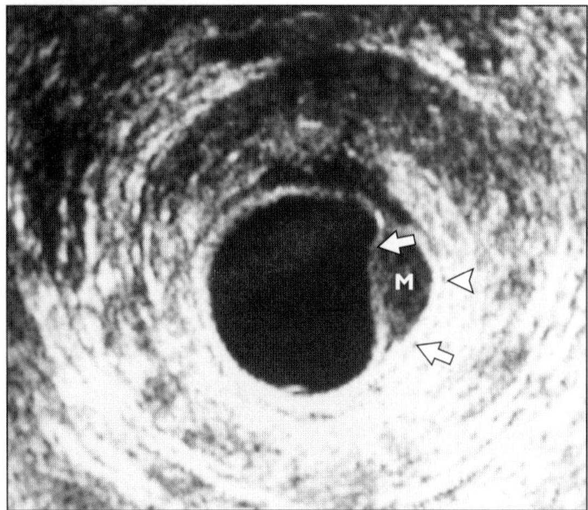

Figure 2.12. *Transrectal sonography identifies a well-circumscribed mucosal carcinoma (M). The echogenic interface (arrows) between the mucosa and the muscularis propria (arrowhead) is unbroken, indicating that this is a T1 lesion.*

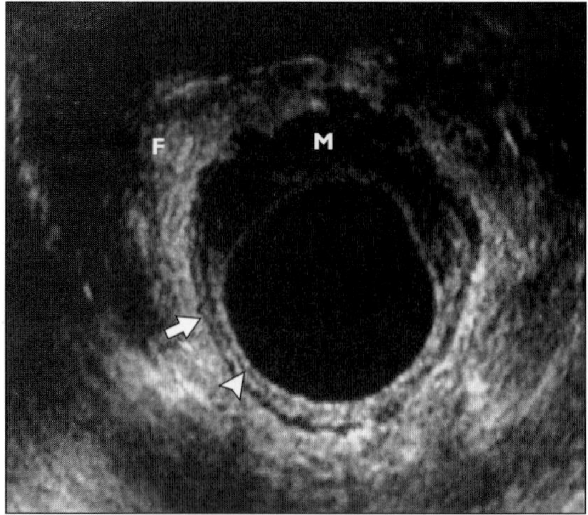

Figure 2.13. *Transrectal sonography in a patient with a large anteriorly positioned tumour (M) shows tumour disruption of the first (arrowhead) and second (arrow) hypoechoic stripes, indicating that the tumour has passed through the muscularis propria. Invasion of the hyperechoic fat (F) is evident in this patient, diagnostic of a T3 lesion.*

reported by Hulsmans *et al.*,[51] ultrasound examiners have interpretative difficulties differentiating between stage T2 (tumour infiltrates the muscularis propria but does not cross into the perirectal fat) and stage T3 (tumour has passed beyond the rectal wall into the perirectal fat). In their series, in the 16 patients overstaged as T3, the pathologists commented on macroscopic examination of the gross specimen that the outer contour of the rectum was irregular. However, microscopic examination revealed either inflammation or desmoplasia, rather than carcinoma, as the cause of the irregularity. In the authors' practice, biopsy of the primary cancer was routinely performed a few days before ultrasound staging. Understaging, which occurs far less frequently, is probably due to the limitation of spatial resolution, so that tiny extrarectal deposits are not detected.

Application of this sonographic method requires considerable experience, and most studies have indicated that staging accuracy increases substantially after experience is gained. Other practical problems with the method are that it is not technically feasible in some stenotic lesions;[62] very bulky tumours may prohibit an adequate examination of the wall near the lesion site, and very proximal rectal tumours may not be reached with rigid proctoscopic equipment.

N-staging

High-resolution (7 MHz) sonographic equipment has spatial resolution in the order of 0.5 mm; accordingly, it is possible to identify small lymph nodes within the field of view (Figure 2. 14). Unfortunately, this has not translated into an increase in the accuracy with which metastatic deposits have been detected. Of the recent studies cited above (in the section on T-staging), several addressed the problem of N-staging as well.[26,27,40,50,53–56,59,60] The range of accuracies reported in these studies was 58–81%. The study by Nielsen *et al.*[52] set the limits of detectability using currently available equipment; the authors performed scanning *in vitro* of 20 resected specimens, in which 205 lymph nodes were found by pathological examination. Sonography *in vitro* detected only 64 total nodes, which represented only 56% of the nodes involved with malignant tumour spread.

Apart from failure to detect nodes, the major factor producing errors in N-staging by sonography is the inability reliably to distinguish benign from malignant lymph node enlargement. It is generally true, however, that hyperechoic nodes are inflammatory,

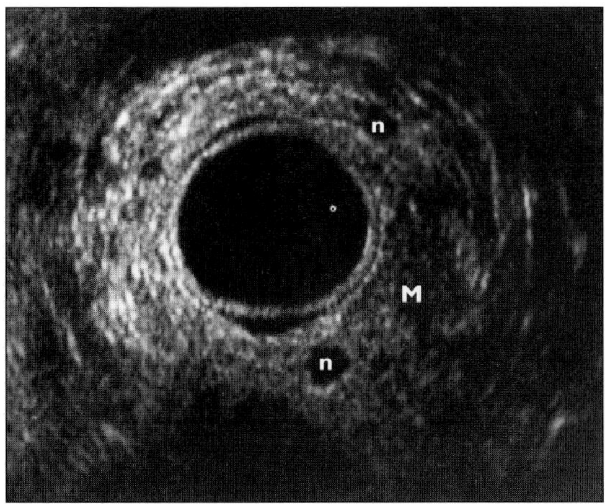

Figure 2.14. *Transrectal sonography in a patient with a large T3 lesion (the origin of the mass, M, is shown on sections taken lower in the rectum) shows two 5 mm hypoechoic lymph nodes (n) which proved to contain tumour.*

and that hypoechoic nodes are more likely to be malignant. This problem could be addressed in part by performing needle aspiration biopsies of nodes within the perirectal fat.[56,63]

Detection of recurrence

Although the major thrust of endosonography is staging at the time of tumour discovery, several groups [64–66] have studied patients with intraluminal ultrasound following curative surgery. Although the study by Romano *et al.*[65] suggested that CT was more sensitive than ultrasound to recurrences, the other studies indicated that ultrasound detected all proven disease, and was often the only method that was successful in this regard.

A recent study[67] assessed whether colour Doppler imaging adds substantially to the staging information gathered by grey-scale sonography alone. In the 24 patients referred for preoperative staging, there was no advantage in demonstrating the increased vascularity associated with malignant infiltration; however, in patients with previously resected cancers, the addition of colour Doppler allowed the interpreter to differentiate between recurrent cancer and postoperative scarring. Further studies are necessary to determine whether intraluminal ultrasound, with or without colour Doppler, is effective in detecting small localized recurrent cancer.

IMMUNOSCINTIGRAPHY AND POSITRON EMISSION TOMOGRAPHY

One of the major problems with the cross-sectional imaging techniques discussed in previous sections is that, as currently used, they are capable only of displaying morphology. The clinical success of these methods has been a result of the technical refinements that have allowed that morphology to be displayed with increasingly better spatial resolution. However, morphology alone is insufficient to predict the presence of tumour involvement, so that all methods in clinical use today have in common an insensitivity to small but tumour-positive deposits, and an unavoidable false-positive rate related to large but tumour-negative nodes. Immunoscintigraphy provides an attractive solution to these difficulties.

Radio-immunoscintigraphy has been the beneficiary of a number of technical advances in both immunology and nuclear radiology in the last two decades, including the hybridoma technique for producing monoclonal antibodies, and the discovery of methods to link radionuclides with attractive clinical properties (such as indium-111) to antibodies without appreciably affecting their avidity to tumour antigen sites. Introduction of single photon emission computed tomography (SPECT) has allowed the data to be displayed with moderate spatial resolution.[68–70]

The majority of the successful clinical trials have used a monoclonal antibody that recognises either CEA[71–81] or a glycoprotein resembling mucin, that is associated with a number of epithelial malignant tumours, including colorectal, breast, ovary and non-small cell lung carcinomas (TAG-72).[82–85] Other surface antigens have also formed the basis for investigations.[86,87] Studies have investigated whole antibodies and antibody fragments; these molecules have been labelled with technetium-99m, indium-111, and both iodine-123 and iodine-131.

Radio-immunoscintigraphy is a method in evolution, so that it is premature to draw conclusions about the results reported to date; however, there is considerable enthusiasm about the potential for this technique. In a recent study comparing CT and immunoscintigraphy, there was a trend (not statistically significant in the sample size studied) toward the superiority of antibody scanning in tumour detection and in negative predictive value.[84] Most studies indicate that standard cross-sectional imaging techniques are superior to scintigraphy in detecting liver metastases, but immunoscintigraphy is complementary to CT or MRI in evaluating the extrahepatic abdomen and the pelvis.

Studies reported in the sections above have documented the relative insensitivity of cross-sectional imaging methods to recurrent carcinoma, specifically in the operative bed of an anteroposterior resection. Early results of immunoscintigraphy in postoperative patients are highly encouraging, and suggest that this method is fruitful in patients at high risk for locoregional recurrence.

A few institutions have investigated the use of radio-immuno-guided surgery (RIGS).[88–91] In this technique, patients with known primary or recurrent colorectal cancers are injected with a monoclonal antibody labelled with a radioactive agent having a relatively long physical half-life. Two to three weeks after the injection, surgical resection of the tumour is combined with exploration of the abdomen assisted by a hand-held gamma counter. Areas with higher than background activity are sampled. Although the method has been successful in identifying sites not likely to be detected by standard methods, including surgical inspection, there have not yet been published randomized, multi-institutional studies validating the technique.

Finally, there has been recent well-justified enthusiasm for the application of PET scanning to the clinical questions arising in colorectal carcinoma (Figure 2.15).[92–97] These investigators have employed fluorine-18 (the positron emitter) linked to a glucose analogue, fluoro-2–deoxy-*d*-glucose (FDG), to assess the metabolic utilization of glucose throughout the whole body. Imaging depends on the fact that FDG competes for glucose receptors at cell membrane sites, enters the cell as the phosphorylated FDG-6–phosphate (owing to the action of the enzyme hexokinase), but, once inside the cell, cannot undergo glycolysis. Escape of the labelled compound occurs when the FDG-6-phosphate is dephosphorylated by the enzyme glucose-6-phosphatase. This biodistribution has an important imaging consequence: unlike the radio-immunoscintigraphic techniques, background uptake of FDG in the normal liver is not a significant problem. Viable tumour cells are relatively rich in hexokinase, but deficient in glucose-6-phosphatase, so the label tends to accumulate rapidly within tumours. In contrast, normal hepatocytes are rich in glucose-6-phosphatase, and successfully clear the label soon after it enters the cell.

False-positive 18-FDG-PET scans are relatively infrequent, but occur in inflammatory processes, in which cellular metabolism increases to mimic that of neoplasia. False-negative scans occur when the affected area is very small, so that the increase in tracer uptake is masked by background noise, and when the tumour is either very well differentiated (as in fibrolamellar hepatoma) or completely necrotic, so that its glucose kinetics are reduced.

In practice, 18–FDG-PET scanning for staging at presentation or for detection of recurrence remains a project for specialty research centres, since the imaging technology is expensive and the cyclotron-produced radiolabel is not easily acquired. However, the results reported by current investigators are highly encouraging, and suggest that the technique will find a place in the management of colorectal cancer patients in the near future.

Hepatic metastases from colorectal cancer: radiological detection

The detection of hepatic metastases is of special importance in the management of colorectal cancer patients. First, and most obviously, the presence of hepatic metastases confirms the systemic nature of the disease; accordingly, radical local surgical approaches are unwarranted. Secondly, there is growing evidence that it is of particular importance to detect limited metastatic disease (usually defined as fewer than four deposits); many studies have shown that hepatic metastasectomy is associated with a 5–year survival in the range of 20%.[98] The problem is to find a method (preferably one that is preoperative and minimally invasive) that is capable of predicting not only the presence of hepatic metastases but also their precise number and distribution.

The problem is compounded by the high

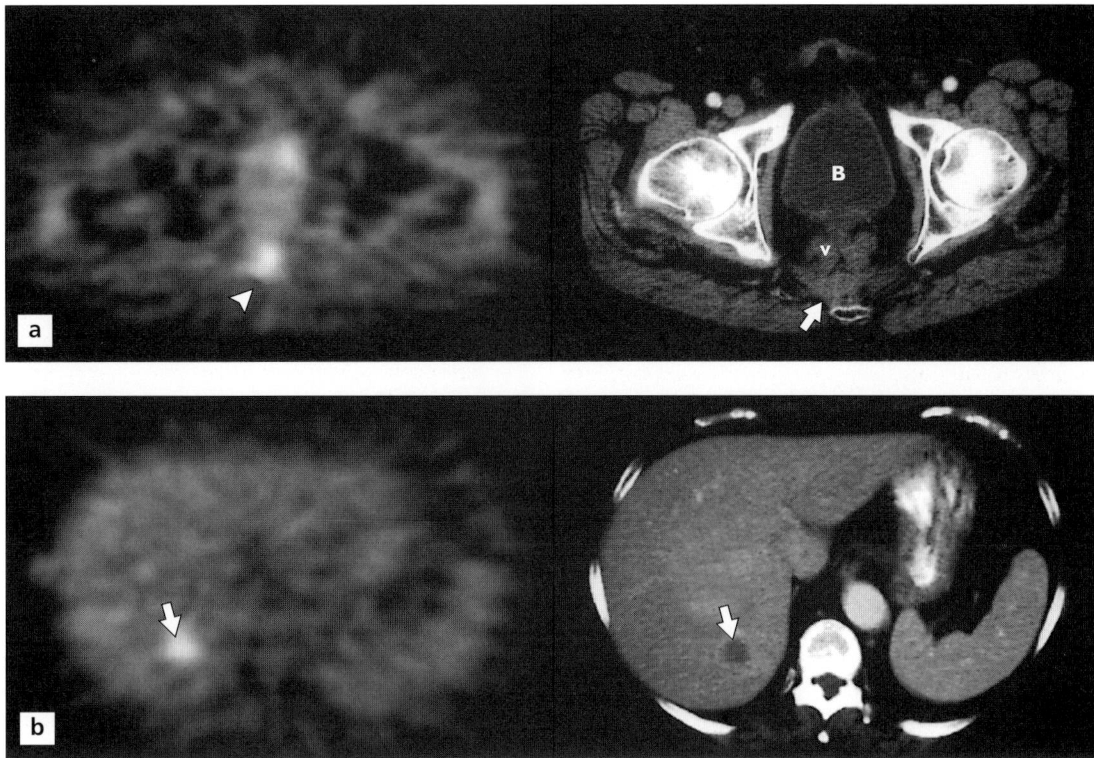

Figure 2.15. *Position emission tomography (PET) in evaluating recurrent tumour. (a) Patient with increasing sacral pain 16 months after abdominoperineal resection. CT (right) shows diffuse high-attenuation material (arrow) in the presacral region. This appearance had not changed appreciably from a scan obtained several months previously (v, seminal vesicle; B, bladder). PET scan performed the next day (left) shows marked increased activity (arrowhead) on the left side of the sacrum. Biopsy confirmed recurrent adenocarcinoma; (b) in the same patient the CT (right) showed a new low-attenuation mass (arrow) in the posterosuperior segment of the right hepatic lobe (Couinaud segment 7). PET scan (left) shows increased activity (arrow) precisely corresponding to the mass.*

frequency of hepatic metastases in patients with colorectal primary cancers (Figure 2.16). It is estimated that about 20% of patients will have detectable liver metastases at the time they first present with cancer, while another 30% will develop clinical evidence of hepatic disease within 24 months. This latter group almost certainly had occult metastases at the time of original presentation.

Many of these figures have probably changed since the introduction of higher-resolution preoperative screening techniques, such as CT, MRI and sonography. The fact remains, however, that no screening technique now in use adequately informs the surgical team about the status of the liver.

Because of the importance of this problem, numerous studies have been performed evaluating the performance of imaging methods in assessing the liver in patients with colorectal carcinoma. The following paragraphs review the most recent studies of non-invasive methods—CT, MRI, and transabdominal sonography (US)—and the minimally invasive methods—CT during angioportography and intra-operative sonography.

COMPUTED TOMOGRAPHY

Imaging of liver metastases from colorectal cancer using CT has evolved considerably during the last 20 years. Virtually all of the blood supply to hepatic metastases is derived from the hepatic artery, while the hepatic parenchyma receives blood from both the hepatic artery and the portal vein. Accordingly, imaging strategies

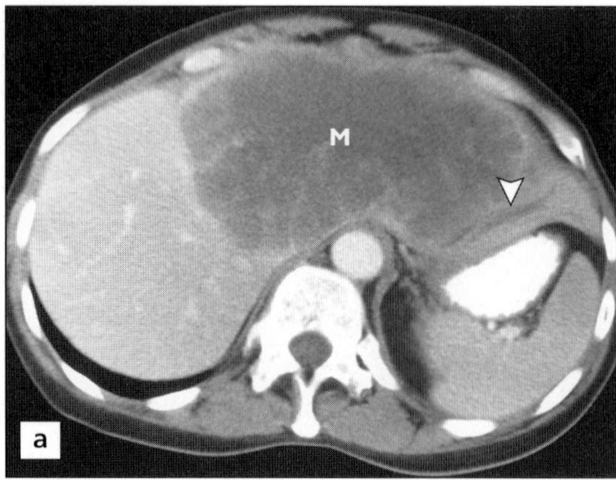

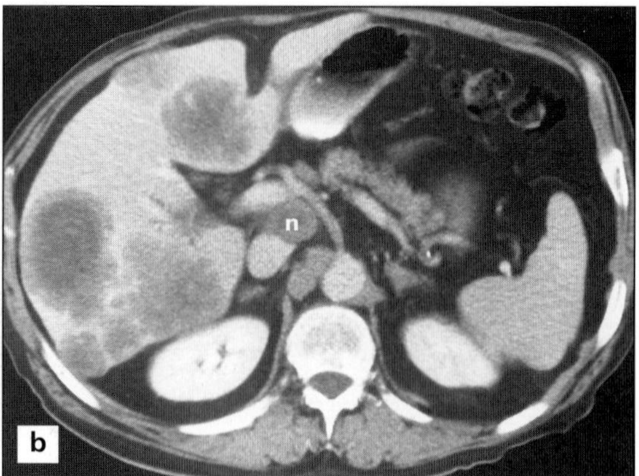

Figure 2.16. *Hepatic metastasis from colorectal cancer: CT detection. (a) CT section through the upper abdomen shows a large solitary liver metastasis (M) replacing the majority of the medial segment of the left hepatic lobe (Couinaud segment 4). The tumour has caused thrombosis of the portal vein to the lateral segment (arrowhead); (b) CT section in another patient shows innumerable hepatic metastases; in addition, a large node (n) in the hepatic chain is observed.*

aimed to detect metastases utilize a bolus of iodinated intravenous contrast material, and images are timed to coincide with the portal venous phase of contrast enhancement (generally 40–60 seconds after the beginning of the bolus). This strategy maximizes the attenuation difference between colorectal cancer metastases and normal liver parenchyma; in most cases, the metastases have attenuation values 50 to 80 Hounsfield units (HU) less than that of the liver. However, as time elapses after bolus administration, metastases increase in attenuation while liver slowly decreases; during this equilibrium phase, the attenuation difference may become so small that lesions are missed. Spiral (helical) CT allows rapid data collection during a single vascular phase, which minimizes the likelihood that a lesion will be missed because the section is sampled too late.

The most recently published study to consider a population comprising colorectal cancer patients is the RDOG collaborative study authored by Zerhouni *et al.*[29] In this study, follow-up examinations were rigorously obtained in an effort to document false-negative imaging studies. The sensitivity of CT in this report was 62%. This is consistent with other studies using modern CT equipment,[22,99–101] in which sensitivities range from 68 to 79%. Studies have uniformly shown that the detection rate for liver metastases from all primaries is size dependent, and that CT is insensitive to metastatic lesions under 1 cm in diameter.

An invasive preoperative technique, CT angioportography (CTAP) has been utilized in patients who are considered candidates for liver metastasectomy.[102–112] It is accomplished by positioning an angiographic catheter in the superior mesenteric or splenic artery, and then performing a hepatic CT scan during continuous infusion of iodinated intravenous contrast material. This results in intense enhancement of hepatic parenchyma and essentially no enhancement of the hepatic metastases, achieving attenuation differences in excess of 150 HU. This has led to vastly improved detection rates compared with other preoperative imaging methods, particularly for lesions in the 5–10 mm range. Unfortunately, all lesions that produce an interruption of portal venous flow will be associated with a region of diminished attenuation, so that the specificity of CTAP is quite low. This has reduced the potential impact of CTAP in the population of patients considered for metastasectomy.

MAGNETIC RESONANCE IMAGING

Because the sensitivity of CT for small metastatic deposits is too low to be an adequate guide for management decisions, other imaging methods have been studied. Of these, MRI is the most promising (Figure 2.17). The major advantage of MRI is its exquisite contrast sensitivity; even without contrast agents, the signal intensity of hepatic metastases from colorectal

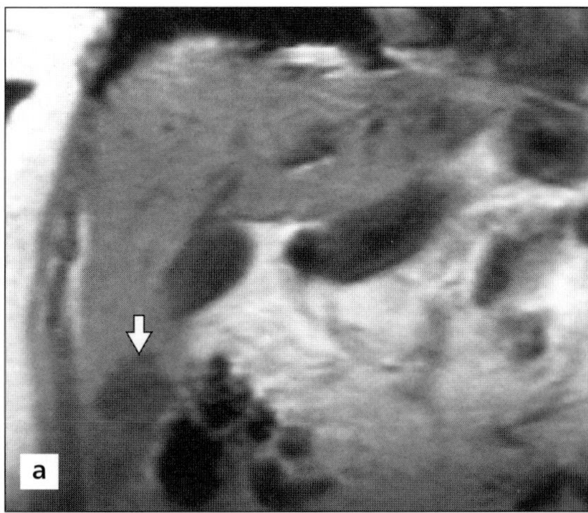

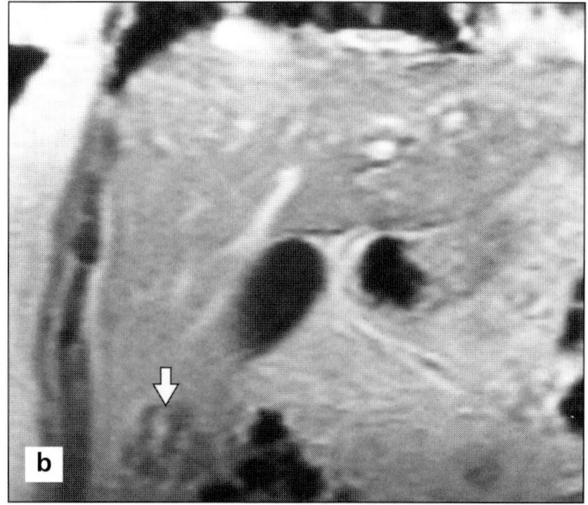

Figure 2.17. *Hepatic metastasis from colorectal cancer: MRI. (a) Coronal T1-weighted MR image obtained in a patient with prior resection of colorectal carcinoma shows low-intensity nodular lesion (arrow) in the anterior inferior segment of the right hepatic lobe (Couinaud segment 5); (b) after intravenous administration of Gd-DTPA, there is central irregular increase in intensity within the mass.*

carcinoma is markedly different from that of normal hepatic parenchyma. Almost all recent studies comparing MRI and CT have shown a statistically insignificant trend toward superiority of MRI.[29,99] It is hoped that the addition of hepatocyte-specific contrast agents will translate to clear improvement of the ability of MRI to detect metastases, and it is likely that technical advances will allow the spatial resolution of MRI to become comparable to that of CT. At present, however, CT is the preferred non-invasive method to detect hepatic metastases, for several reasons: (1) it is more easily scheduled in most centres, (2) it is capable of studying the entire abdomen and pelvis in a very short time, and (3) it seems to be more sensitive to lymphadenopathy and alimentary tract lesions than is MRI.

ULTRASOUND

Transabdominal sonography for the detection of liver metastases has, in most studies, been inferior to both CT and MRI,[99–101,111–114] with sensitivities ranging from 48 to 76%. However, there are two relatively recent innovations which may prove useful in clinical practice. Intra-operative sonography (IOUS) has been widely utilized as an eleventh hour staging manoeuvre, in patients who apparently qualify for resection of limited hepatic metastases (Figure 2.18).[101,114,115–117] No study has yet been reported in which the intra-operative sonographer has been blinded to the results of the preoperative imaging studies, so its true performance is hard to gauge. However, in most recent studies, IOUS demonstrated sensitivity of more than 95% for liver metastases present at the time of surgery. The drawbacks to this procedure are that it requires that laparotomy be performed and that it is very time-intensive for all involved.

A very interesting series of reports by Leen suggests a potentially important use for sonography.[118–123] It has been reported on dynamic nuclear scintigraphy that, in patients who ultimately develop overt clinical liver metastases, the relative ratio of hepatic artery to portal venous blood supply to the hepatic parenchyma is increased.[124] The reason for this phenomenon is not completely clear, but may be related to a vasoactive tumour-associated peptide that causes splanchnic constriction. Although it is technically difficult to perform reproducibly, Doppler sonography can determine the relative flow rates within the hepatic artery and portal vein, allowing calculation of a Doppler perfusion index (DPI). In a recent study of 80 patients with colorectal carcinoma who were followed for a minimum of 2 years, 97% of patients with a normal DPI survived, whereas 78% of patients with an abnormally elevated DPI developed recurrent disease or died.[120] This technique clearly has important implications, but the results have yet to be reproduced in other centres.

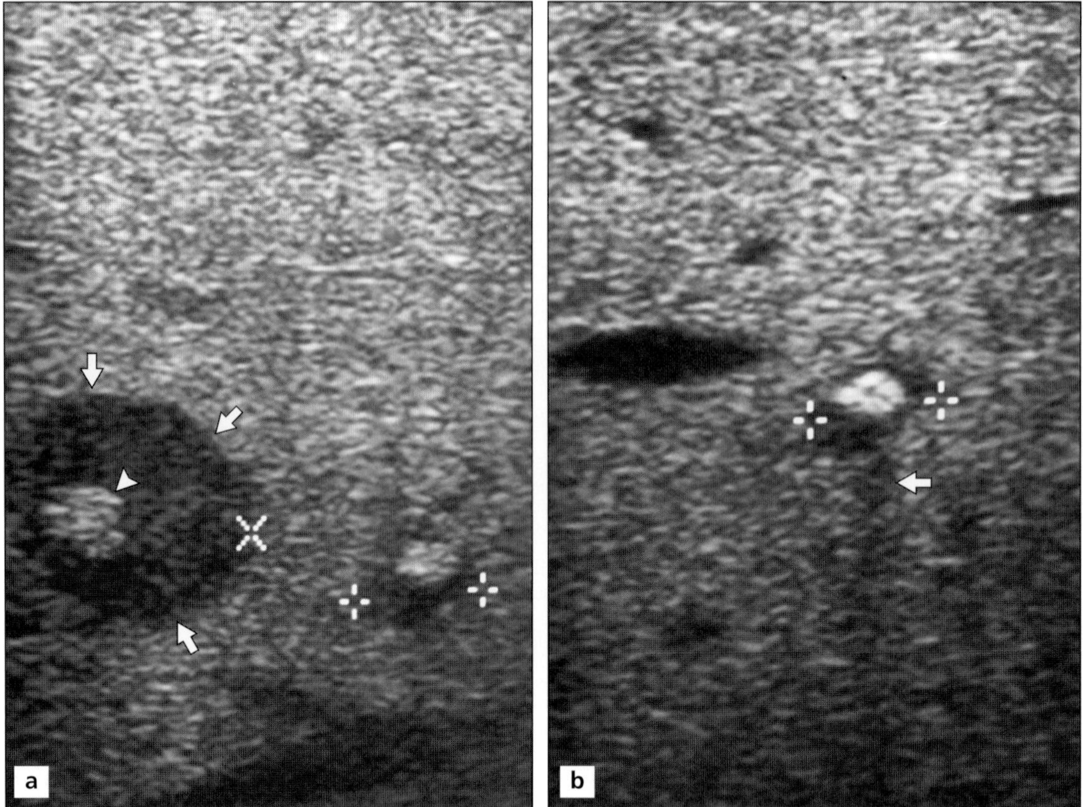

Figure 2.18. *Intra-operative sonography for liver metastases. (a) Intra-operative sonogram obtained during hepatic resection for localized metastases shows a 1.5 cm, chiefly hypoechoic, lesion (arrows) with eccentrically located hyperechoic centre (arrowhead). The 7 mm lesion adjacent to it (outlined by crosshairs) had not been detected on preoperative imaging; (b) image obtained of the smaller lesion (outlined by crosshairs) shows shadowing (arrow) due to lesional calcification.*

Summary

- As there are more treatment options for rectal cancer, there is more reason to obtain staging information than in colon cancer.
- At present, early detection of recurrent disease in asymptomatic patients has been proved to be of value only in isolated local recurrence in rectal cancer and for well-circumscribed, small volume hepatic or lung deposits.
- The accuracy of CT and MRI (using a standard body coil) is approximately equivalent in T- and N-staging rectal cancer. Both are relatively inaccurate in detecting pericolic infiltration and the accuracy for lymph node detection is about 60–65%.
- EUS is the most accurate imaging technique for the staging of early rectal cancer, but has not improved the accuracy for N-staging.
- Immunoscintigraphy and PET offer exciting prospects for increased sensitivity in the detection of disease undetected in cross-sectional imaging and also, particularly, in detecting extrahepatic recurrent disease.
- A relatively large number of patients with colorectal cancer will have liver metastases at presentation, of which a substantial number will be undetected initially.
- No screening technique now in use is adequately sensitive for the detection of liver metastases but, for several reasons, CT is the preferred non-invasive method.

References

1. Cohen AM. Preoperative evaluation of patients with primary colon cancer. *Cancer* 1992; 70: 1328–1332

2. Steele G Jr. Accomplishment and promise in the understanding and treatment of colorectal cancer. *Lancet* 1993; 342: 1092–1096

3. Izbicki JR, Blöchle C. Colorectal carcinoma: impact of staging on surgical treatment. *Endoscopy* 1993; 25: 117–124

4. Kronborg O. Staging and surgery for colorectal cancer. *Eur J Cancer* 1993; 29: 575–583

5. McGinnis L. Surgical treatment options for colorectal cancer. *Cancer* 1994; 74: 2147–2150

6. Moertel CG. Accomplishments in surgical adjuvant therapy for large bowel cancer. *Cancer* 1992; 70: 1364–1371

7. Mehta S, Johnson RJ, Schofield PF. Staging of colorectal cancer. *Clin Radiol* 1994; 49: 515–523

8. Sexe R, Miedema BW. Rectal cancer: treatment advances that reduce recurrence rates and lengthen survival. *Postgrad Med* 1993; 94: 183–190

9. Kemeny N, Lokich JJ, Anderson N, Ahlgren JD. Recent advances in the treatment of advanced colorectal cancer. *Cancer* 1993; 71: 9–18

10. Steele G Jr. Standard postoperative monitoring of patients after primary resection of colon and rectum cancer. *Cancer* 1993; 71: 4225–4235

11. Kelly CJ, Daly JM. Colorectal cancer: principles of postoperative follow-up. *Cancer* 1992; 70: 1397–1408

12. Wang JY, Tang R, Chiang JM. Value of carcinoembryonic antigen in the management of colorectal cancer. *Dis Colon Rectum* 1994; 37: 272–277

13. McCall JL, Cox MR, Wattchow DA. Analysis of local recurrence rates after surgery alone for rectal cancer. *Int J Colorect Dis* 1995; 10: 126–132

14. Benotti P, Steele G Jr. Patterns of recurrent colorectal cancer and recovery surgery. *Cancer* 1992; 70: 1409–1413

15. Zavadsky KE, Lee Y-T. Liver metastases from colorectal carcinoma: incidence, resectability, and survival results. *Am Surg* 1994; 60: 929–933

16. Stevenson GW. Radiology and endoscopy in the pretreatment diagnostic management of colorectal cancer. *Cancer* 1993; 71: 4198–4206

17. Mayes GB, Zornoza J. Computed tomography of colon carcinoma. *AJR* 1980; 135: 43–46

18. Thoeni RF, Moss AA, Schnyder P, Margulis AR. Detection and staging of primary rectal and rectosigmoid cancer by computed tomography. *Radiology* 1981; 141: 135–138

19. van Waes PFGM, Koehler PR, Feldberg MAM. Management of rectal carcinoma: impact of computed tomography. *AJR* 1983; 140: 1137–1142

20. van Waes PFGM, Koehler PR, Feldberg MAM. CT of rectal cancer: its accuracy and effect on patient management. *RadioGraphics* 1984; 4: 801–819

21. Freeny PC, Marks WM, Ryan JA, Bolenn JW. Colorectal carcinoma evaluation with CT: preoperative staging or detection of post-operative recurrence. *Radiology* 1986; 158: 347–353

22. Balthazar EJ, Megibow AJ, Hulnick D, Naidich D P. Carcinoma of the colon: detection and preoperative staging by CT. *AJR* 1988; 150: 301–306

23. Shank B, Dershaw DD, Caravelli J *et al.* A prospective study of the accuracy of preoperative computed tomographic staging of patients with biopsy-proven rectal carcinoma. *Dis Colon Rectum* 1990; 33: 285–290

24. Guinet C, Buy J-N, Ghossain MA *et al.* Comparison of magnetic resonance imaging and computed tomography in the preoperative staging of rectal cancer. *Arch Surg* 1990; 125: 385–388

25. Butch RJ, Stark DD, Wittenberg J *et al.* Staging rectal cancer by MR and CT. *AJR* 1986; 146: 1155–1160

26. Rifkin MD, Ehrlich SM, Marks G. Staging of rectal carcinoma: prospective comparison of endorectal US and CT. *Radiology* 1989; 170: 319–322

27. Holdsworth PJ, Johnston D, Chalmers AG *et al.* Endoluminal ultrasound and computed tomography in the staging of rectal cancer. *Br J Surg* 1988; 75: 1019–1022

28. Beynon J, Mortensen NJ, Foy DM *et al.* Pre-operative assessment of local invasion in rectal cancer: digital examination, endoluminal sonography or computed tomography? *Br J Surg* 1986; 1015–1017

29. Zerhouni EA, Rutter C, Hamilton SR *et al.* CT and MR imaging in the staging of colorectal carcinoma: report of the Radiology Diagnostic Oncology Group II. *Radiology* 1996; 200: 443–451

30. Angelelli G, Macarini L, Lupo L *et al.* Rectal carcinoma CT staging with water as contrast medium. *Radiology* 1990; 177: 511–514

31. Gazelle GS, Gaa J, Saini S, Shellito P. Staging of colon carcinoma using water enema CT. *J Comput Assist Tomogr* 1995; 19: 87–91

32. Nishioka T, Shimizu T, Shirato H *et al.* Relation between preoperative CT findings in rectal cancer and local recurrence rate. *Acta Oncol* 1993; 32: 555–558

33. Thoeni RF, Rogalla P. CT for the evaluation of carcinomas in the colon and rectum. *Semin Ultrasound*, CT, MRI 1995; 16: 112–126

34 Lee JKT, Stanley RJ, Sagel SS, *et al.* CT appearance of the pelvis after abdomino-perineal resection for rectal carcinoma. *Radiology* 1981; 141: 737–741

35. Reznek RH, White FE, Young JWR, Kelsey Fry I. The appearances on computed tomography after abdomino-perineal resection for carcinoma of the rectum: a comparison between the normal appearances and those of recurrence. *Br J Radiol* 1983; 56: 237–240

36. McCarthy SM, Barnes D, Deveney K *et al.* Detection of recurrent rectosigmoid carcinoma: prospective evaluation of CT and clinical factors. *AJR* 1985; 144: 577–579

37. Sugarbaker PH, Gianola FJ, Dwyer A, Neuman NR. A simplified plan for follow-up of patients with colon and rectal cancer supported by prospective studies of laboratory and radiological test results. *Surgery* 1987; 102: 79–87

38. Méndez RJ, Rodrígue R, Kovacevich T *et al.* CT in local recurrence of rectal carcinoma. *J Comput Assist Tomogr* 1993; 17: 741–744

39. de Lange EE, Fechner RE, Edge SB, Spaulding CA. Preoperative staging of rectal carcinoma with MR imaging: surgical and histopathologic correlation. *Radiology* 1990; 176: 623–628

40. Thaler W, Watzka S, Martin F *et al.* Preoperative staging of rectal cancer by endoluminal ultrasound vs magnetic resonance imaging: preliminary results of a prospective, comparative study. *Dis Colon Rectum* 1994; 37: 1189–1193

41. Chan TW, Kressel HY, Milestone B *et al.* Rectal carcinoma: staging at MR imaging with endorectal surface coil: work in progress. *Radiology* 1991; 181: 461–467

42. Schnall MD, Furth EE, Rosato EF, Kressel HY. Rectal tumor stage: correlation of endorectal MR imaging and pathologic findings. *Radiology* 1994; 190: 709–714

43. Pegios W, Vogl THJ, Mack MG *et al.* MRI diagnosis and staging of rectal carcinoma. *Abdom Imag* 1996; 21: 211–218

44. Joosten FBM, Jansen JB, Joosten HJ, Rosenbusch G. Staging of rectal carcinoma using MR double surface coil, MR endorectal coil, and intrarectal ultrasound: correlation with histopathologic findings. *J Comput Assist Tomogr* 1995; 19: 752–758

45. de Lange EE, Fechner RE, Wanebo HJ. Suspected recurrent rectosigmoid carcinoma after abdominoperineal resection: MR imaging and histopathologic findings. *Radiology* 1989; 170: 323–328

46. Pema PJ Bennett WF, Bova JG, Warman P. CT vs MRI in diagnosis of recurrent rectosigmoid carcinoma. *J Comput Assist Tomogr* 1994; 18: 256–261

47. Fedyaev EB, Volkova EA, Kuznetsova EE. Transrectal and transvaginal ultrasonography in the preoperative staging of rectal carcinoma. *Eur J Radiol* 1995; 20: 35–38

48. Anderson BO, Hann LE, Enker WE *et al.* Transrectal ultrasonography and operative selection for early carcinoma of the rectum. *J Am Coll Surg 1994*; 179: 513–517

49. Harnsberger JR, Charvat P, Longo WE *et al.* The role of intrarectal ultrasound (IRUS) in staging of rectal cancer and detection of extrarectal pathology. *Am Surg* 1994; 60: 571–577

50. Rafaelsen SR, Kronborg O, Fenger C. Digital rectal examination and transrectal ultra sonography in staging of rectal cancer. *Acta Radiol* 1994; 35: 300–304

51. Hulsmans F-JH, Tio TL, Fockens P *et al.* Assessment of tumor infiltration depth in rectal cancer with transrectal sonography: caution is necessary. *Radiology* 1994; 190: 715–720

52. Nielsen MB, Qvitzau S, Pedersen JF. Detection of pericolonic lymph nodes in patients with colorectal cancer: an *in vitro* and *in vivo* study of the efficacy of endosonography. *AJR* 1993; 161: 57–60

53. Sentovich SM, Blatchford GJ, Falk PM *et al.* Transrectal ultrasound of rectal tumors. *Am J Surg* 1993; 166: 638–642

54. Herzog U, von Flüe M, Tondelli P, Schuppisser JP. How accurate is endorectal ultrasound in the preoperative staging of rectal cancer? *Dis Colon Rectum* 1993; 36: 127–134

55. Lindmark G, Elvin A, Pählman L, Glimelius B. The value of endosonography in preoperative staging of rectal cancer. *Int J Colorect Dis* 1992; 7: 162–166

56. Milsom JW, Lavery IC, Stolfi VM *et al.* The expanding utility of endoluminal ultrasonography in the management of rectal cancer. *Surgery* 1992; 112: 832–841

57. Katsura Y, Yamada K, Ishizawa T *et al.* Endorectal sonography for the assessment of wall invasion and lymph node metastasis in rectal cancer. *Dis Colon Rectum* 1992; 35: 362–368

58. Fleshman JW, Myerson RJ, Fry RD, Kodner IJ. Accuracy of transrectal ultrasound in predicting pathologic stage of rectal cancer before and after preoperative radiation therapy. *Dis Colon Rectum* 1992; 35: 823–829

59. Tio TL, Coene PP, van Delden OM, Tytgat GN. Colorectal carcinoma: preoperative TNM classification with endosonography. *Radiology* 1991; 179: 165–170

60. Dershaw DD, Enker WE, Cohen AM, Sigurdson ER. Transrectal ultrasonography of rectal carcinoma. *Cancer* 1990; 66: 2336–2340

61. Reading CC. Endorectal sonography. *Crit Rev Diagn Imag* 1992; 33: 1–28

62. Hawes RH. Endoscopic ultrasound. *Cancer* 1993; 71: 4207–4213

63. Tempero M, Brand R, Holdeman K, Matamoros A. New imaging techniques in colorectal cancer. *Semin Oncol* 1995; 22: 448–471

64. Ramirez JM, Mortensen NJ McC, Takeuchi N, Smilgin Humphreys MM. Endoluminal ultrasonography in the follow-up of patients with rectal cancer. *Br J Surg* 1994; 81: 692–694

65. Romano G, Esercizio L, Santangelo M *et al.* Impact of computed tomography vs. intrarectal ultrasound on the diagnosis, resectability, and prognosis of locally recurrent rectal cancer. *Dis Colon Rectum* 1993; 36: 261–265

66. Tschmelitsch J, Glaser K, Schwarz C *et al.* Endosonography (ES) in the diagnosis of recurrent cancer of the rectum. *J Ultrasound Med* 1992; 11: 149–153

67. Sudakoff GS, Gasparaitis A, Mechelassi F *et al.* Endorectal color Doppler imaging of primary and recurrent rectal wall tumors: preliminary experience. *AJR* 1996; 166: 55–61

68. Ryan JW. Immunoscintigraphy in primary colorectal cancer. *Cancer* 1993; 71: 4217–4224

69. Abdel-Nabi H, Doerr RJ. Radiolabeled monoclonal antibody imaging (immunoscintigraphy) of colorectal cancers: current status and future perspectives. *Am J Surg* 1992; 163: 448–456

70. Abdel-Nabi H, Doerr RJ. Clinical applications of indium-111–labeled monoclonal antibody imaging in colorectal cancer patients. *Semin Nucl Med* 1993; 23: 99–113

71. Stomper PC, D'Souza DJ, Bakshi SP *et al.* Detection of pelvic recurrence of colorectal carcinoma: prospective, blinded comparison of Tc-99m-IMMU-4 monoclonal antibody scanning and CT. *Radiology* 1995; 197: 688–692

72. Rodriguez-Bigas MA, Bakshi S, Stomper P *et al.* 99mTc-IMMU-4 monoclonal antibody scan in colorectal cancer: a prospective study. *Arch Surg* 1992; 127: 1321–1324

73. Lechner P, Lind P, Binter G, Cesnik H. Anticarcinoembryonic antigen immuno scintigraphy with a 99mTc-Fab' fragment (Immu 4TM) in primary and recurrent colorectal cancer: a prospective study. *Dis Colon Rectum* 1993; 36: 930–935

74. Patt YZ, Podoloff DA, Curley S *et al.* Monoclonal antibody imaging in patients with colorectal cancer and increasing levels of serum carcino-embryonic antigen. *Cancer* 1993; 71: 4293–4297

75. Patt YZ, Podoloff AD, Curley S *et al.* Technetium 99m-labeled IMMU-4, a monoclonal antibody against carcinoembryonic antigen, for imaging of occult recurrent colorectal cancer in patients with rising serum carcinoembryonic antigen levels. *J Clin Oncol* 1994; 12: 489–495

76. Gasparini M, Buraggi GL, Regalia E *et al.* Comparison of radioimmunodetection with other imaging methods in evaluating local relapses of colorectal carcinoma. *Cancer* 1994; 73: 846–849

77. Buraggi GL, Gasparini M, Seregni E. Immunoscintigraphy of colorectal carcinoma with an anti-CEA monoclonal antibody: a critical review. *Nucl Med Biol* 1991; 18: 45–50

78. Abdel-Nabi H, Schwartz AN, Goldfogel G *et al.* Colorectal tumors: scintigraphy with In-111 anti-CEA monoclonal antibody and correlation with surgical, histopathologic, and immuno-histochemical findings. *Radiology* 1988; 166: 747–752

79. Lamki LM, Patt YZ, Rosenblum MG *et al.* Metastatic colorectal cancer: radioimmunoscintigraphy with a stabilized In-111–labeled F(ab')2 fragment of an anti-CEA monoclonal antibody. *Radiology* 1990; 174: 147–151

80. Corbisiero RM, Yamauchi DM, Williams LE *et al.* Comparison of immunoscintigraphy and computerized tomography in identifying colorectal cancer: individual lesion analysis. *Cancer Res* 1991; 51: 5704–5711

81. Takenoshita S-I, Hashizumee T, Asao T *et al.* Immunoscintigraphy using 99mTc-labeled anti-CEA monoclonal antibody for patients with colorectal cancer. *Anticancer Res* 1995; 15: 471–476

82. Abdel-Nabi H, Doerr RJ, Chan H-W *et al.* In-111–labeled monoclonal antibody immunoscintigraphy in colorectal carcinoma: safety, sensitivity, and preliminary clinical results. *Radiology* 1990; 175: 163–171

83. Doerr RJ, Abdel-Nabi H, Krag D, Mitchell E. Radiolabeled antibody imaging in the management of colorectal cancer: results of a multi-center clinical study. *Ann Surg* 1991; 214: 118–124

84. Collier BD, Abdel-Nabi H, Doerr RJ *et al.* Immunoscintigraphy performed with In-111–labeled CYT-103 in the management of colorectal cancer: comparison with CT. *Radiology* 1992; 185: 179–186

85. Petersen BM Jr, Bass BL, Bates HR *et al.* Use of the radiolabeled murine monoclonal antibody, 111In-CYT-103, in the management of colon cancer. *Am J Surg* 1993; 165: 137–143

86. Philpott GW, Siegel BA, Schwarz SW *et al.* Immunoscintigraphy with a new indium-111-labeled monoclonal antibody (MAb 1A3) in patients with colorectal cancer. *Dis Colon Rectum* 1994; 37: 782–792

87. Granowska M, Mather SJ, Britton KE *et al.* 99mTc radioimmunoscintigraphy of colorectal cancer. *Br J Cancer* 1990 62: 30–33

88. Arnold MW, Hitchcock CL, Young DC *et al.* Intra-abdominal patterns of disease dissemination in colorectal cancer identified using radioimmuno-guided surgery. *Dis Colon Rectum* 1996; 39: 509–513

89. Roselli M, Guadagni F, Buonomo O *et al.* Intraoperative radioimmunolocalization of an anti-CEA MAb F(Ab')2 (F023C5) in CEA serum-negative colorectal cancer patients. *Anticancer Res* 1996; 16: 883–889

90. Arnold MW, Schneebaum S, Berens A *et al.* Radioimmunoguided surgery challenges traditional decision making in patients with primary colorectal cancer. *Surgery* 1992; 112: 624–630

91. Arnold MW, Young DC, Hitchcock CL *et al.* Radioimmunoguided surgery in primary colorectal carcinoma: an intraoperative prognostic tool and adjuvant to traditional staging. *Am J Surg* 1995; 170: 315–318

92. Goldberg MA, Lee MJ, Fischman AJ *et al.* Fluorodeoxyglucose PET of abdominal and pelvic neoplasms: potential role in oncologic imaging. *RadioGraphics* 1993; 13: 1047–1062

93. Gupta N, Bradfield H. Role of positron emission tomography scanning in evaluating gastrointestinal neoplasms. *Semin Nucl Med* 1996; 26: 65–73

94. Strauss LG, Clorius JH, Schlag P. *et al.* Recurrence of colo-rectal tumors: PET evaluation. *Radiology* 1989; 170: 329–332

95. Ito K, Kato T, Tadokoro M *et al.* Recurrent rectal cancer and scar: differentiation with PET and MR imaging. *Radiology* 1992; 182: 549–552

96. Beets G, Penninckx F, Schiepers C *et al.* Clinical value of whole-body positron emission tomography with [18F] fluorodeoxyglucose in recurrent colorectal cancer. *Br J Surg* 1994; 81: 1666–1670

97. Falk PM, Gupta NC, Thorson AG *et al.* Positron emission tomography for preoperative staging of colorectal carcinoma. *Dis Colon Rectum* 1994; 37: 153–156

98. Hughes KS, Rosenstein RB, Songhorabodi S *et al.* Resection of the liver for colorectal carcinoma metastases: a multi-institutional study of long-term survivors. *Dis Colon Rectum* 1988; 31: 1–4

99. Wernecke K, Rummeny E, Bongartz G *et al.* Detection of hepatic masses in patients with carcinoma: comparative sensitivities of sonography, CT and MR imaging. *AJR* 1991; 157: 731–739

100. Soyer P, Levesque M, Elias D *et al.* Preoperative assessment of resectability of hepatic metastases from colonic carcinoma: CT portography vs sonography and dynamic CT. *AJR* 1992; 159: 741–744

101. Paul MA, Sibinga Mulder L, Cuesta MA *et al.* Impact of intraoperative ultrasonography on treatment strategy for colorectal cancer. *Br J Surg* 1994; 81: 1660–1663

102. van Ooijen B, Oudkerk M, Schmitz PIM, Wiggers T. Detection of liver metastases from colorectal carcinoma: is there a place for routine computed tomography arteriography? *Surgery* 1996; 119: 511–516

103. Langmo LS, Dagher AP Mehard WB *et al.* Does CTAP prior to hepatic resection improve patient survival rates? *Abdom Imag* 1994; 19: 317–319

104. Baron RL. Detection of liver neoplasms: techniques and outcomes. *Abdom Imag* 1994; 19: 320–324

105. Lundstedt C, Ikberg H, Hederström *et al.* Radiologic diagnosis of liver metastases in colo-rectal carcinoma. *Acta Radiol* 1987; 28: 431–438

106. Yamaguchi A, Ishida T, Nishimura G *et al.* Detection by CT during arterial portography of colorectal cancer metastases to liver. *Dis Colon Rectum* 1991; 34: 37–40

107. Heiken JP, Weyman PJ, Lee JKT *et al.* Detection of focal hepatic masses: prospective evaluation with CT, delayed CT, CT during arterial portography, and MR imaging. *Radiology* 1989; 171: 47–51

108. Soyer P, Levesque M, Elias D *et al.* Detection of liver metastases from colorectal cancer: comparison of intraoperative US and CT during arterial portography. *Radiology* 1992; 183: 541–544

109. Chezmar JL, Bernardino ME, Kaufman SH, Nelson RC. Combined CT arterial portography and CT hepatic angiography for evaluation of the hepatic resection candidate: work in progress. *Radiology* 1993; 189: 407–409

110. Nelson RC, Thompson GH, Chezmar JL *et al.* CT during arterial portography: diagnostic pitfalls. *RadioGraphics* 1992; 12: 705–718

111. Matsui O, Takashima T, Kadoya M *et al.* Liver metastases from colorectal cancers: detection with CT during arterial portography. *Radiology* 1987; 165: 65–69

112. Ward BA, Miller DL, Frank JW *et al.* Prospective evaluation of hepatic imaging studies in the detection of colorectal metastases: correlation with surgical findings. *Surgery* 1989; 105: 180–187

113. Peterson MS, Baron RL, Dodd GD III *et al.* Hepatic parenchymal perfusion defects detected with CTAP: imaging-pathologic correlation. *Radiology* 1992; 185: 149–1550

114. Rafaelson SR, Kronborg O, Larsen C, Fenger C. Intraoperative ultrasonography in detection of hepatic metastases from colorectal cancer. *Dis Colon Rectum* 1995; 38: 355–360

115. Brower ST, Dumitrescu O, Rubinoff S *et al.* Operative ultrasound establishes resectability of metastases by major hepatic resection. *World J Surg* 1989; 13: 649–657

116. Meijer S, Paul MA, Cuesta MA, Blomjous J. Intra-operative ultrasound in detection of liver metastases. *Eur J Cancer* 1995; 31: 1210–1211

117. Clarke MP, Kane RA, Steele G Jr *et al.* Prospective comparison of preoperative imaging and intraoperative ultrasonography in the detection of liver tumors. *Surgery* 1989; 106: 849–855

118. Leen E, Goldberg JA, Robertson J *et al.* The use of duplex sonography in the detection of colorectal hepatic metastases. *Br J Cancer* 1991; 63: 323–325

119. Leen E, Goldberg JA, Robertson J *et al.* Early detection of occult colorectal hepatic metastases using duplex colour Doppler sonography. *Br J Surg* 1993; 80: 1249–1251

120. Leen E, Angerson WG, Cooke TG, McArdle C S. Prognostic power of Doppler perfusion index in colorectal cancer. *Ann Surg* 1996; 223: 199–203

121. Leen E, Angerson WJ, Wotherspoon H *et al.* Detection of colorectal liver metastases: comparison of laparotomy, CT, US, and Doppler perfusion index and evaluation of postoperative follow-up results. *Radiology* 1995; 195: 113–116

122. Shuman WP. Liver metastases from colorectal carcinoma: detection with Doppler US-guided measurements of liver blood flow–past, present, future. *Radiology* 1995; 195: 9–10

123. Leen E, Angerson WJ, O'Gorman P *et al.* Intraoperative ultrasound in colorectal cancer patients undergoing apparently curative surgery: correlation with two year follow-up. *Clin Radiol* 1996; 51: 157–159

124. Hemingway DM, Cooke TG, McCurrach G *et al.* Clinical correlation of high activity dynamic hepatic scintigraphy in patients with colorectal cancer. *Br J Cancer* 1992; 65: 781–782

Chapter 3

PATHOLOGY OF COLORECTAL CANCER AND PREMALIGNANT LESIONS*

P. Hermanek with contributions by J. Rüschoff

Introduction

Pathological studies have demonstrated the development of colorectal carcinoma through the dysplasia–carcinoma sequence, the pathways of tumour spread and the significance of morphological prognostic factors. This knowledge provides an important general basis for present-day treatment of colorectal carcinoma. In daily practice, the pathologist should be integrated into the team of clinical oncologists to confirm the diagnosis and provide adequate tumour classification. The latter is today a precondition for proper planning of treatment and for subsequent analysis of treatment results. Furthermore, the cooperation of the pathologist is needed for quality control of diagnosis and treatment of cancer.

Precancerous lesions

PRECANCEROUS LESIONS VS PRECANCEROUS CONDITIONS

Since the end of the nineteenth century it has been known that carcinomas in general do not arise like a bolt from the blue, but develop in certain clinical states and/or tissue changes. This concept of 'precancers' applies also to colorectal carcinoma.

Following the activities of the World Health Organization (WHO) in the 1970s, today it is usual to distinguish between precancerous conditions and precancerous lesions. Precancerous conditions are clinical states which are associated with a significantly increased risk of cancer; precancerous lesions are histopathological abnormalities in which cancer is more likely to occur than in its apparently normal counterpart.[1,2] Neither in precancerous conditions nor in precancerous lesions is the development of malignant tumours inevitable; in fact, only a relatively

*Dedicated to Dr Basil Morson, the father of modern colorectal pathology, whose stimulating ideas live to this day.

small proportion of patients with precancerous conditions develop precancerous lesions. Although carcinomas obviously always arise in precancerous lesions, i.e. dysplasia, this malignant progression is observed only in a small percentage of dysplasias. In other words, precancer does not always become cancer, but nearly always cancer has its precancer.[3]

In Table 3.1 the precancerous lesions are listed. Although up to 10% of all colorectal carcinomas develop in hereditary syndromes, the great majority of colorectal carcinomas are observed in patients without evidence of hereditary syndromes (so-called sporadic carcinomas). The risk of development of carcinomas in precancerous conditions is known only for familial adenomatous polyposis (FAP). If prophylactic removal of the entire colorectal mucosa with its adenomas is not performed, almost invariably carcinomas arise from one or more of the numerous adenomas, usually between the ages of 25 and 40 years, and only in extremely rare cases before puberty. Thus, FAP is the model of an 'obligatory' precancerous condition, the individual adenoma representing 'obligatory' precancerous lesions. In contrast, for other precancerous conditions precise figures on the percentage of carcinoma development are lacking.

Table 3.1. *Precancerous conditions in colorectal carcinoma**

1. Hereditary syndromes with increased risk of carcinoma[†]
   - Polyposis syndromes
   - Neoplastic
     - Familial adenomatous polyposis (FAP)
     - Hereditary flat adenoma syndrome (HFAS)
   - Non-neoplastic
     - Juvenile polyposis
     - (Peutz–Jeghers syndrome)
   - Hereditary non-polyposis colon cancer (HNPCC)
     - Lynch syndrome I (hereditary site-specific non-polyposis colon cancer syndrome)
     - Lynch syndrome II (cancer family syndrome)
   - (Muir–Torre syndrome)
   - (Turcot syndrome)
2. Precancerous conditions in so-called sporadic carcinomas
   - Chronic ulcerative colitis
   - Colorectal carcinoma(s) in first degree relatives (without evidence of hereditary syndromes)
   - Previous colorectal carcinoma
   - Previous colorectal adenoma
   - Synchronous or previous breast, ovary and endometrial carcinoma
   - (Previous urinary conduit into sigmoid colon)
   - (Chronic Crohns disease of the colorectum)
   - (Chronic irradiation colitis)
   - (*Schistosomiasis japonica* colitis)
   - (Familial agammaglobulinaemia)

* Very uncommon conditions in parentheses.

† For details see pp. 71–79.

DYSPLASIA AND DYSPLASIA–CARCINOMA SEQUENCE

The concept that colorectal carcinoma arises from dysplasia is widely accepted nowadays.[2,4,5]

The general definition of dysplasia

In general, in the gastrointestinal tract, dysplasia is defined as unequivocal neoplastic epithelial alteration without invasive growth. A synonymous term is intraepithelial neoplasia. It is characterized by cytological atypia, aberrant differentiation and disorganized architecture.[2] Depending on the extent of deviation from the normal, dysplasia has been classified into mild, moderate and severe. However, today a subdivision into low grade (combining mild and moderate) and high grade is preferred.[4]

Dysplasia vs carcinoma in the colorectum

In contrast to the stomach or the small intestine, a neoplasm in the colon and rectum has metastatic potential only after invasion of at least the submucosa. This is generally explained by Fenoglio's report[6] that lymphatic vessels are found only at the level of, and below, the crypt bases. This explanation is not entirely tenable, however, because in pathological conditions lymph vessels containing tumour cells can be demonstrated between the mucosal crypts.[7] Nevertheless, the irrefutable fact remains that in 'mucosal carcinomas', metastasis does not take place. Thus, for the colorectum in the biological and clinical sense, carcinoma is present only after the submucosa is invaded. Such lesions are termed invasive carcinomas (Table 3.2).

Dysplasia–carcinoma sequence and 'de novo' carcinoma

The most common macroscopic type of dysplasia is polypoid and is traditionally termed adenoma. Thus, in the older literature the 'adenoma–carcinoma sequence' has been in the foreground of the discussion on the formal pathogenesis of colorectal carcinoma. Subsequently, flat dysplasia in chronic inflammatory bowel disease, predominantly in ulcerative colitis and, only in the 1980s, so-called flat adenomas (i.e. flat dysplasia in mucosa without inflammation) have been described.[9] Consequently, the concept of the adenoma–carcinoma sequence was extended to that of the dysplasia–carcinoma sequence (Table 3.3, Figure 3.1), which explains the formal pathogenesis for all clinical presentations of carcinoma.

The concept of the dysplasia–carcinoma sequence primarily was developed from conventional microscopy and clinical epidemiology. It could be confirmed by experimental pathology, DNA analysis and sophisticated histopathological methods such as mucin, enzyme and immunohistochemistry. With all these modern methods the stepwise transition from normal mucosa to dysplasia of increasing grade and lastly to invasive carcinoma can be observed (for references see the review by Lewin *et al.*[5]). Lastly, molecular pathology has shown that, in dysplasia, changes similar to those in carcinomas are present and that during the dysplasia–carcinoma sequence an accumulation of these molecular changes takes place.[11–13]

Diagnosis

PRETREATMENT MICROSCOPIC DIAGNOSIS

The microscopic diagnosis of invasive carcinoma requires the histological examination of tissue from the submucosa because only in this manner can the decisive criterion of invasion of submucosa be determined. Therefore, cytology is not useful for pretreatment microscopic diagnosis of the primary lesion.

The procedure for obtaining tissue from the submucosa differs according to the gross fea-

Table 3.2. *Nomenclature of dysplasia–carcinoma sequence*

Nomenclature	Intraepithelial	Invasion of lamina propria and muscularis mucosae	Invasion of submucosa
Terms used in literature	Intraepithelial neoplasia	Mucosal carcinoma	Invasive carcinoma
	Carcinoma *in situ*	Intramucosal carcinoma	
	High-grade dysplasia	Focal carcinoma	
		High-grade dysplasia	
UICC 1997 (ref. 8)	----------pTis Carcinoma *in situ*----------		pT1 carcinoma
Preferred nomenclature	----------High-grade dysplasia---------- (Non-invasive carcinoma)		Invasive carcinoma

Table 3.3. *Formal pathogenesis of colorectal carcinoma*

Origin of carcinoma	Former concept	Present concept
Polypoid adenoma (Figure 3.1a)	Adenoma–carcinoma sequence	Dysplasia–carcinoma sequence
Flat ademoma (Figure 3.1b)	Carcinoma *de novo*	
FAP	–	
IBD	–	

FAP, familial adenomatous polyposis; IBD, inflammatory bowel disease.

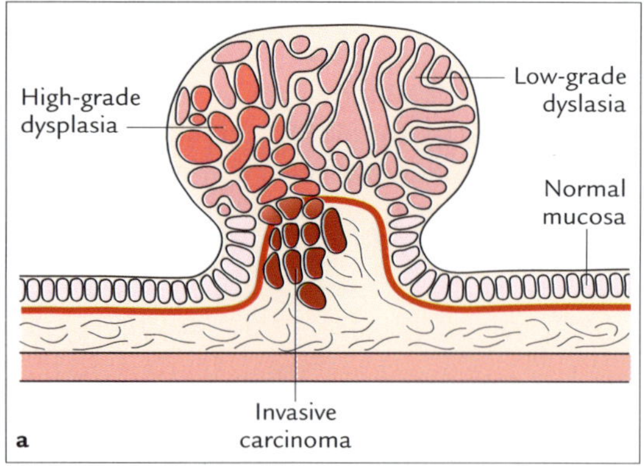

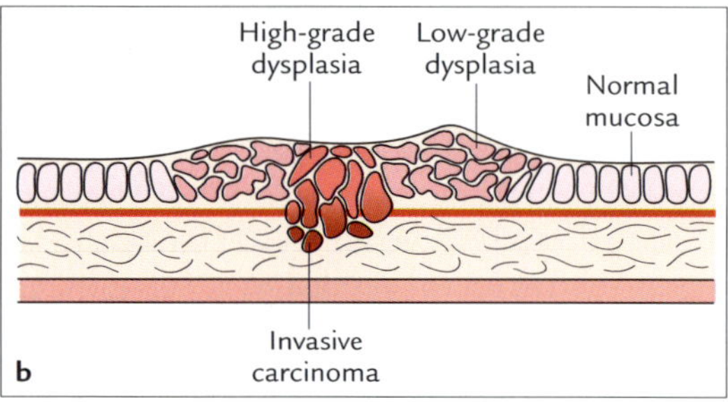

Figure 3.1. *Graphic representation of dysplasia–carcinoma sequence: (a) polypoid dysplasia; (b) flat dysplasia. Modified from ref. 10.*

ture of the suspicious lesion. If there is ulceration, tissue of different sites of the ulcer should be removed by (not too superficial) forceps biopsies. In polypoid, elevated or flat lesions, forceps biopsies often reveal only tissue from the mucosa. In such cases only a differentiation between non-neoplastic mucosa and neoplastic epithelium (dysplasia) is possible. In this case the following summary is recommended: 'A definitive assessment of the biopsied growth, in particular a differentiation between dysplasia and invasive carcinoma, will be possible only after microscopic examination of the completely removed lesion'.[14] In such cases, endoscopic polypectomy or mucosal resection, and sometimes surgical local excision, is indicated. The result of the histological examination then shows definitively whether there is invasive carcinoma. The further procedure for carcinoma depends on the results of the tumour classification (see pp. 61–64).

DIAGNOSIS OF FAMILIAL ADENOMATOUS POLYPOSIS (FAP) AND HEREDITARY NON-POLYPOSIS COLON CANCER (HNPCC) SYNDROME BY J. Rüschoff

Less than 1% of colorectal carcinomas arise in FAP. The diagnostic hallmark is the development of hundreds of adenomas within the large bowel and rectum by the third to fourth decades of life. The underlying gene defect has been shown to be a germline mutation within the adenomatous polyposis gene (*APC*) on chromosome 5q21.Thus, the diagnosis of FAP is made by clinical findings, histological confirmation of the adenomatous type of polyps and molecular tests. Affected patients are essentially diagnosed by sigmoidoscopy and histology. Molecular analysis on blood samples, however, is indicated for carcinoma risk assessment in asymptomatic individuals. For details see pp. 72–75.

HNPCC accounts for about 5–8% of colorectal carcinomas. Since patients lack any clear-cut precursor lesion, such as adenomatosis seen in FAP, diagnosis is primarily based upon family history. According to the so-called Amsterdam criteria, HNPCC kindred should meet the following criteria: (1) at least three family members out of two generations should be affected by colorectal carcinoma, two of whom are first-degree relatives; (2) one individual should be diagnosed before the age of 50 years. Recently, the molecular pathogenesis of HNPCC has been linked to mismatch repair genes on chromosome 2 (*hMSH2, MSH6, hPMS1*), chromosome 3 (*hMLH1*), and chromosome 7 (*hPMS2*) (see pp. 75–78). According to these molecular data, new guidelines for the diagnosis of HNPCC, the so-called Bethesda criteria, have most recently been established.[15] At first, clinical features suggestive of HNPCC should be examined, including Amsterdam criteria, occurrence of colorectal carcinoma before the age of 40 years or incidence of HNPCC-associated extracolonic cancers especially those in endometrium, stomach, upper urinary tract and ovary. If HNPCC is clinically suspected, carcinoma should be tested for microsatellite instability. If genetic instability is found, repair genes (*hMSHS2, hMLH1*) must be analysed in blood samples of the patient by direct sequencing or RNA-based tests.

International standardization in pathology

The international efforts to standardize tumour classification were focused by the WHO and the Union Internationale Contre le Cancer (UICC).

PRESENT TUMOUR CLASSIFICATION

At present, the histomorphology (type, grade) is classified according to the WHO International Histological Classification of Tumours.[4] It is the basis for coding by the ICD-O[16] (Table 3.4).

The anatomical extent of carcinoma is classified according to the fifth edition of the UICC TNM classification,[8] which has been agreed upon by all national TNM Committees (Table 3.5). The TNM (clinical) and the pTNM (pathological) classifications describe the anatomical extent without considering treatment. The residual tumour (R) classification deals with the tumour status after treatment; it reflects the effects of therapy. Although the R classification is considered optional by the UICC because of historical reasons, it is absolutely necessary for decisions on further therapeutic procedure following tumour resection, for estimating prognosis and for analysis of treatment results[17] (see pp. 65–67).

FEATURES TO BE RECORDED IN PATHOLOGY REPORTS

Specific recommendations for the content of surgical pathology reports have been published since the 1980s in several countries. In 1991, an International Documentation System for Colo-Rectal Carcinoma (IDS for CRC) has been achieved by an International Working Group[18] and has recently been updated.[19] In Table 3.6 the relevant pathological features to be recorded are shown.

Pathology and therapy

LOCAL THERAPY OR RADICAL RESECTION?

In local therapy of colorectal carcinoma the primary tumour is completely removed, however, the regional lymph nodes are not dissected. Thus, for use of local treatment in curative intention, the main problem is to estimate the risk of lymph node metastasis already present. If this risk is lower than the increased risk of surgical mortality of radical resection in comparison to that of local therapy, the latter is to be preferred.[7,20,21]

About 30–40% of lymph nodes involved in

Table 3.4. *Histological typing and grading of colorectal carcinoma according to WHO classification*[4]

Histological type	Description	ICD-O-code[16]	Grading system G1–4	Low/high (L/H)
Adenocarcinoma	Glandular epithelium, tubular and/or villous	8140/3	1–3	L/H
Mucinous adenocarcinoma	More than 50% extracellular mucin	8480/3	1–3	L/H
Signet ring cell carcinoma	More than 50% signet ring cells (intracytoplasmatic mucin)	8490/3	3	H
Squamous cell carcinoma	Exclusively squamous differentiation	8070/3	1–3	L/H
Adenosquamous carcinoma	Adenocarcinoma and squamous cell carcinoma	8560/3	1–3	L/H
Small cell carcinoma	Similar to small-cell carcinoma of the lung (neuroendocrine)	8041/3	4	H
Undifferentiated carcinoma	No glandular structure or other features to indicate definite differentiation (may be uniform or pleomorphic)	8020/3	4	H

Table 3.5. *Classification of anatomical extent of carcinoma according to UICC*[8]

A. Anatomical extent before treatment

TNM CLINICAL CLASSIFICATION

T – Primary tumour

TX	Primary tumour cannot be assessed
T0	No evidence of primary tumour
Tis	Carcinoma *in situ*: intraepithelial or invasion of lamina propria*
T1	Tumour invades submucosa
T2	Tumour invades muscularis propria
T3	Tumour invades through muscularis propria into subserosa or into non-peritonealized pericolic or perirectal tissues
T4	Tumour directly invades other organs or structures† and/or perforates visceral peritoneum

Notes:
* Tis includes cancer cells confined within the glandular basement membrane (intraepithelial) or lamina propria (intramucosal) with no extension through muscularis mucosae into submucosa
† Direct invasion in T4 includes invasion of other segments of the colorectum by way of the serosa, e.g. invasion of the sigmoid colon by a carcinoma of the caecum

N – Regional lymph nodes

The regional lymph nodes are the pericolic and perirectal and those located along the ileocolic, right colic, middle colic, left colic, inferior mesenteric, superior rectal (haemorrhoidal), and internal iliac arteries.

NX	Regional lymph nodes cannot be assessed
N0	No regional lymph node metastasis
N1	Metastasis in 1–3 regional lymph nodes
N2	Metastasis in four or more regional lymph nodes

Note:
A tumour nodule greater than 3 mm in diameter in perirectal or pericolic adipose tissue without histological evidence of a residual lymph node in the nodule is classified as regional perirectal/pericolic lymph node metastasis. However, a tumour nodule up to 3 mm in diameter is classified in the T category as discontinuous extension, e.g. T3.

M – Distant metastasis

MX	Distant metastasis cannot be assessed
M0	No distant metastasis
M1	Distant metastasis

pTNM PATHOLOGICAL CLASSIFICATION

The pT, pN, and pM categories correspond to the T, N, and M categories.
pN0: Histological examination of a regional lymphadenectomy specimen will ordinarily include 12 or more lymph nodes.

Stage grouping

Stage 0	Tis	N0	M0
Stage I	T1,2	N0	M0
Stage II	T3,4	N0	M0
Stage III	Any T	N1,2	M0
Stage IV	Any T	Any N	M1

B. Anatomical extent after treatment = residual tumour (R) classification

RX	Presence of residual tumour cannot be assessed
R0	No residual tumour
R1	Microscopic residual tumour
R2	Macroscopic residual tumour

Note:
In the R classification, not only is locoregional tumour to be taken into consideration, but also distant residual tumour in the form of remaining distant metastases.

In case of R1 and R2, the site of residual tumour should be stated.

Table 3.6. *Features to be recorded in pathology reports, with inclusion of the recommendations of the updated international Documentation System for Colorectal Carcinoma[19] and with consideration of the new 5th edition of TNM[8]*

Basic patient information	Feature
• Number of primary colorectal carcinomas	
• Measurements at tumour site	• Bowel wall transverse measurement • Maximal tumour size: transverse, longitudinal (fresh specimen), thickness (fixed specimen) • Distal clearance margin (bowel) (fresh unstretched specimen/fixed specimen)
• Serosal surface involved (macroscopically)	
• Associated pathology	• None/ulcerative colitis/Crohn disease/familial adenomatous polyposis (FAP)/radiation colitis/schistosomiasis/contiguous adenoma/separate adenomas (give number)
• Histological tumour type	See Table 3.4
Data of proven prognostic significance	**Feature**
• Anatomical extent of tumour	See Table 3.5A • Local spread (pT) • Regional lymph nodes: pN/number of nodes examined/Number of nodes involved/apical node status • Distant metastasis (pM)
• Residual tumour (R) classification	See Table 3.5B In case of R1,2: site of residual tumour (local: bowel resection line/local: circumferential resection line/distant metastasis/local and distant)
• Venous involvement	Intramural/extramural
• Histological pattern of infiltrating margin	Expanding (well-circumscribed)/diffusely infiltrating
• Histological grade of differentiation	See Table 3.4
Data of probable prognostic significance	**Feature**
• Tumour perforation	Spontaneous/surgical
• Mixed inflammatory-cell infiltrate	Not conspicuous/conspicuous
• Lymphoid aggregates	None/present

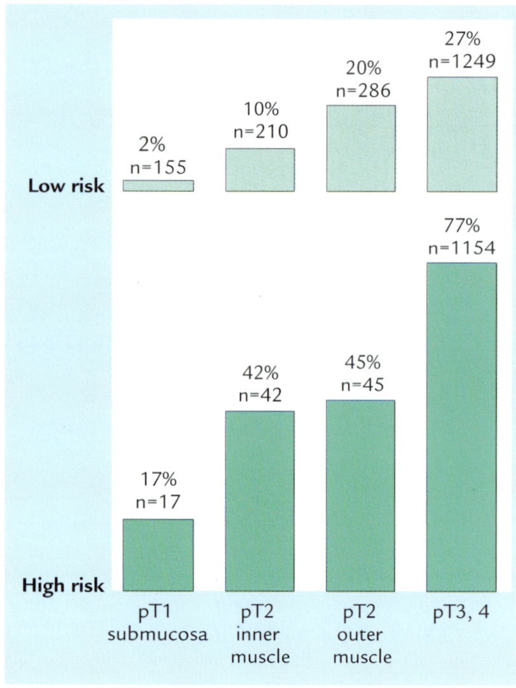

Figure 3.2. *Colorectal carcinoma/frequency of regional lymph node metastasis. Patients with radical resection for cure (R0), Department of Surgical Pathology, University of Erlangen, 1970–1990 (*n *= 3241: 1900 low risk; 1258 high risk; classification not possible in 83). Low-risk: G1, 2 (low grade) and L0 (no lymphatic invasion). High-risk: G3, 4 (high grade) or L1 (lymphatic invasion).*

colorectal carcinoma are 4 mm or less in greatest dimension.[22–24] This explains why imaging procedures, including endoluminal ultrasonography, are not sufficiently sensitive to detect regional lymph node metastasis. However, pathological features of the primary tumour are reliable when estimating the risk of lymph node metastasis.

Careful examination of radical tumour resection specimens has shown that lymphatic spread is dependent not only on the depth of invasion and grade of differentiation but also on the presence or absence of histological invasion of lymphatics in the primary tumour region.[20] Therefore, with regard to lymphatic spread we distinguish between low-risk and high-risk histology,[7,25] where low risk is indicated by a low grade of differentiation (G1, G2) *and* absence of histological invasion of lymphatics (L0), and high risk is associated with a high grade (G3,G4) *or* lymphatic invasion (L1). On the basis of histomorphology and depth of invasion it is possible to define a patient group for which the risk of lymph node metastasis already present is 3% or less (Figure 3.2)—namely, patients with low-risk histology carcinomas limited to the submucosa (pT1). For all other patients (except those with very high surgical risk), radical resection with *en bloc* dissection of the regional lymph nodes is the appropriate surgical treatment.

EXTENT OF SURGERY IN RADICAL RESECTION

The extent of surgery in radical resection is predominantly determined by lymphatic spread—in rectal carcinoma in addition by the discontinuous local spread. Continuous longitudinal local spread within the bowel wall is limited,[26] at least in curable patients, and causes problems only in carcinomas of the lowest part of the rectum.

In colon carcinoma, the central lymphatic spread to nodes along the supplying vascular trunks requires their central ligature. In consequence, the bowel resection includes in most cases the area of lymphatic spread along the marginal circulation (7 cm or less!).[24]

In carcinomas of the hepatic and splenic flexures and the adjacent thirds of the transverse, ascending and descending colon, a bidirectional lymph drainage is observed;[27,28] for example, in a carcinoma of the hepatic flexure, metastases may be found in nodes along the right colic artery as well as the middle colic artery. Thus, for such tumours with bidirectional lymph drainage, extended colonic resections such as right and transverse colectomy (extended right hemicolectomy), left and transverse colectomy (extended left hemicolectomy) or subtotal colectomy are appropriate.

In rectal carcinoma, tumour nodules in the perirectal tissue (mesorectum), separated from the primary tumour, up to 3 mm, without histological evidence of a residual lymph node, and designated as tumour deposits or satellites, are today considered as discontinuous local extension of the primary tumour.[8] Such satellites may be found in the mesorectum, not only at the height of the tumour but also distal to its lower margin.[29–31] Therefore, in carcinomas of the lower and middle third of the rectum, total mesorectal excision (in a distal direction until the pelvic floor) is necessary for removal of all satellites. This explains the drastic reduction in local recurrence attendant on total mesorectal excision since the 1980s.[32–35]

In carcinomas of the upper rectal third, satellites may be completely removed if the distal margin of clearance in the mesorectum is 5 cm measured *in situ* (corresponding to about 3 cm on the fresh, unstretched specimen) and if the distal resection line is radially at 90 degrees to the rectal wall (without coning) (so-called partial mesorectal excision).[19,36]

Histological examination of rectal carcinomas in curable stages demonstrates that the continuous distal local spread in the rectal wall proper extends usually not more than a few millimetres beyond the grossly recognizable margin of the tumour. Thus, the margin of clearance within the proper wall of the rectum may be limited to 1 cm *in situ* except in case of high-grade tumours or cases with extensive lymphatic spread, which require a 2 cm distal margin.[37]

In the case of adherence of a tumour to adjacent organs, gross inspection or palpation cannot distinguish between adherence by peritumorous inflammation or neoplastic invasion of the adjacent organ. In such cases, *en bloc* multivisceral resection (removal of the carcinoma together with the adherent part of the adjacent organ) is indicated if curative surgery seems possible. Biopsies from the adherence should be avoided because, in cases of tumour invasion, local tumour cell dissemination results and locoregional recurrences are observed with increased frequency.[38,39]

Pathology and analysis of results of treatment

Where there are differences in the results of treatment, it is always necessary to exclude differences in the distribution of patients' prognostic factors. Thus, any analysis of treatment results requires the consideration of proven (and, preferably, also the probable) prognostic factors of the patient population.

Prognostic factors differ for patients with residual tumour and for those with complete tumour resection.[40]

PROGNOSTIC FACTORS FOR PATIENTS WITH RESIDUAL TUMOUR (R1, R2)

Median survival times of 10–11 months are reported; the 5-year survival rates are about 5%. Significant prognostic factors are presence or absence of distant metastases and the localization of residual tumour, whereas local spread (T) and lymph node metastasis (N) have no influence on prognosis in these patients. For patients with multiple distant metastases, the performance status influences survival time; other possible factors have not been proven.

PROGNOSTIC FACTORS FOR PATIENTS WITH COMPLETE RESECTION OF TUMOUR (NO RESIDUAL TUMOUR, R0)

In Table 3.7 the proven and probable prognostic factors are listed. By far the most important factors are the anatomical extent of carcinoma, as described by the TNM system (Table 3.8), and the individual surgeon and his technique. It is now well documented that the surgeon influences not only short-term prognosis (i.e. surgical mortality) but also the frequency of locoregional recurrences and thus survival (Table 3.9).

NEW PROBABLE OR POSSIBLE BIOLOGICAL AND MOLECULAR PROGNOSTIC FACTORS J. Rüschoff

Colorectal carcinoma is one of the most widely accepted models for a molecular understanding of carcinogenesis. This process involves not only mutational changes within oncogenes and tumour suppressor genes but also a variety of molecular alterations leading to disturbances of cell proliferation, differentiation, apoptosis, angiogenesis and metastatic spread. Using immunohistochemistry, as well as molecular biological techniques such as *in situ* hybridization and polymerase chain reaction, a series of these tumour parameters can readily be assessed even in routinely formalin-fixed specimens. However, the prognostic value of most of these new factors remains to be established.[40]

The prognostic value of well-known tumour parameters such as ploidy and proliferation activity has not yet been shown conclusively. Data regarding ploidy are still contradictory, and it seems that ploidy, DNA index or S-phase fraction are of predictive value

Table 3.7. *Prognostic factors* for patients with colorectal carcinoma resected for cure (R0)*

Prognostic factors	Tumour related	Patient related	Treatment related
Proven	Anatomical extent: pTNM and stage group (higher category) Histological grade (high grade) Venous invasion (present, predominantly extramural)	–	Surgeon
Probable	Anatomical site of primary (lower rectum)	Gender (male)	Technique of tumour mobilization (other than 'no touch')
	Tumour perforation/ obstruction (present) Lymphatic and perineural invasion (present) Histological pattern of tumour margin (infiltrating) Peritumorous mixed cell infiltrate (not conspicuous) Lymphoid aggregates (absent)	CEA serum level (> 5 ng/ml)	

Modified from ref. 40.
* Unfavourable level of covariates in parentheses.
CEA, carcinoembryonic antigen.

only within subgroups with defined tumour stages. Similarly, the so-called proliferation markers, such as Ki-67/Mib-1, PCNA and AgNOR, have been shown to be relevant for the assessment of the tumour aggressiveness. However, the prognostic value for Ki-67/Mib-1 staining has not yet been shown unequivocally. In this respect, AgNOR analysis (which, in contrast to Ki-67, is a measure of the rapidity of cell growth) seems to be of greater importance.[41]

At present, there is a rush into studies dealing with disseminated single tumour cells, especially within bone marrow aspirates. Accordingly, epithelial cells can be detected by specific antibodies (e.g. against cytokeratins) in about 30–60% of patients with colorectal carcinoma patients.[42,43] Although there is growing evidence that these patients have a shorter relapse-free (as well as overall) survival time, multicentre studies with long-term follow-up data are still lacking.

The process of tumour invasion and metastasis has recently been studied in more detail with respect to its molecular mechanisms and their probable prognostic implications. The expression of cell adhesion molecules (such as E-cadherin) and of splice variants of CD44 (v6, v8–10) seems to predict patients' outcome. Of particular interest is the expression of proteases (metalloproteases, cathepsin B and D as well as urokinase plasminogen activator), their receptors and inhibitors. Some of these (MMP-1, uPA and PAI-1) appear to have an independent prognostic value in colorectal carcinoma.[44,45]

Today, most studies concerning the prognostic value of genetic alterations that are involved in the carcinogenesis of colorectal carcinoma have been performed for activation of the oncogene k-*ras* and for inactivation of tumour-suppressor genes such as *DCC* (deleted in colon cancer gene), *p53* and *nm23*. About 40% of colorectal carcinomas overexpress the mutated k-*ras* oncogene product *p21*. Mutations of k-*ras* at codons 12 and 13 seem to indicate a shorter 5-year relapse-free survival time in univariate analyses. In contrast, mutations of *p53* and *DCC* have been shown to be of prognostic value even in multivariate analyses. This holds true for mutations of exon 5–8 of the *p53* gene, as well as for losses of heterozygosity (LOH) at the *p53* or *DCC* gene locus. However, the prognostic value of immunohistochemistry demonstrating an accumulation of the *p53* protein has not consistently been proven. Recently, it has been shown that reduced expression of the metastasis-suppressor gene

Table 3.8. *Observed 5-year survival rates after resection for cure (R0)*

Patient group (UICC 1997)(ref. 8)	Patients (*n*)	Observed 5-year survival rates (%) with 95% confidence interval (surgical mortality not excluded)
pTl	164	77 (70–84)
pT2	349	72 (67–77)
pT3	1119	54 (51–57)
pT4	201	32 (25–39)
pN0	1016	69 (66–72)
pN1	417	48 (43–53)
pN2	326	30 (25–35)
(p)M0	1722	58 (56–60)
(p)M1	61	18 (6–26)
Stage I	424	76 (72–81)
Stage II	646	65 (61–69)
Stage III	702	42 (38–45)
• pN1	404	49 (44–54)
• pN2	295	32 (26–37)
Stage IV	61	18 (6–26)

Data of the German SGCRC (Study Group Colo-Rectal Carcinoma) prospective multicentre study.

Table 3.9. *Variations in the rate of locoregional recurrences and 5-year survival: patients with radical resection for cure (R0), without distant metastasis*

	Inter-institutional variation (%)	Inter-surgeon variation (%)
Rate of locoregional recurrence		
Colon carcinoma	4–11	0–18
Rectal carcinoma	9–23	4–54
Observed 5-year survival rates (surgical mortality excluded)		
Colon carcinoma	64–77	50–90
Rectal carcinoma	54–69	45–79

Data of the German SGCRC study, three departments with the greatest number of patients.

nm23-H1 seems to be another molecular marker indicative of aggressive colorectal cancer. The prognostic benefit has, however, not yet been shown clearly.[46]

Pathology and quality management

Quality management is needed for diagnostic activities in pathology departments,[47] as well as for treatment of cancer and clinical studies. In particular, some pathology findings in resection specimens indicate the oncological quality of surgery.[48] This applies to the following:

- Completeness of tumour resection (RO resections);
- No evidence of local spillage of tumour cells: tumour resection *en bloc* without transection of tumour tissue, no surgically induced tumour perforation;

- Length of resected bowel: limited (segmental) resection or radical resection with ligature of the trunk of the supplying vessels;
- In cases of colon carcinoma with bidirectional lymph drainage: dissection of one or two lymph drainage areas;
- Number of lymph nodes removed (provided that there is adequate node-examination technique);
- In rectal carcinoma of the upper third: distal margin of clearance in muscular wall as well as in mesorectum (no coning) not less than 5 cm *in situ* corresponding to about 3 cm measured on the fresh, unstretched, resection specimen;
- In rectal carcinoma of the middle and lower third: incomplete or total mesorectal excision? Careful gross inspection of the surface of the specimen: bilobed appearance of the correctly mobilized mesorectum with intact smooth surface.[49,50]

In clinical trials of adjuvant and neoadjuvant therapy, up-to-date adequate quality assurance of surgery and pathology never has been realized.[51] It is one of the most important tasks for the future to start new clinical trials to redefine the place of adjuvant therapy in modern optimized surgery,[19,52] and to introduce careful quality management of surgery and pathology into such trials.

References

1. Morson BC, Sobin LH, Grundmann E *et al.* Precancerous conditions and epithelial dysplasia of the stomach. *J Clin Pathol* 1980; 33: 231–240

2. Morson BC, Jass JR, Sobin LH. *Precancerous lesions of the gastrointestinal tract.* London: Baillière Tindall, 1985

3. Bauer K-H. *Das Krebsproblem*, 2nd edn. Berlin: Springer-Verlag, 1963

4. Jass JR, Sobin LH. *Histological typing of intestinal tumours*, 2nd edn. (WHO International Histological Classification of Tumours). Berlin: Springer-Verlag, 1989

5. Lewin KJ, Riddell RH, Weinstein WM. *Gastrointestinal pathology and its clinical implications.* New York: Igaku-Shoin, 1992

6. Fenoglio CM, Kaye GI, Lane N. Distribution of human colonic lymphatics in normal, hyperplastic and adenomatous tissues. *Gastroenterology* 1973; 64: 51–66

7. Hermanek P. Malignant polyps–pathological factors governing clinical management. *Curr Top Pathol* 1990; 81: 278–293

8. UICC. *TNM classification of malignant tumours*, 5th edn. (Sobin LH, Wittekind Ch, eds). New York: Wiley and Sons, 1997

9. Owen DA. Flat adenoma, flat carcinoma, and de novo carcinoma of the colon. *Cancer* 1996; 77: 3–6

10. Hermanek P, Wittekind C. Präkanzeröse Bedingungen und Läsionen des Verdauungstraktes. In: Hahn EG, Riemann JF (eds) Klinische *Gastroenterologie*, 3rd edn. Stuttgart: Georg Thieme, 1996, pp. 1920–1947

11. Cho KR, Vogelstein B. Genetic alterations in the adenoma–carcinoma sequence. *Cancer* 1992; 70: 1727–1731

12. Scott N, Quirke P. Molecular biology of colorectal neoplasia. *Gut* 1993; 34: 289–292

13. Jen J, Powell SM, Papadopoulos N *et al.* Molecular determinants of dysplasia in colorectal lesions. *Cancer Res* 1994; 54: 5523–5526

14. Hermanek P. Colorectal carcinoma: histopathological diagnosis and staging. *Baillière's Clin Gastroenterol* 1989; 3: 511–529

15. Kuska B. New diagnostic criteria for HNPCC are on the way. *J Natl Cancer Inst* 1997; 89: 11–12

16. Percy C, van Holten V, Muir C (eds). *International classification of diseases for oncology (ICD-O)*, 2nd edn. Geneva: World Health Organization, 1990

17. Hermanek P, Wittekind C. Residual tumour (R) classification and prognosis. *Semin Surg Oncol* 1994; 10: 12–20

18. Fielding LP, Arsenault PA, Chapuis PH *et al.* Clinicopathological staging for colorectal cancer: an international documentation system (IDS) and an international comprehensive anatomic terminology (ICAT). *J Gastroenterol Hepatol* 1991; 6: 325–344

19. Soreide O, Norstein J, Fielding LP, Silen W. International standardization and documentation of the treatment of rectal cancer. In: Soreide O, Norstein J (eds) *Rectal cancer surgery. Optimisation – Standardisation – Documentation.* Berlin: Springer, 1997, pp. 405–445

20. Hermanek P, Marzoli GP (eds). *Lokale Therapie des Rektumkarzinoms.* Berlin: Springer-Verlag, 1994

21. Hermanek P. Local tumour surgery: the pathologist's point of view. *Min Invas Ther Allied Technol* 1996; 5: 197–201

22. Dworak O. Number and size of lymph nodes and node metastases in rectal carcinomas. *Surg Endosc* 1989; 3: 96–99

23. Rodriguez-Bigas MA, Maamoun S, Weber TK *et al.* Clinical significance of colorectal cancer: metastases in lymph nodes <5 mm in size. *Ann Surg Oncol* 1996; 3: 124–130

24. Hida J, Yasutomi M, Maruyama T *et al.* The extent of lymph node dissection for colon carcinoma: the potential impact on laparoscopic surgery. *Cancer* 1977; 80: 188–192

25. Hermanek P. On the diagnosis of colorectal polyps. *Beitr Pathol* 1977; 161: 203–205

26. Cross SS, Bull AD, Smith JHF. Is there any justification for the routine examination of bowel resection margins in colorectal adenocarcinomas? *J Clin Pathol* 1989; 42: 1040–1042

27. Enker WE. Extent of operations for large bowel cancer. In: DeCosse JJ (ed). *Large bowel cancer.* Edinburgh: Churchill Livingstone, 1981, pp. 78–93

28. Jatzko G, Lisberg P, Wette V. Improving survival rates for patients with colorectal cancer. Br J Surg 1992; 79: 588–591

29. Heald RJ, Husband EM, Ryall RDH. The mesorectum in rectal cancer surgery – the clue to pelvic recurrence? *Br J Surg* 1982; 69: 613–616

30. Scott N, Jackson P, Al-Jaberi T *et al.* Total mesorectal excision and local recurrence: a study of tumour spread in the mesorectum distal to rectal cancer. *Br J Surg* 1995; 82: 1031–1033

31. Reynolds JV, Joyce WP, Dolan J *et al.* Pathological evidence in support of total mesorectal excision in the management of rectal cancer. *Br J Surg* 1996; 83: 1112–1115

32. MacFarlane JK, Ryall RDH, Heald RJ. Mesorectal excision for rectal cancer. *Lancet* 1993; 341: 457–460

33. Enker WE, Thaler HT, Cranor ML, Polyak T. Total mesorectal excision in the operative treatment of rectal cancer. *J Am Coll Surg* 1995; 181: 335–346

34. Heald RJ. Rectal cancer: the surgical options. *Eur J Cancer* 1995; 31A: 1189–1192

35. Arbman G, Nilsson E, Hallböök O, Sjödahl R. Local recurrence following total mesorectal excision for rectal cancer. *Br J Surg* 1996; 83: 375–379

36. Aitkin RJ. Mesorectal excision for rectal cancer. *Br J Surg* 1996; 83: 214–216

37. Hohenberger W, Hermanek P Jr, Hermanek P, Gall FP. Decision-making in curative rectum carcinoma surgery. *Onkologie* 1992; 15: 209–220

38. Hunter JA, Ryan JA Jr, Schultz P. En bloc resection of colon cancer adherent to other organs. *Am J Surg* 1987; 154: 67–71

39. Hermanek P Jr. Multiviszerale Resektion beim kolorektalen Karzinom. Erfahrungen der SGKRK-Studie. *Langenbecks Arch Chir* 1992; Suppl: 95–100

40. Hermanek P, Sobin LH. Colorectal carcinoma. In: Hermanek P, Gospodarowicz MK, Henson DE, Hutter RVP, Sobin LH (eds) *Prognostic factors in cancer.* Berlin: Springer, 1995, pp. 64–79

41. Hofstädter F, Knüchel R, Rüschoff J. Cell proliferation in oncology – Meeting report. *Virchoros Archiv* 1995; 427: 323–341

42. Lindemann F, Schlimock G, Dirschedel P, Witte J, Riethmüller G. Prognostic significance of micrometastatic tumour cells in bone marrow of colorectal cancer patients. *Lancet* 1992; 340: 685–689

43. Braun S, Pantel K. Immunodiagnosis and immunotherapy of isolated tumour cells disseminated to bone marrow of patients with colorectal cancer. *Tumori* 1995; 81, Suppl: 78–83

44. Murray GI, Duncan ME, O'Neil P *et al.* Matrix metalloproteinase-1 is associated with poor prognosis in colorectal cancer. *Nature Med* 1996; 2: 461–462

45. Streit M, Schmidt R, Hilgenfeld RU *et al.* Adhesion receptors in malignant transformation and dissemination of gastrointestinal tumours. *J Mol Med* 1996; 74: 253–268

46. Quirke P, Cawkwell L. Potential of molecular biology in preoperative evaluation. In: Soreide O, Norstein J (eds) *Rectal cancer surgery. Optimisation – Standardisation – Documentation.* Berlin: Springer, 1997, pp. 101–114

47. Rosai J. *Ackerman's surgical pathology*, 8th edn. St. Louis: Mosby, 1996

48. Hermanek P. Qualitätsmanagement bei Diagnose und Therapie kolorektaler Karzinome. *Leber Magen Darm* 1996; 26: 20–24

49. Heald RJ. The 'Holy Plane' of rectal surgery. *J R Soc Med* 1988; 81: 503–508

50. Quirke P. Limitations of existing systems of staging for rectal cancer: the forgotten margin. In: Soreide O, Norstein J (eds) *Rectal cancer surgery. Optimisation – Standardisation – Documentation.* Berlin: Springer, 1997, pp. 63–81

51. Hermanek P. Data collection aspects for the design of adjuvant treatment protocols in colorectal carcinoma. *Onkologie* 1991; 14: 491–497

52. Enker WE. Designing the optimal surgery for rectal carcinoma. *Cancer* 1996; 78: 1847–1850

Chapter 4

GENETICS OF COLORECTAL CANCER

S.R. Brown and D.T. Bishop

Introduction

Dramatic advances in our understanding of the pathogenesis of colorectal cancer have occurred over the past 20 years, and the fundamental concept leading to these advances has been the recognition of cancer as a genetic disorder.[1] This is manifested at two different levels – that of the person and that of the tumour. Different people have different levels of risk of bowel cancer because of their genetic make-up. A small proportion of bowel cancer cases (probably less than 5%) and an even smaller proportion of the general population have a hereditary syndrome such as familial adenomatous polyposis (FAP) or hereditary nonpolyposis colorectal cancer (HNPCC). Individual mutation carriers with either of these two syndromes have a particularly high risk of bowel cancer.

Outside these syndromes, perhaps 15–20% of patients report a family history of colorectal cancer.[2–4] These families are not consistent with either FAP or HNPCC but the extent of family aggregation supports a role for either more-common lower-risk inherited susceptibility, shared environmental exposures to risk factors, or interactions between the two. Because of the population prevalence of bowel cancer, within individual families the occurrence of multiple cancer cases by chance is usually not distinguishable from the presence of one or more causal agents.

At the level of the tumour, molecular genetic analysis shows that particular genetic changes in cells are associated with increasing degrees of pathology from normal cells initially to adenomas and eventually to invasive carcinomas. These genetic changes appear to be consistent across the hereditary syndromes, as well as in tumours in those without a recognized hereditary predisposition. This commonality reflects in part the central role of the adenoma in the oncogenesis of bowel cancer. In fact, this serves as a useful way of categorizing bowel cancer syndromes – those associated with adenomas and those not. Of particular note is the increased risk of bowel cancer in those with adenoma-associated syndromes.

This chapter outlines the salient features of hereditary colorectal cancer syndromes, followed by current theories on the genetics of familial colorectal cancer and finally discussing the genetic alterations arising in the colorectal carcinogenesis pathway. Although the focus of this chapter is on genetic factors, it is imperative to recognize the importance of non-genetic factors, primarily diet, in the aetiology of bowel cancer. The strongest support for the role of non-genetic factors comes from studies of migrants, especially those of migrants from low-risk areas (for instance, Japan) to high-risk areas (for instance, the United States) (reviewed in ref. 5). Such migrants incur an increase in risk, which is compatible only with a role of non-genetic factors. The challenge for the next decade is to bring together the interaction of a variety of exposures with genetic predisposition.

Hereditary syndromes predisposing to colorectal cancer

The hereditary syndromes and their respective genes that predispose to colorectal cancer are listed in Table 4.1

FAMILIAL ADENOMATOUS POLYPOSIS

Clinical features

Although easily recognized clinically, familial adenomatous polyposis coli (FAP) is, in fact, rare, accounting for less than 1% of all colorectal cancers[6] (see Figure 4.1 for an example of an FAP pedigree). The hallmark of the syndrome is the appearance of colonic polyps which are usually tubular, sessile, and distributed evenly throughout the large bowel.[7] Although the original definition of FAP described at least 100 of these polyps,[8] it has now become evident that, in certain affected individuals, there may be a great deal fewer. Clinically, FAP is first manifest during the second decade as the development of these colonic polyps which increase in size and number with time until, if untreated, malignant change occurs in the fourth or fifth decade.[9,10]

FAP does not only affect the large intestine and this becomes all too apparent in patients treated by total removal of colonic mucosa: These individuals tend to develop upper small bowel polyps in their fifties, and duodenal tumours are now a major cause of death in FAP.[10] Polyps have also been noted in the stomach, mainly the gastric body, and also the biliary tree.[7]

A variety of other extracolonic manifestations occur in FAP.[7] Tissues affected include

Table 4.1. *Hereditary syndromes and respective genes involved in predisposition to colorectal cancer*

Syndrome	Gene responsible	Chromosome location
Polyposis		
Familial adenomatous polyposis	*APC*	5q
Gardner's	*APC*	5q
'Non-polyposis'		
Hereditary non-polyposis colorectal cancer	*hMSH2, GTBP hMLH1, hPMS1, hPMS2*	2p, 3p, 2q, 7p
Hereditary flat adenoma	*APC*, ?mismatch repair genes	5q, (?2p, 2q, 3p, 7p)
Attenuated adenomatous polyposis coli	*APC* (5′ end)	5q
Muir–Torre	*hMSH2, hMLH1*, ? other mismatch repair genes	2p, 3p, (?2q, 7p)
Miscellaneous		
Cowden's	*PTEN*	10q
Peutz–Jeghers	?	?
Hereditary mixed polyposis		6q
Turcot's	*APC, hMLH1, hPMS2*	5q, 3p, 7p

liver (resulting in hepatoblastoma), bone (leading to osteomas, particularly in the mandible), teeth (resulting in various dental abnormalities) and fibrous tissue (resulting in desmoid tumours). Desmoid tumours are worthy of particular mention as they are common and tend to run in families.[11] They usually occur in retroperitoneal tissues or, less frequently, the abdominal wall, and are characteristically seen as a mass of firm, pale, rounded tissue expanding around and between other structures. They are difficult to treat surgically, being very vascular and tending to recur.

Other FAP manifestations affect the eye, skin and endocrine glands. In the eye, multiple patches of congenital hypertrophy of retinal pigment epithelium (CHRPE) is seen in the majority of affected individuals.[12] Skin lesions were first recognized by Gardner and consist of epidermal cysts of the skin, usually of the face and usually multiple.[13] Patients with these lesions are classified as having Gardner's syndrome. Finally there is a slight increase in the incidence of endocrine tumours in FAP, particularly papillary carcinoma of the thyroid.[14]

Genetic features

Genetically, FAP is inherited as an autosomal dominant trait,which means that only a single copy of the aberrant gene is necessary for clinical presentation and that a parent with FAP has a 50:50 chance of passing on the aberrant gene to each offspring (Figure 4.1). Initial genetic research into FAP concentrated on the search for the responsible gene(s) through linkage analysis, whereby the inheritance of DNA markers with precise chromosomal locations is tracked though a single family and correlated with the presence of affected and unaffected family members. A tight correlation implies that a gene for FAP lies close to that marker. The first breakthrough in the search came with the recognition of a patient with Gardner's syndrome and mental retardation, who was found to have a deletion of chromosome 5q.[15] Investigation of FAP families found linkage to this region[16] and subsequently the tumour-suppressor gene, termed *APC* (for 'adenomatous polyposis coli') was cloned and sequenced (Figure 4.2).[17,18]

APC consists of 15 exons, and codes for a

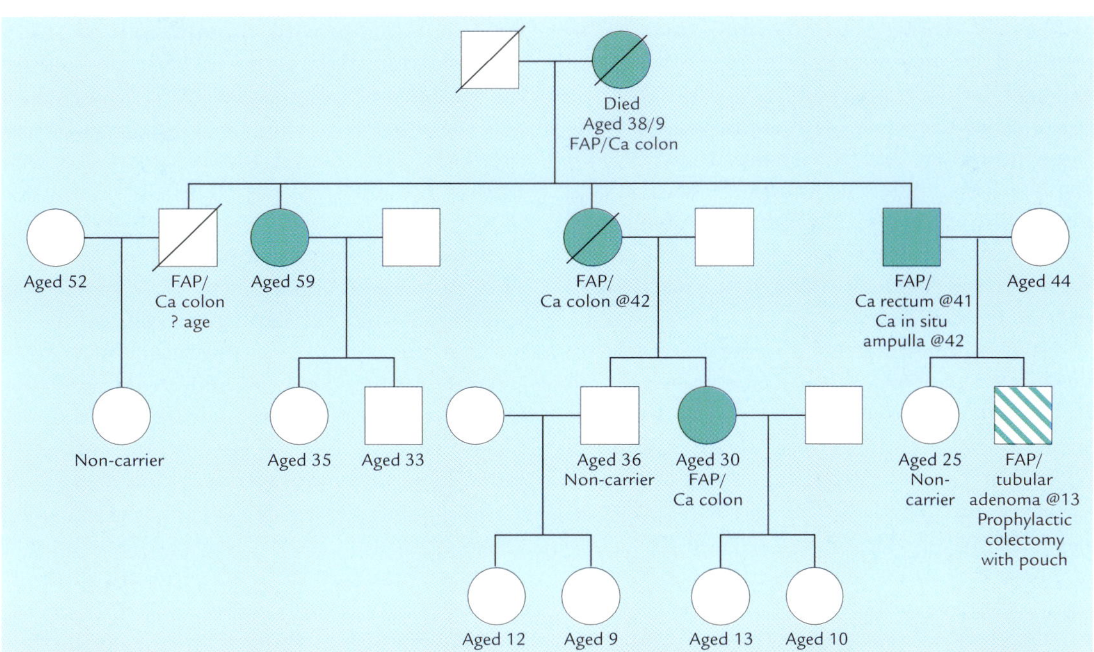

Figure 4.1. *Example of an FAP pedigree showing autosomal dominant inheritance. The pedigree also shows one affected member who developed carcinoma of the duodenal papilla after total colectomy for carcinoma. His son was found to be a carrier and underwent prophylactic colectomy before the age of 20.*

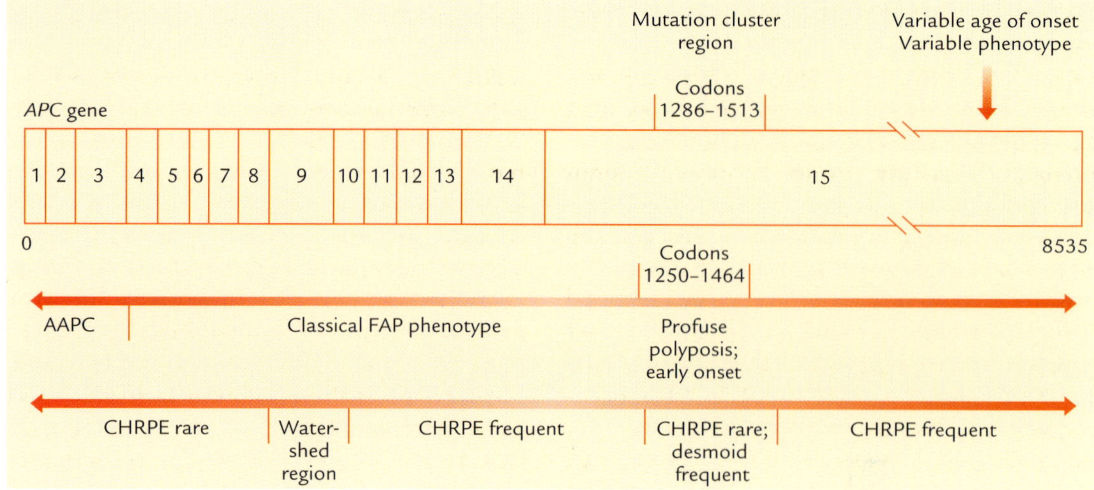

Figure 4.2. *Diagrammatic representation of the APC gene showing correlations with site of mutation and clinical manifestations. (Adapted from ref. 99.)*

protein product which appears to be involved in cell adhesion and possibly intercellular communication.[19] FAP is due to the disruption of the *APC* gene, which occurs most frequently by mutations that create premature stop codons and result in a truncated protein product.[20] Studies of these germline mutations have found that they are distributed throughout the gene but with the majority occurring in the first half of the gene.[20] Few families show the same mutation, and this makes screening for the particular germline mutation in a family time-consuming and laborious.[21] However, as most mutations result in a truncated protein product, functional assays have been developed that detect this defect.[21,22]

It is becoming clear from further work on germline mutations, that there is some correlation with the clinical features of FAP in a particular family and the site of the mutation within *APC*. For instance, the commonly observed feature of CHRPE tends to occur in patients with mutations in exons 9–15, whereas mutations which produce a smaller protein are associated with a normally pigmented retina.[23] Further work has found that mutations occurring in the regions between codons 1445 and 1578 in exon 15 do not induce the CHRPE phenotype.[24] However, these patients do develop desmoid lesions confirming the clinical observation of an inverse relationship between the presence of CHRPE lesions and desmoid tumours.[25]

The number of polyps also varies according to the site of mutation, with profuse polyposis occurring in individuals with mutations between codons 1250 and 1464 on exon 15, whereas patients with mutations near the 5′ end have minimal polyposis.[26] In these families the number of polyps may be as low as 5–10 and these patients have been classified as having AAPC (attenuated adenomatous polyposis coli).[27]

Screening and treatment for FAP

The purpose of clinical screening in patients with family histories of FAP is to allow prophylactic treatment against colorectal cancer to be offered. Regular sigmoidoscopy, commencing at puberty, has been the mainstay of diagnosis for individuals from FAP families for many years.[9] Each individual from an FAP family has a 50% chance of inheriting the defective gene. Blind screening of all family members will therefore result in 50% undergoing unnecessary screening. Prophylactic surgery is recommended for those who develop polyps and this takes the form of either a total colectomy and ileorectal anastomosis and regular rectal surveillance, or a proctocolectomy with either ileostomy or pouch formation in order to remove all colorectal mucosa. With the identification of a germline mutation, family members can be classified as either carriers or noncarriers, resulting in focused screening and more precise recommendations for prophylactic surgery. There also exists the possibility of prenatal screening using chorionic villous sampling.[28]

The observed genotype–phenotype correlations may have important clinical implications, although these remain to be tested. For instance, those with mutations that predict profuse polyposis may well benefit from a total proctocolectomy to remove all at-risk mucosa rather than a rectal-sparing operation with rectal surveillance. In addition, the presence or absence of CHRPE or desmoid tumours acts as a guide for any causative mutation search, thereby limiting the laborious and time-consuming analyses and providing more rapid results.

HEREDITARY NON-POLYPOSIS COLORECTAL CANCER

Clinical features

Hereditary nonpolyposis colorectal cancer (HNPCC) is characterized by early onset of predominantly right-sided colorectal cancer and the tendency to develop multiple primary cancers, both of the colorectum and extracolonic lesions.[29] As its name suggests, polyposis is not a prominent feature and, unlike FAP, there is no obvious clinical marker of disease. Diagnosis has therefore relied upon a family history of early-onset bowel cancer suggestive of an autosomal dominant pattern of inheritance (Figure 4.3). In an effort to standardize the mainly descriptive criteria for diagnosis of HNPCC and, in particular to facilitate the comparison of research studies, the Amsterdam criteria were put forward as the minimum factors required for a diagnosis (Table 4.2).[30] Using these criteria, the frequency of HNPCC has been estimated at between 1 and 5% of all colorectal cancers.[31,32]

Clinically, HNPCC often presents as cancer occurring before the age of 45–50 years. Large bowel tumours are the commonest malignancy and over 70% are proximal to the splenic flexure, compared with only 30% seen in sporadic cancers.[33] Multiple colorectal cancers are also common at presentation, with one study finding over 18% with synchronous lesions.[33] More significantly, the same study showed a 10-year cumulative incidence of metachronous cancer

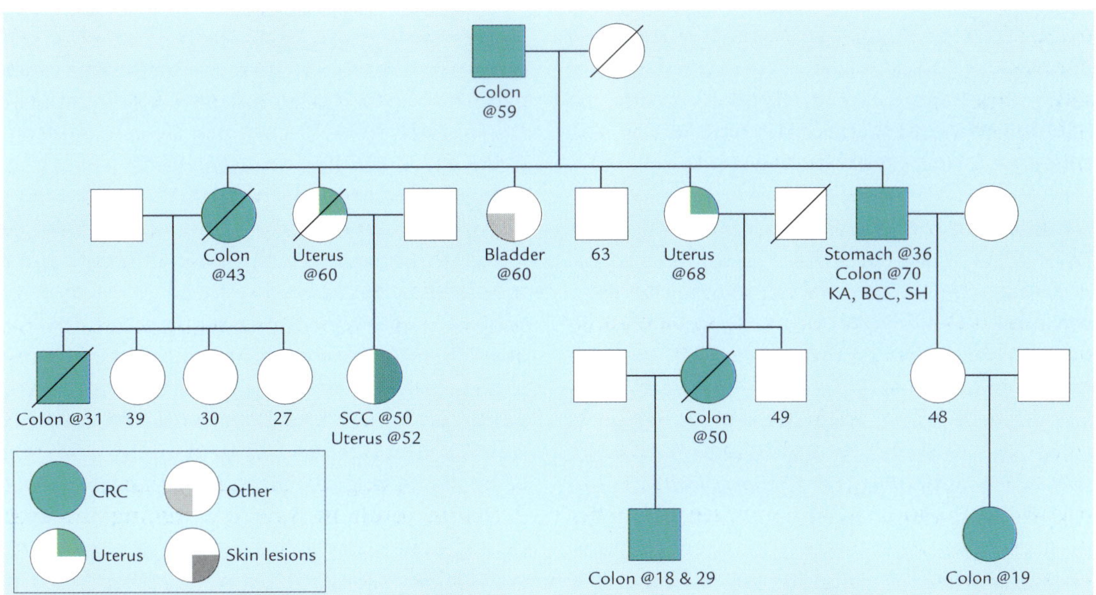

Figure 4.3. *Typical HNPCC pedigree showing autosomally dominantly inherited susceptibility to early-onset colorectal cancer (CRC) as well as a variety of extracolonic cancers. This pedigree also illustrates some skin features of Muir–Torre syndrome. A germline mutation exists in hMSH2 in this family.BCC, basal cell carcinoma; KA, Keratoacanthoma; SH, sebaceoushyperplasia; SCC, squamous cell carcinoma.*

Table 4.2. *Amsterdam criteria for diagnosis of HNPCC*

- Histologically verified colorectal cancer in three relatives, one a first-degree relative of the other two
- One colorectal cancer diagnosed before age 50 years
- Two or more generations affected
- Familial adenomatous polyposis excluded

of 40%. Adenomatous polyps do occur in HNPCC but not with the same frequency or extent as in FAP; it seems, instead, that those that do occur have an increased malignant potential.[34]

Extracolonic neoplasms occurring at increased frequency in HNPCC families compared with the general population include tumours from the stomach, small bowel, uterus, ovary and urinary tract.[35] In addition, there are two subsets of HNPCC deserving particular mention when considering extracolonic tumours. As with FAP and Gardner's syndrome, these have become known by alternative eponyms. Muir–Torre syndrome is one, characterized by the combination of multiple visceral adenocarcinomas with the development of cutaneous sebaceous tumours.[36] Turcot syndrome is another, characterized by the development of colon cancer in association with certain brain tumours, particularly glioblastoma multiforme.[37] Of interest is that some other families with Turcot's syndrome have been found to have *APC* mutations and therefore form part of the FAP syndrome.

Genetic features

HNPCC is again inherited as an autosomal dominant trait, so that the approach to identify the responsible gene(s) has followed the linkage analysis route described for FAP. After an extensive analysis of two large kindreds, linkage was first found with markers on chromosome 2p.[38] However, an important observation was made concurrently: the markers used in this study consisted of short repeat sequences of nucleotide bases known as microsatellites. These are found throughout the DNA genome and show great variability between individuals with this variability being inherited in a stable manner. Thus, analysis of microsatellite markers allows accurate tracing of inheritance and 'genetic fingerprinting'. In the initial study confirming linkage to 2p, it became evident that these DNA microsatellites were unstable in tumour material, so that tumours showed novel alleles not present in the germline.[39,40] Specifically, the length of these microsatellite sequences varied between tumour and normal tissue from the same individual (Figure 4.4). This variation occurred throughout the genome and suggested a widespread defect. Analysis of additional HNPCC patients showed this instability in over 85% of patients compared with only 10–15% of apparently sporadic cases,[40] and suggested a novel mechanism of oncogenesis in these tumours.

This phenomenon became known as microsatellite instability or replication error (RER) and had been noted in bacteria and yeast as a result of defects in DNA mismatch repair genes,[41,42] a system of genes responsible for repairing defects occurring in DNA during replication. Noting this observation, researchers designed primers to conserved regions of the bacterial mismatch repair gene *mutS*,[43] This resulted in rapid progress, and successful cloning of the candidate gene on chromosome 2p soon followed. The gene was subsequently named *hMSH2* to reflect its phylogeny. Further progress was also rapid, with the discovery of *hMLH1* localized on chromosome 3p, *hPMS1* on 2q and *hPMS2* on 7p, all located using the same technique.[44,45] More recently, a possible further mismatch repair gene has been discovered near and related to the *hMSH2* gene.[46] This has been called the *GTBP* (G–T binding protein) gene because of the protein's affinity for specific G–T nucleotide mismatches.

Germline mutations in a number of genes involved in the mismatch repair pathway have subsequently been discovered in HNPCC families. The majority occur in the *hMSH2* gene, accounting for of the order of one half of all families.[47] Unfortunately, no mutational 'hot spot' is observed and this, coupled with the large size of the mismatch repair genes (as well as the possibility of further, as yet undiscovered genes) makes design of a screening test difficult. In addition, studies so far have failed to show any correlation with phenotypic expression and site of mutation as seen in the *APC* gene.

The presumed mechanism of oncogenesis for HNPCC is that a mismatch repair gene

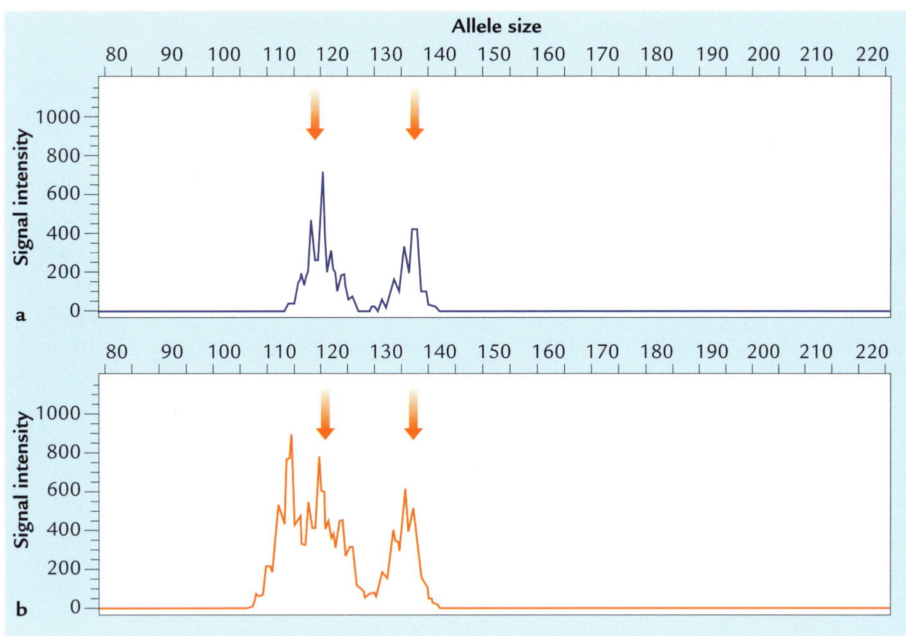

Figure 4.4. *Microsatellite instability. The figure represents a cross-sectional image of the electrophoresed product of a polymerase chain reaction. In (a), the two normal alleles can be seen (arrowed). These are represented in (b), the tumour tissue graph, but with an additional preceding novel allele.*

mutation results in inefficient repair of DNA errors that may arise during cell division and replication. Such errors occurring in microsatellites are, in general, insignificant, since such sequences occur in non-coding DNA. However, occasional mutations will affect crucial genes. For instance, tumours showing RER frequently have mutations in transforming growth factor beta (TGF-β) type II receptor gene, consistent with a mismatch repair defect.[48] Growing evidence supports the speculation that the mismatch repair genes act as tumour-suppressor genes, with inactivation of the wild-type (normal) allele being required for tumour development; analysis of tumours from HNPCC patients with a germline *hMLH1* mutation shows frequent loss of heterozygosity at this locus similar to the behaviour of other tumour-suppressor genes.[49]

Screening and treatment for HNPCC

Screening for HNPCC involves recognition of potential families. Any patient with early-onset, or multiple colorectal, or colorectal and extracolonic lesions should have a detailed family history taken. If there is a strong family history of colorectal cancer, and other hereditary syndromes such as FAP have been excluded clinically, the family is potentially HNPCC.

As HNPCC patients are most likely to develop colorectal cancer, colonoscopy is the screening method of choice.[29] This is started at an early age and, because of evidence of the aggressive nature of any polyps occurring, should be repeated at frequent intervals. The management of affected individuals with colorectal cancer should include a subtotal colectomy with rectal surveillance because of the risk of synchronous and metachronous lesions. In addition, a woman should be considered for prophylactic oöphorectomy and hysterectomy, particularly if she has completed her family or is postmenopausal.

Genetic testing may be considered for these potential HNPCC families. As with FAP, this will allow more accurate risk assessment for individuals in a family if a germline mutation is identified. In addition, the possibility of prophylactic subtotal colectomy may be considered for patients with the defect.

Screening of sites outside the colorectum is

more controversial with regard to potential benefit. Endometrial cancer is the second-commonest cancer found in HNPCC,[35] but an international study showed that this tumour is an infrequent cause of death.[50] Although several screening procedures, including transvaginal sonography and vacuum aspiration, have been advocated in HNPCC families for a long time, the value of such screening programmes is still unknown. Many, however, still recommend such screening, to include the ovaries, in well-defined large HNPCC families.[29,51] Urological cancers tend to be prevalent in certain families. If there is evidence of a preponderance in a particular pedigree then many recommend screening in the form of urinalysis, urine cytology and ultrasonography. In the same way some advocate upper gastrointestinal endoscopy for screening for gastric cancer in families with a preponderance of such cancers.[29] Although the relative risk of developing small bowel cancer is extremely high in HNPCC, the lifetime risk is low (about 4%) and therefore probably does not warrant screening.[51]

Other syndromes

Other hereditary syndromes are rare and, as a result, genetic analysis is difficult. Again, they are all autosomal dominantly inherited. Some of the relatively more common syndromes are discussed briefly.

Hereditary flat adenoma syndrome is so called because patients tend to develop multiple, slightly elevated, colonic mucosal lesions, occurring mainly in the proximal colon[52] and at an age of onset later than that seen in FAP and HNPCC. These lesions have a malignant potential. Linkage of some families with these clinicopathological features has been localized to the *APC* gene, whereas others have flat adenomas as a variant of HNPCC.[53]

Cowden's disease is characterized by hamartomatous lesions affecting multiple organ systems, but mainly predisposing to mucocutaneous and gastrointestinal polyps which are essentially harmless.[54] Recently the syndrome has been linked to 10q.[55] The importance of recognition of the syndrome is for differentiation from other more sinister syndromes.

Peutz–Jeghers syndrome results in gastrointestinal hamartomas associated with mucocutaneous macules.[56] Polyps occur mainly in the small intestine where they increase progressively in size. Although polyps are non-neoplastic there is evidence that they predispose to cancer in a few individuals.[57]

Juvenile polyps are again non-neoplastic hamartomas and are the most common type of polyp in children.[58] Some are associated with the presence of adenomatous epithelium[59] and are therefore associated with increased cancer risk. A possibly related disorder, termed hereditary mixed polyposis syndrome, has recently been found to be linked to chromosome 6q.[60]

Familial colorectal cancer

Mainly epidemiological studies provide the evidence that genetic factors may play a role in susceptibility to bowel cancer in families with no obvious hereditary disorder. Studies consistently show that relatives of colorectal cancer patients are at increased risk of developing colorectal cancer themselves when compared with a controlled group of relatives of patients with no cancer (reviewed in ref. 61). This risk is between two and three times the population risk for first-degree relatives and is increased further if more than one family member is affected, or if the affected proband is young[4] (see Figure 4.5). This increased risk has also been observed in close relatives of patients with adenomatous polyps, providing further evidence of the importance of adenoma in the development of colorectal cancer.[62]

A number of studies have attempted to identify specific genes involved in determining this increased susceptibility. The most obvious candidates would be mutations within genes already known to be involved in colorectal cancer, but perhaps resulting in more subtle and less destructive changes. For instance, an *APC* gene mutation may result in a protein product that is almost normal but is less effective. Alternatively, mutation of a modifier gene elsewhere in the genome may result in dysfunction of an otherwise normal protein product.

The phenomenon of microsatellite instability is a feature of most HNPCC tumours. However, 10–15% of apparently sporadic tumours also show instability.[40] It is conceivable that some of these cases may represent familial can-

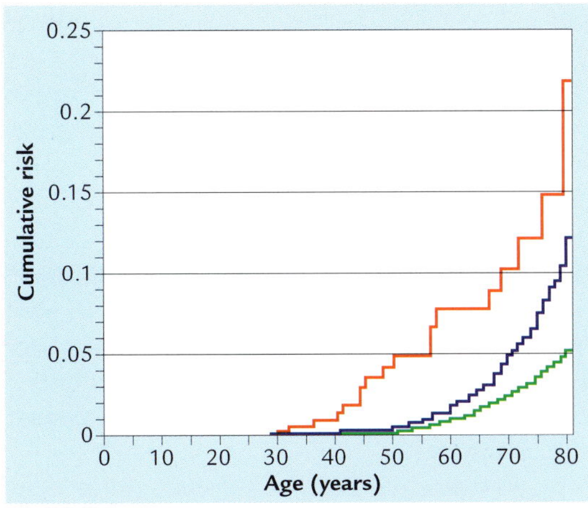

Figure 4.5. *Life-table analysis for relatives of three groups of probands. The lower plot shows the lifetime accumulative risk for colorectal cancer for the general population. Relatives of colorectal cancer patients are represented by the middle plot, while the relatives of early-onset colorectal cancer patients (<45 years at onset of cancer in this analysis) are at the most risk (upper plot).*

cer or, indeed, may even be unrecognized HNPCC. However, several studies disprove this theory, showing no correlation between incidence of instability and strength of family history, even in families with several affected individuals.[63,64] Furthermore, only about 10% of these sporadic RER-positive cases have been found to harbour a mutation on one of the known mismatch repair genes.[65] Thus simple mismatch repair gene mutations are also unlikely to explain the mechanism of oncogenesis in these families.

Environmental factors

Epidemiological studies not only provide evidence of genetic influence in colorectal cancer but also strongly suggests that environmental factors, particularly diet, have a significant role.[5] Observational studies on diet have consistently shown an inverse association between consumption of vegetables and fruit and colorectal cancer.[66] With regard to specific nutrients, the data are, so far, inconsistent, although there is a suggestion that fibre may have a protective effect whereas diets high in protein and fat are associated with increased cancer rates.[5]

Non-dietary environmental factors include cigarette smoking and the effect of chemopreventive agents such as aspirin. Studies of cigarette smoking have shown a weak positive association with colorectal cancer risk.[67] Most studies of aspirin have shown it to have a protective effect against colorectal cancer (reviewed in ref. 68). Associated with this, and operating in a similar way, is the effect of non-steroidal anti-inflammatory drugs such as sulindac, which has been shown to decrease the number of polyps in patients with FAP.[69]

How cells respond to this plethora of environmental agents is a predominant factor in cancer development, and cells and tissues are able to recruit a number of defence mechanisms.[70] It follows, therefore, that interindividual variation in the genes involved influences susceptibility.[71] Possible candidate genes include those coding for the drug or xenobiotic metabolizing enzymes (XMEs). These enzymes have important endogenous roles in intermediary metabolism but, in addition, they are active in the detoxification of a wide variety of xenobiotic compounds. On the basis of knowledge so far, the most important enzymes to consider are the cytochromes *p*450, the glutathione-*S*-transferases, and the *N*-acetyltransferases.

A number of cytochromes *p*450 involved in xenobiotic metabolism are now known to be variably expressed in some patients and in the general population.[72] In relation to colon cancer, CYP1A2 has been implicated in the activation of dietary heterocyclic amines into potent procarcinogens.[73] The glutathione-*S*-transferases are a family of enzymes which have a central role in carcinogen detoxification by conjugating glutathione with a wide variety of substrates, facilitating excretion in urine or bile.[74] As with the cytochromes *p*450, there is considerable variation of expression of these enzymes and associations have been observed with the glutathione-*S*-transferase M1 null genotype and increased colorectal cancer incidence.[74] The *N*-acetyltransferase (NAT) group of enzymes are responsible for acetylation of amino groups ubiquitous to animals. They also have the capacity to activate or detoxify carcinogens, mainly acrylamine carcinogens present in cooked protein.[75] Again, there is individuality in expression of these enzymes as a result of genetic variation: individuals can be classified as 'rapid' or 'slow' acetylators depending on a polymorphism determined by a single gene locus and inherited as an autosomal recessive trait.[76,77]

Further work has allowed isolation of the NAT protein products and indicate that two functional enzymes exist.[77] It is a genetic defect on the NAT-2 gene that results in the polymorphism. These NAT proteins appear to activate aromatic amines to reactive electrophiles and it is these compounds that have been implicated in the aetiology of colorectal cancer. 'Slow' acetylators are therefore afforded some degree of protection from these compounds, whereas there is a statistically significant increase in the incidence of colon cancer among fast acetylators, especially in those eating large quantities of meat.[78]

Genetic events in sporadic colorectal cancer

Histological and epidemiological observations indicate that most bowel cancers arise from pre-existing adenomas.[79] This adenoma--carcinoma sequence is related to a specific sequence of genetic mutations, even in apparently sporadic colorectal cancers. These sequential mutations result in both loss of tumour-suppressor genes and activation of oncogenes (Figure 4.6).[80,81]

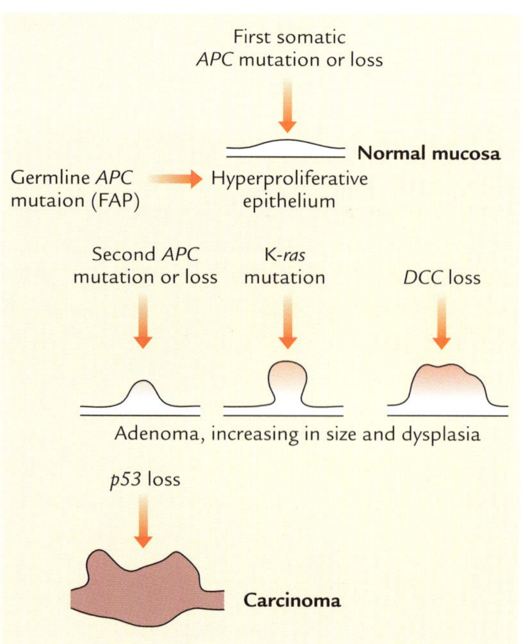

Figure 4.6. *Multistep process of carcinogenesis. (Adapted from ref. 99.)*

The first of these mutations occurs in the *APC* tumour-suppressor gene. As with FAP, mutations result in mucosal cell proliferation and the formation of polyps. These mutations are found in 60–80% of cases of sporadic colorectal cancer.[80]

As the adenomas progress and become more polypoid they accumulate mutations on the k-*ras* oncogene[81] found in approximately 50% of all sporadic colorectal cancers.[80] The family of ras proteins are involved in signal transduction and point mutations of k-*ras* result in protein overactivity and a growth advantage over non-mutated cells.

The next mutation is deletion of the *DCC* gene on chromosome 18q22. This codes for a cellular adhesion molecule.[83] The *DCC* gene is mutated in approximately 50% of late adenomas and 70% of sporadic colorectal carcinomas.[80] Mutation tends to occur before the development of invasion and *DCC* expression may therefore be important for maintaining cell adhesion.[84]

The final mutation in the sporadic colorectal cancer model occurs in the *p53* tumour-suppressor gene. Mutation within this gene is almost ubiquitous to human tumour development,[85] occurring in about 70% of sporadic colorectal cancers.[80] The function of the p53 protein is such that it has been described as 'the guardian of the genome'.[86] It serves to prevent a cell from undergoing further mitotic division should its DNA be damaged in any way. Mutation results in a failure of this mechanism, and DNA damage may then be copied and propagated to the progeny of the cell. Alternatively, it may mean that damaged cells persist in novel environments such as sites of metastasis.

Although this pathway explains oncogenesis in the majority of colorectal cancer, not all cancers arise in this way, as the highest frequency of mutation at any of these loci is about 70%. This suggests that other oncogenes or tumour suppressors – or, indeed, other pathways – may be involved in carcinogenesis and account for the remaining 30% or that other types of mutations remain to be found in the already identified genes.

There is evidence for other involved genes with potential tumour suppressor genes discovered on chromosomes 1p, 7q, 8p, 14q, 17q and 22q.[87–92] Alternatively, tumorigenesis may occur by alterations in genes that result in modification of known tumour suppressors. This modifier effect has been mentioned earlier.

Apart from additional oncogenes/tumour-suppressor genes and possible modifier genes, there is a possibility of an alternative pathway to explain oncogenesis. The observation of replication errors in 10–15% of sporadic colorectal cancers[40] suggests a possible mechanism of defective mismatch repair for this alternative pathway. There is evidence for this alternative pathway, but there may be considerable overlap with the accepted model of carcinogenesis. Thus, loss of mismatch repair may be just one event resulting in acceleration of tumorigenesis down the same cancer pathway. However, in some sporadic RER-positive tumours, mismatch repair deficiency may allow mutation of a different growth-regulating gene, promoting a completely alternative pathway. A possible candidate gene is the type II TGF-β,[93] found to be mutated in over 90% of such patients.[48]

Final thoughts

Bowel cancer is an important model for the genetic analysis of common cancer. The investigation of the inherited syndromes together with the elucidation of the genetic changes in the adenoma–carcinoma sequence and, specifically, the finding of consistency between the two lines of enquiry compellingly show the power of modern genetic analysis. Currently, however, this knowledge has not translated into any benefit for the patient with bowel cancer. The initial benefit of such developments will be for members of families with either FAP or HNPCC. However, there are opportunities for a much broader impact into common (or 'sporadic') bowel cancer through not only improved diagnosis and screening but also more effective chemoprevention and therapy.

Within families with HNPCC with a recognized mutation, DNA testing allows the identification of those family members predisposed to bowel cancer. This, in turn, allows more focused screening. In some FAP families, DNA testing will add reassurance to those individuals who are polyp free and past the age of usual presentation, that intensive screening is not necessary.

Other benefits of the knowledge of the precise genetic events will probably arise most immediately through improvements in screening and potentially customizing treatment. One such example is provided by Vogelstein and colleagues,[94] who looked for cells with k-*ras* mutations in the stools of patients with bowel cancer and showed that they could detect such cells, which were thought to have been sloughed off from the tumour. If this is, in fact, the case then this would provide a screening test that is both more sensitive than faecal occult blood testing and less invasive than endoscopy. This study showed that such cells were detectable from cancer patients with known mutations in k-*ras*; if this approach is to work then such cells must be detectable from the late-adenoma–early-carcinoma stages when the precise mutations are not known *a priori*.

A second analysis which merits discussion is an examination by Nakamura and colleagues[95] of lymph nodes from patients with bowel cancer. Although pathological analysis of lymph nodes is standard for the detection of widespread disease, the analysis of DNA from cells contained in the lymph nodes rather than simple histological examination provided greater predictive knowledge of the state of the individual's disease.

A final example of potential benefits from developments in this field is the observation that RER positive tumours (characteristic of HNPCC but not confined to this syndrome) respond poorly to alkylating anticancer agents.[96] Assessing RER status before therapy may be a useful way of predicting response, while strategies aimed at restoring mismatch repair may in the future broaden chemotherapeutic options.

One of the major challenges for epidemiologists is to reconcile the genetic and epidemiological information. Specifically, the compelling evidence that diet has a role in determining disease incidence must relate to the disease progression model described above. The failure to identify DNA mutations in bowel tumours which are characteristic of specific exposures has led some authors[97] to conclude that sufficient mutations arise in the bowel as a matter of course and that the role of diet is to impact cell replication rates. Such hypotheses require further investigation especially if appropriate dietary modifications could eventually be formulated for either the general population or a subset of predisposed individuals. Finally, the similarity in genetic changes between those with an hereditary syndrome involving adenomas (FAP and HNPCC) and 'sporadic' bowel cancer suggests that individuals with these syndromes might aid the investigation of dietary and other non-genetic exposures. One such study, the CAPP study, is aimed at investigating dietary supplementation of resistant starch and aspirin in those predisposed individuals.[98]

References

1. Bodmer W. Cancer genetics. *Br Med Bull* 1994; 50: 517–526
2. Ponz de Leon M, Sassatelli R, Sacchetti C *et al.* Familial aggregation of tumours in the three-year experience of a population based colorectal cancer registry. *Cancer Res* 1989; 49: 4344–4348
3. Stephenson B, Finan P, Gascoyne J *et al.* Frequency of familial colorectal cancer. *Br J Surg* 1991; 78: 1162–1166
4. St John DJB, McDermott FT, Hopper JL *et al.* Cancer risk in relatives of patients with common colorectal cancer. *Ann Intern Med* 1993; 118: 785–790
5. Potter JD, Slattery ML, Bostick RM, Gatspur SM. Colon cancer: a review of the epidemiology. *Epidemio Rev* 1993; 15: 499–545
6. Jarvinen HJ. Epidemiology of familial adenomatous polyposis in Finland: impact of family screening on the colorectal cancer rate and survival. *Gut* 1992; 33: 357–360
7. Talbot I. Pathology of FAP. In: Phillips R, Spigelman A, Thomson J (eds) *Familial Adenomatous Polyposis and Other Polyposis Syndromes,* 1st edn. London: Edward Arnold, 1994, pp. 15–25
8. Bussey HJR. *Familial Polyposis Coli.* Baltimore: Johns Hopkins University Press, 1975
9. Northover J, Murday VA. Familial colorectal cancer and familial adenomatous polyposis. *Baillieres Clin Gastroenterol* 1989; 3: 593–613
10. Spigelman AD, Williams CB, Talbot IC *et al.* Upper gastrointestinal cancer in patients with familial adenomatous polyposis. *Lancet* 1989; ii: 783–785
11. Klemmer S, Pascoe L, DeCosse J. Occurrence of desmoids in patients with familial adenomatous polyposis of the colon. *Am J Med Genet* 1987; 28: 385–392
12. Chapman PD, Church W, Burn J, Gunn A. The detection of congenital hypertrophy of retinal pigment epithelium (CHRPE) by indirect ophthalmoscopy: a reliable clinical feature of familial adenomatous polyposis. *Br Med J* 1989; 298: 353–354
13. Gardner EJ, Richards RC. Multiple cutaneous lesions occurring simultaneously with hereditary polyposis and osteomatosis. *Am J Hum Genet* 1953; 5: 139–148
14. Plail RO, Bussey HJR, Glazer G, Thomson JPS. Adenomatous polyposis: an association with carcinoma of the thyroid. *Br J Surg* 1987; 74: 377–380.
15. Herrera L, Kakati S, Gibas L *et al.* Brief clinical report: Gardner syndrome in a man with an interstitial deletion of 5q. *Am J Med Genet* 1986; 25: 473–476
16. Bodmer WF, Bailey CJ, Bodmer J *et al.* Localisation of the gene for familial adenomatous polyposis on chromosome 5. *Nature* 1987; 328: 614–616
17. Groden J, Thliveris A, Samowitz W *et al.* Identification and characterization of the familial adenomatous polyposis coli gene. *Cell* 1991; 66: 589–600
18. Kinzler KW, Nilbert MC, Su L-K *et al.* Identification of FAP locus genes from chromosome 5q21. *Science* 1991; 253: 661–665.

19. Su L-K, Vogelstein B, Kinzler KW. Association of the *APC* tumor suppressor protein with catenins. *Science* 1993; 262: 1734–1737

20. Miyoshi Y, Ando H, Nagase H *et al.* Germ-line mutations of the *APC* gene in 53 familial adenomatous polyposis patients. *Proc Natl Acad Sci USA* 1992; 89: 4452–4456

21. Powell SM, Petersen GM, Krush AJ *et al.* Molecular diagnosis of familial adenomatous polyposis. *N Eng J Med* 1993; 329: 1982–1987

22. Van der Luijt RB, Meera Khan P, Vasen H *et al.* Rapid detection of translation-terminating mutations at the adenomatous polyposis coli (*APC*) gene by direct protein truncation test. *Genomics* 1994; 20: 1–4

23. Oschwang S, Tiret A, Laurent-Puig P *et al.* Restriction of ocular fundus lesions to a specific group of *APC* mutations in adenomatous polyposis coli patients. *Cell* 1993; 75: 959–967

24. Caspari R, Olschwang S, Friedl W *et al.* Familial adenomatous polyposis: desmoid tumours and lack of ophthalmic lesions (CHRPE) associated with *APC* mutations beyond codon 1444. *Hum Mol Genet* 1995; 4: 337–340.

25. Hodgson SV, Bishop DT, Jay B. Genetic heterogeneity of congenital hypertrophy of the retinal pigment epithelium (CHRPE) in families with familial adenomatous polyposis. *J Med Genet* 1994; 31: 55–58

26. Nagase H, Miyoshi Y, Horii A *et al.* Correlation between the location of germline mutations in the *APC* gene and the number of colorectal polyps in familial adenomatous polyposis patients. *Cancer Res* 1992; 52: 4055–4057

27. Spirio L, Otterud B, Stauffer D *et al.* Linkage of a variant or attenuated form of adenomatous polyposis coli to the adenomatous polyposis coli (*APC*) locus. *Am J Hum Genet* 1992; 51: 92–100

28. Hodgson SV, Spigelman AD. Genetics of FAP. In: Phillips R, Spigelman A, Thomson J (eds) *Familial Adenomatous Polyposis and Other Polyposis Syndromes*, 1st edn. London: Edward Arnold, 1994, pp. 26–35

29. Lynch H, Smyrk T. Hereditary nonpolyposis colorectal cancer. An updated review. *Cancer* 1996; 78: 1149–1167

30. Vasen HFA, Mecklin J-P, Meerakhan P, Lynch HT. The international collaborative group on hereditary nonpolyposis colorectal cancer. *Dis Colon Rectum* 1991; 34: 424–425

31. Ponz de Leon M. Prevalence of hereditary nonpolyposis colorectal cancer (HNPCC). *Ann Med* 1994; 26: 209–214

32. Mecklin J, Jarvinen HJ, Hakkiluoto A *et al.* Frequency of hereditary nonpolyposis colorectal cancer: a prospective multicentre study in Finland. *Dis Colon Rectum* 1995; 38: 588–593

33. Lynch HT, Watson P, Kriegler M *et al.* Differential diagnosis of hereditary nonpolyposis colorectal cancer (Lynch syndrome I and Lynch syndrome II). *Dis Colon Rectum* 1988; 31: 372–377

34. Sankila R, Aaltonen LA, Jarvinen HJ, Mecklin J. Better survival rates in patients with MLH 1 associated hereditary colorectal cancer. *Gastroenterology* 1996; 110: 682–687

35. Watson P, Lynch HT. Extracolonic cancer in hereditary nonpolyposis colorectal cancer. *Cancer* 1993; 71: 677–685

36. Cohen PR, Kohn SR, Kurzrock R. Association of sebaceous gland tumours and internal malignancy: the Muir–Torre syndrome. *Am J Med* 1991; 90: 606–613

37. Hamilton S, Liu B, Parsons R *et al.* The molecular basis of Turcot's syndrome. *N Eng J Med* 1995; 332: 839–847

38. Peltomaki P, Aaltonen LA, Sistonen P *et al.* Genetic mapping of a locus predisposing to human colorectal cancer. *Science* 1993; 260: 810–812

39. Aaltonen LA, Peltomaki P, Leach FS *et al.* Clues to the pathogenesis of familial colorectal cancer. *Science* 1993; 260: 812–816

40. Aaltonen LA, Peltomaki P, Mecklin J-P *et al.* Replication errors in benign and malignant tumours from hereditary nonpolyposis colorectal cancer patients. *Cancer Res* 1994; 54: 1645–1648

41. Cox E. Bacterial mutator genes and the control of spontaneous mutation. *Ann Rev Genet* 1976; 10: 135–136

42. Strand M, Prolla TA, Liskay RM, Petes TD. Destabilization of tracts of simple repetitive DNA in yeast by mutations affecting DNA mismatch repair. *Nature* 1993; 365: 274–276

43. Fishel R, Lescoe MK, Rao MRS *et al.* The human mutator gene homolog *MSH2* and its association with hereditary nonpolyposis colon cancer. *Cell* 1993; 75: 1027–1038

44. Bronner CE, Baker SM, Morrison PT *et al.* Mutation in the DNA mismatch repair gene homologue *hMLH1* is associated with hereditary non-polyposis colon cancer. *Nature* 1994; 368: 258–261

45. Nicolaides NC, Papadopoulos N, Liu B *et al.* Mutations of two PMS homologues in hereditary nonpolyposis colon cancer. *Nature* 1994; 371: 75–80

46. Palumbo F, Gallinori P, Iaccarino I *et al. GTBP* a 160-kilodalton protein essential for mismatch-binding activity in human cells. *Science* 1995; 268: 1912–1914

47. Liu B, Parsons RE, Hamilton SR *et al. hMSH2* mutations in hereditary nonpolyposis colorectal cancer kindreds. *Cancer Res* 1994; 54: 4590–4594

48. Parsons R, Myeroff LL, Liu B *et al.* Microsatellite instability and mutations of the transforming growth factor beta type II receptor in colorectal cancer. *Cancer Res* 1995; 55: 5548–5550

49. Hemminki A, Peltomaki P, Mecklin J-P *et al.* Loss of the wild type MLH1 gene is a feature of hereditary nonpolyposis colorectal cancer. *Nature Genet* 1994; 8: 405–410

50. Vasen HFA, Mecklin J-P Meera Khan P, Lynch HT. Screening for hereditary colorectal cancer. *Lancet* 1994; 344: 877

51. Vasen HFA, Wijnen JT, Menko FH *et al.* Cancer risk in families with hereditary nonpolyposis colorectal cancer diagnosed by mutation analysis. *Gastroenterology* 1996; 110: 1020–1027

52. Lynch H, Smyrk T, Watson P *et al.* Hereditary flat adenoma syndrome: a variant of familial adenomatous polyposis? *Dis Colon Rectum* 1992; 35: 411–421

53. Wanabe T, Muto T, Sawada T, Miyaki M. Flat adenoma as a precursor of colorectal carcinoma in hereditary nonpolyposis colorectal cancer. *Cancer* 1996; 77: 627–634

54. Galt S, Cricklow R. Cowden disease. In: Watne AL (ed) *Problems in General Surgery: Vol. 10. Colonic Polyposis*, Philadelphia: Lippincott,1993, pp. 695–698

55. Nelen MR, Padberg GW, Peeters EA *et al.* Localisation of the gene for Cowden disease to chromosome 10q22–23. *Nature Genet* 1996; 13: 114–116

56. Jeghers H, McKusick VA, Katz KH. Generalized intestinal polyposis and melanin spots of the oral mucosa, lips and digits. *N Eng Med* 1949; 241: 993–1005

57. Perzin K, Bridge M. Adenomatous and carcinomatous changes in hamartomatous polyps of the small intestine (Peutz–Jeghers syndrome): report of a case and review of the literature. *Cancer* 1982; 49: 971

58. Herrera L, Iwama T, Davidson B, Goedde T. Endoscopic diagnosis and treatment of gastric, duodenal and small intestinal polyps. In: Watne AL (ed) *Problems in General Surgery: Vol. 10. Colonic Polyposis*. Philadelphia: Lippincott, 1993, pp. 731–741

59. Rozen P, Baratz M. Familial juvenile colonic polyposis with associated colon cancer. *Cancer* 1982; 49: 1500–1503

60. Thomas H, Whitelaw S, Cotrell S *et al.* Genetic mapping of the hereditary mixed polyposis syndrome to chromosome 6q. *Am J Hum Genet* 1996; 58: 770–776

61. Bishop DT, Thomas HJW. The genetics of colorectal cancer. *Cancer Surv* 1990; 9: 585–604

62. Winawer S, Zauber A, Gerdes H *et al.* Risk of colorectal cancer in the families of patients with adenomatous polyps. *N Eng J Med* 1996; 334: 82–87

63. Lothe RA, Peltomaki P, Meking GI *et al.* Genomic instability in colorectal cancer: relationship to clinicopathological variables and family history. *Cancer Res* 1993; 53: 5849–5852

64. Samowitz W, Slattery M, Kerber R. Microsatellite instability in human colonic cancer is not a useful indicator of familial colorectal cancer. *Gastroenterology* 1995; 109: 1765–1771

65. Liu B, Nicolaides N, Markowitz S *et al.* Mismatch repair gene defects in sporadic colorectal cancers with microsatellite instability. *Nature Genet* 1995; 9: 48–55

66. Howe G, Benito E, Castelleto R *et al.* Dietary intake of fibre and decreased risk of cancers of the colon and rectum: evidence from the combined analysis of thirteen control studies. *J Nat Cancer Inst* 1992; 84: 1887–1896.

67. Heineman E, Zahm S, McLaughlin J *et al.* Increased risk of colorectal cancer among smokers: results of a 26 year follow-up of US veterans and a review. *Int J Cancer* 1995; 59: 728–738

68. Berkel HJ, Holcombe RF, Middlebrooks M, Kannan K. Nonsteroidal antiinflammatory drugs and colorectal cancer. *Epidemiol Rev* 1996; 18: 205–217

69. Giardiello F, Hamilton S, Krush A *et al.* Treatment of colonic and rectal adenomas with Sundilac in Familial Adenomatous Polyposis. *N Engl J Med* 1993; 328: 1313–1316.

70. Doll R, Peto R. Causes of Cancer. Oxford: Oxford University Press, 1981

71. Weinberg R. *Oncogenes and the Molecular Origins of Cancer.* Cold Spring Harbor: Cold Spring Harbor Press, 1990

72. Smith C, Smith G, Wolf CR *et al.* Genetic polymorphisms in xenobiotic metabolism. *Eur J Cancer* 1994; 30A: 1921–1934

73. Boobis A, Lynch A, Murray S *et al.* CYP1A2 catalysed conversion of dietary heterocyclic amines to their proximate carcinogens is their major route of metabolism in humans. *Cancer Res* 1994; 54: 89–94

74. Zhong S, Wyllie AH, Barnes D *et al.* Relationship between the GSTM1 genetic polymorphism and susceptibility to bladder, breast and colon cancer. *Carcinogenesis* 1993; 14: 1821–1824

75. Grant D. Molecular genetics of the N-acetyl transferases. *Pharmacogenetics* 1993; 3: 45–50

76. Cartwright R. Historical and modern epidemiological studies in populations exposed to N-substituted aryl compounds. *Environ Health Perspect* 1983; 49: 13–19

77. Grant D, Lottspiech F, Meyer UA. Evidence for two closely related isoenzymes of arylamine N-acetyltransferase in human liver. *FEBS Lett* 1989; 244: 203–207

78. Roberts-Thompson, Ryan P, Khoo KK *et al.* Diet, acetylator phenotype and risk of colorectal neoplasia. *Lancet* 1996; 347: 1372–1374

79. Morson BC. The evolution of colorectal carcinoma. *Clin Radiol* 1984; 35: 425–431

80. Vogelstein B, Fearon ER, Hamilton SR *et al.* Genetic alterations during colorectal-tumor development. *N Engl J Med* 1988; 319: 525–532

81. Fearon ER, Vogelstein B. A genetic model for colorectal tumorigenesis. *Cell* 1990; 61: 759–767

82. Powell SM, Zilz N, Beazer-Barclay Y *et al.* *APC* mutations occur early during colorectal tumorigenesis. *Nature* 1992; 359: 235–237

83. Hedrick L, Cho K, Fearon E, Wu T *et al.* The DCC gene product in cellular differentiation and colorectal tumorigenesis. *Genes Dev* 1994; 8: 1174–1183

84. Stallmach A, von-Lampe B, Orzechowski HD *et al.* Increased fibronectin- receptor expression in colon carcinoma derived HT 29 cells decreases tumorigenicity in nude mice. *Gastroenterology* 1994; 106: 19–27

85. Greenblatt M, Bennett W, Hollstein M, Harris C. Mutations in the p53 tumour suppressor gene: clues to cancer aetiology and molecular pathogenesis. *Cancer Res* 1994; 54: 4855–4878

86. Lane D. *p53*, guardian of the genome. *Nature* 1992; 358: 15–16

87. Bravard A, Luccioni C, Muleris M, Lefrancois DBD. Relationships between UMPK and PGD activities and deletions of chromosome 1p in colorectal cancers. *Cancer Genet Cytogenet* 1991; 56: 45–56

88. Atkin N, Baker M. Chromosome 7q deletions: observations on 13 malignant tumours. *Cancer Genet Cytogenet* 1993; 67: 123–125

89. Keleman PR, Yaremko ML, Kim AH *et al.* Loss of heterozygosity in 8p is associated with microinvasion in colorectal carcinoma. *Genes Chromosomes Cancer* 1994; 11: 195–198

90. Young J, Leggett B, Ward M *et al.* Frequent loss of heterozygosity on chromosome 14 occurs in advanced colorectal carcinomas. *Oncogene* 1993; 8: 671–675

91. Leggett B, Young J, Buttenshaw R *et al.* Colorectal carcinomas show frequent allelic loss on the long arm of chromosome 17 with evidence for a specific target region. *Br J Cancer* 1995; 71: 1070–1073

92. Yana I, Kurahashi H, Nakamori S *et al.* Frequent loss of heterozygosity at telomeric loci on 22q in sporadic colorectal cancers. *Int J Cancer* 1995; 60: 174–177

93. Markowitz S, Wong J, Myeroff L *et al.* Inactivation of the type II TGF-beta receptor in colon cancer cells with microsatellite instability. *Science* 1995; 268: 1336–1338

94. Sidransky D, Tokino T, Hamilton SR *et al.* Identification of ras oncogene mutations in the stool of patients with curable colorectal tumours. *Science* 1995; 256: 102–105

95. Hayashi N, Ito I, Kato Y *et al.* Genetic diagnosis of lymph node metastases in colorectal cancer. *Lancet* 1995; 345: 1257–1259

96. Branch P, Aquina G, Bignami M, Karran P. Defective mismatch binding and a mutator phenotype in cells tolerant to DNA damage. *Nature* 1993; 362B: 652–654

97. Bodmer W, Bishop T, Karran P. Genetic steps in colorectal cancer. *Nature Genet* 1994; 6, 217–219

98. Burn J, Chapman PD, Mathers J *et al.* The protocol for a European double- blind trial of aspirin and resistant starch in familial adenomatous polyposis: the CAPP study. *Eur J Cancer A Gen Topics* 1995; 31/7–8: 1385–1386

99. Bishop DT, Hall NR. The genetics of colorectal cancer. *Eur J Cancer* 1994; 30A: 1946–1956

Chapter 5

SCREENING FOR COLORECTAL CANCER

J. Cuzick

Introduction

The goal of screening is to reduce disease morbidity and mortality by earlier detection of cancer or identification of high-risk precancerous lesions. In many cases the latter is a more effective strategy, since cure rates approach 100% and screening intervals can be longer.

It is crucial not only that screening tests identify lesions at an early stage but that this extra 'lead time' is enough to ensure that the natural history can be favourably altered. Clearly, there is little point in identifying cancer at an earlier stage if the natural history cannot be affected. In fact, such an outcome would be detrimental since individuals with cancer would merely be informed of an inexorable process without any added hope of mitigation.

Thus, it is clear that the basic requirement of screening is to have an effective test capable of detecting abnormalities at a time when it is possible to influence the course of disease favourably. Of almost equal importance is to achieve a high compliance in the target population. Several factors are relevant for accomplishing this. First, the test must be acceptable to the population towards which it is targeted. This involves consideration of ease of use, lack of discomfort, social acceptability, and (to some extent) cost. The other key feature is proper organization of the screening programme so that the population is accurately informed about the importance of being screened, individuals are actively invited to participate by a respected individual (GP), with adequate flexibility to be convenient, and results are made available so that appropriate follow-up and reassurance takes place.

EVALUATION OF SCREENING

Screening can be evaluated at a number of different levels, and a number of potential problems exist which can lead to erroneous conclusions.

Ultimately, one is looking for a health gain, which for cancer usually is reduced mortality. However, it is useful to look at a number of short-term indicators as well. Generally speaking, these short-term indicators are necessary requirements to achieve longer-term mortality gains, but satisfying them does not guarantee that the longer-term goals will also be achieved.

Screening results can often be summarized as a 2 × 2 table and tests can be evaluated in at least two different ways (Figure 5.1). A major difficulty is deciding what constitutes the disease state, especially when precursor lesions are being screened for. Some lesions are clearly more important to detect than others. One approach is in terms of sensitivity and specificity. Sensitivity is the percentage of individuals with disease who are positive on the test. Since additional work-up is not done on individuals with negative tests, 'false negative' tests, are not discovered immediately, and interval cancers occurring within 6 or 12 months are often used to determine sensitivity. An alternative approach is to focus on the ratio of the interval cancer rate in the immediate 1–2 year period after screening divided by the expected number of cancer rate in the absence of screening.[1] Specificity is the percentage of individuals without disease who are test negative, and is more readily determined.

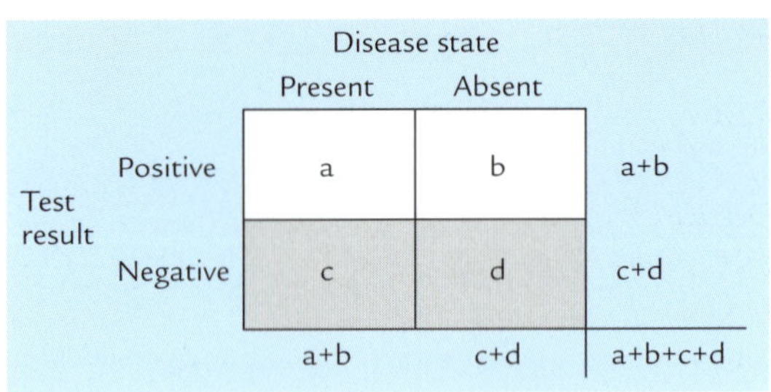

Figure 5.1. Parameters used for evaluating a screening test. The values of a, b, c and d are the numbers of screened individuals in the given category. Sensitivity is estimated by a/(a+c); false-negative rate by c/(a+c); specificity by d/(b+d); false-positive rate by b/(b+d); positive predictive value by a/(a+b); negative predictive value by d/(c+d); detection rate by a/(a+b+c+d), and odds ratio by ad/bc.

Another method of evaluation is referred to the other marginal total in Figure 5.1. Positive predictive value (PPV) is the percentage of test positives who have disease, whereas negative predictive value (NPV) refers to the proportion of test-negative individuals who are disease free. PPVs are readily computed, but NPVs have the same problem as sensitivities in that 'false negatives' can be difficult to determine.

The ultimate goal of cancer screening is to reduce mortality. Simple approaches, such as comparing the stage distribution or survival times of screen-detected cancers with symptomatic cancers are subject to serious biases and are not valid. The two most important biases are lead-time bias – in which screening detects cancers at an earlier stage, so that survival will be longer, even if the natural history is unaffected – and length bias – in which slower-growing cancers are more likely to be detected at screening and faster-growing cancer to present symptomatically between screening intervals. The only reliable way to determine mortality benefits from screening is to follow up cohorts of screened and unscreened populations. Ideally, these should be randomized, but non-randomized cohorts and case–control studies can give useful information, although they are also subject to some biases.[2]

Ultimately, a screening programme needs to be evaluated, not only in terms of benefits but also of costs, by some form of cost–benefit ratio. Once valid data exist on the benefits, this can usually be done by modelling exercises, but the availability of valid 'benefit' data is paramount if these exercises are to be useful.

Screening tests

DIGITAL RECTAL EXAMINATION

Digital palpation of the rectum is part of a routine physical examination in some parts of the world. It is more commonly used in men, where the prostate can also be palpated. The sensitivity of this test is severely limited by the short region (10 cm of distal rectum) that can be investigated, and by the crudeness of the method.

GUAIAC-BASED OCCULT BLOOD TESTS

The concept of occult blood detection by chemical means is usually credited to Van Dean, who in 1864 used gum guaiac. Benzidine and orthotoluidines have also been evaluated, but have proved too sensitive for clinical use, since there is a normal amount of gastrointestinal blood loss. In 1901, Boas first emphasized the value of occult blood testing for the detection of bowel cancer, but little interest was shown in this until the mid-1960s (see refs 3–5 for historical reviews). Greegor[6] developed guaiac-impregnated slides for home use and reported the detection of several asymptomatic cases of colorectal cancer by this means. This was the basis of the Hemoccult test, which has been widely marketed and evaluated since the early 1970s. Modification took place around 1977, which led to the current Hemoccult II test. This test consists of three cards, each of which contains two windows of guaiac-impregnated paper. For three successive bowel movements a small amount of stool is applied to each of the two windows on a single slide, using a supplied wooden applicator. It is usually recommended that the test be performed annually or biennially, beginning around age 50.

This test depends upon the oxidation of a phenolic compound to a quinone structure, resulting in a colour change. Hydrogen peroxide facilitates the oxidation process, which is catalysed by a number of naturally occurring peroxidases and catalyses, including haemoglobin. For the Hemoccult test, gum guaiac is impregnated in a test paper and hydrogen peroxide is provided in a developing solution: the resultant phenolic oxidation in the presence of blood yields a blue colour. Guaiac tests detect haem in any form, provided that the iron has not been removed from the porphyrin ring and will react to any peroxidase. The haem in haemoglobin can be modified by the gut microflora, leading to a removal of iron and a loss of detectability; this can reduce the sensitivity of the test, especially for proximal cancers. Other products will also catalyse the reaction, including animal blood, drugs and certain fresh fruits and vegetables containing peroxidases. This can lead to false positives and, to improve specificity, positive results are often repeated following dietary restriction of red meat and sometimes dark fish (salmon, sardines), dark poultry (e.g. pheasant), and certain peroxidase-rich fresh fruits (e.g. melons) and vegetables or boiled turnips or horseradish. Oral iron preparations and aspirin can also lead to false-positive results, and the antioxidant activity of high-dose vitamin C supplementation may lead to a false-negative result by interfering with the peroxidase reaction. It is usually advised to stop these for at least 2 days before performing the test. A test is conventionally considered positive if at least one window turns blue. Test positivity has been noticed to decrease with storage time.[7] Positivity can be greatly increased by rehydration of samples with a drop of water before processing.[8] However, the added sensitivity appears to be outweighed by the loss of specificity,[9,10] and this is usually no longer done. A number of other commercial tests using guaiac have been marketed, but none are as popular as Hemoccult II. A more sensitive and easily read version of the test (HemoccultSENSA) has also been evaluated. A version for home use in which the reagents are impregnated in toilet paper and a colour change is seen when placed in the toilet bowl is available in some countries, including the United States. These tests have not been evaluated in terms of sensitivity and specificity and may provide false reassurance; they cannot be recommended until they have been properly evaluated.

OTHER OCCULT BLOOD TESTS

Other chemical tests based on oxidation of phenolic compounds have been developed using orthotoluidine (Hematest) and tetramethylbenzidine (Hemo-Fec), but are not used for screening.

Newer tests have attempted to be more selective for haemoglobin and its degradation products. HemoQuant is a haem–porphyrin test which detects not only intact haem but also degraded de-ironed haems (haem-derived porphyrins), which was predicted to increase sensitivity, especially for proximal cancers. The test is based on fluorescent detection of dicarboxylic porphyrins derived from haems after iron removal and provides a quantitative output. The test is unaffected by stool dehydration and storage, dietary peroxidases, iron and ascorbic acid, and thus offers potential advantages over guaiac-based tests; however, it is still affected by red meat ingestion and aspirin usage.

Another approach has been to develop immunochemical tests that are immunoreactive with haemoglobin. These tests are the most specific for human blood and detect only human haemoglobin, globin and, perhaps, some early degradation products. At least four versions of this approach have been reported. Most information is available for HemeSelect, which uses haemaggutination with formalin-fixed chicken erythrocytes coated with anti-human haemoglobin antibodies as a detection method.

SIGMOIDOSCOPY

The goal of endoscopic screening differs from that of faecal ocult blood testing (FOBT), which is primarily an early detection measure. For sigmoidoscopy, the primary aim is to detect and remove adenomas, so that the adenoma–carcinoma sequence can be interrupted and cancer prevented. Such an approach, based on the detection of preinvasive precursor lesions, may allow for a much longer interval between screens and a nearly 100% cure rate for detected lesions.

Improvement in the equipment available has made endoscopic examination a much more attractive proposition for screening. Early work was carried out by a 25 cm rigid instrument which allowed visualization of the rectum only. Development of flexible fibre-optic or video scopes has transformed the procedure and made it simpler, quicker, less painful and more complete. Instruments 35 and 60 cm in length are available, in addition to the full-length colonoscopes. The 60 cm scope is the instrument of choice for screening, permitting visualization of the rectum and whole sigmoid colon in approximately 80% of patients. Bowel preparation can be achieved by a single phosphate enema and most polypectomies can be performed at the same visit, unless the polyps are large or present specific difficulties.[11,12] Typically, the examination takes 6–10 minutes. The approach is highly sensitive, allowing reliable detection of polyps of size down to 5 mm.

BARIUM ENEMA

Barium enema is often used for evaluation of symptomatic patients, especially when endoscopy proves difficult. The lower sensitivity of FOBT for proximal lesions and the lack of coverage of the proximal bowel by flexible sigmoidoscopy have led to a suggestion that barium enema might be used as a screening test for this segment, the only alternative being colonoscopy, which is more expensive and more invasive. Eddy[13] has evaluated by simulation a range of possible screening protocols, some of which involve barium enema. As for endoscopy, bowel preparation with an enema is necessary, but it is possible for both procedures to be performed at the same visit. Both single– and double-contrast methods have been used, but the double-contrast method is now more common except for low-risk, seriously ill, or young patients. For the single-contrast method the bowel is filled with a diluted barium suspension, allowing space-filling defects to be visualized. Good technique and colon compression are needed to obtain good films. In high-risk, occult-blood-positive or symptomatic patients, the double-contrast procedure is more often used. It involves a high-density barium suspension and the bowel is then inflated with air to provide a contrast so that the lining can be visualized. Good mucosal coating with the suspension is critical. Typically, four or five large and 8–10 small films are obtained for each technique. In specialist centres, both techniques appear to have similar high sensitivity for cancer and polyps greater than 1 cm (70–90%), but the double-contrast method has greater sensitivity for smaller adenomas. However these results may not translate to routine use and good technique is essential if they are to be achieved. An additional limitation is that a further endoscopic procedure is needed for polypectomy if an adenoma is discovered. Further details can be found in references 14–16.

COLONOSCOPY

The limitation of sigmoidoscopy in the detection of distal bowel lesions has led some to suggest complete colonoscopy of the large bowel as a screening test.[17,18] This is a much more invasive procedure than flexible sigmoidoscopy, with greater costs and higher complication rates, and is currently limited to symptomatic patients or those who have had an adenoma detected in the distal bowel. In good hands the entire large bowel can be visualized in over 80% of patients and all polyps can be removed at the same time. More complete bowel preparation is needed, usually involving overnight oral preparations.

FUTURE APPROACHES

There is much interest in developing less-invasive methods of visualizing the bowel. Virtual colonoscopy, based on helical CT scanning and the use of a thin probe passed up the bowel, is one possibility. Identification of the position of the endoscope within the colon to allow more accurate localization of visualized lesions and extent of coverage is also being developed.[19] Undoubtedly, endoscopic procedures will be much improved in the future.

Screening studies

DIGITAL RECTAL EXAMINATION

Digital rectal examination (DRE) was used in conjunction with flexible sigmoidoscopy in a study of multiphasic health checkups at the Kaiser-Permanante centres in Northern California.[20] It was not possible to determine if any effect was due to DRE. Herrinton *et al.*[21] have recently conducted a case–control study in which cases were those aged over 45 who had died from distal rectal cancer. About one-quarter of controls had undergone such an examination in the past 10 years, but there was no evidence that the test had any value in preventing mortality (odds ratio [OR] = 0.96; 95% confidence interval [CI] = 0.56–1.7).

FAECAL OCCULT BLOOD TESTS (FOBT)

Detection rates: cross-sectional studies

A major concern about these tests is their lack of sensitivity. The vast majority of results relate to Hemoccult. Even for patients with symptomatic bowel cancer, the test is positive only 60–90% of the time (Table 5.1). In these patients, occult bleeding is more often detected in larger, grossly ulcerated and advanced-stage cancers.

There have been many studies of occult blood testing as a screening test. Lower sensitivities have been reported in these studies, typically of the order of 40–70%, although the methods of assessing sensitivity are more variable here, and usually require follow-up for at least 6–12 months to identify interval cancers as false negatives. Most of these studies are uncontrolled and thus cannot be used to assess effects on mortality, because of lead-time bias and length bias; however, they do provide useful information on detection rates, specificity and compliance. A selection of some of the larger studies is given in Table 5.2.

Some of the studies have evaluated more than one method of occult blood testing. In a post-resection group of 1217 patients with previous cancer, Ahlquist *et al.*[22] evaluated Hemoccult II and HemoQuant testing on three stool samples per subject. Patients also received annual endoscopic or radiological follow-up, which yielded 46 patients with new or recurrent cancers and 386 with polyps but no cancer. The sensitivity of Hemoccult for cancers found during surveillance was 26% and the specificity was 95.3%. When the cutoff level of HemoQuant was adjusted to produce the same specificity (2.1 mg Hb/g stool), the sensitivity for cancer for this test was also 26%. Sensitivity for polyps 1 cm or larger was 13% by Hemoccult and 11% by HemoQuant.

St. John *et al.*[23] compared Hemoccult II, HemoccultSENSA, HemoQuant and HemeSelect on 107 patients with symptomatic colorectal cancer and 81 patients with primarily asymptomatic adenomas. HemeSelect and HemoccultSENSA had significantly higher sensitivities for colorectal cancer (97 and 94%, respectively) than either Hemoccult II (89%) or HemoQuant (71%). HemeSelect had the highest sensitivity for adenomas (58%) or large

Table 5.1. *Sensitivity of Hemoccult for bowel cancer*

Study	Year	Sample size	Sensitivity
Griffith *et al.*[50]	1981	28	82
Macrae & St. John[51]	1982	46	69
Doran & Hardcastle[52]	1982	50	70
Farrands & Hardcastle[53]	1983	61	72
McDonald & Goulston[54]	1984	36	53
St. John *et al.*[23]	1993	107	89
Ahlquist *et al.*[55]	1985	11 symptomatic	36
		35 asymptomatic	23
Crowley *et al.*[56]	1983	27	52
Songster *et al.*[57]	1980	150	40
Kapparis & Frommer[58]	1985	40	72
Reilly[59]	1990	51	61

adenomas (76%) (Table 5.3). HemoccultSENSA and HemeSelect tests were also performed on 1355 screened individuals (Table 5.2). In this screening population HemoccultSENSA and HemeSelect had similar positive predictive values for neoplasia (32 vs 33%, respectively) but HemeSelect had a lower positivity rate overall (3.0 vs 5.0%) and better specificity (97.8 vs 96.1%, $P < 0.05$).

Castiglione *et al.*[24] also compared Hemoccult II with HemeSelect in 24,282 screening subjects aged 40–70 years. Dietary restriction of red meat was advised for the day of the test and the preceding 2 days. A 33% compliance rate was achieved for both tests leading to 8008 completed test pairs in patients with a mean age of 54 years. The Hemoccult tests were rehydrated and produced a 6.0% positivity rate. A total of 15 cancers were detected, giving a PPV of 3.7%. HemeSelect was evaluated at two thresholds. The low threshold had a 8.2% positivity rate and detected 21 cancers (PPV = 3.8%), whereas the high threshold had a positivity rate of 3.1% and detected 17 cancers (PPV = 8.4%). Similar relative performances were seen for adenomas (Table 5.2). Better results were also obtained when only individuals aged 50 or more were considered, and the authors were of the opinion that the tests should be used in this group only. Overall, HemeSelect gave better results than Hemoccult, but the appropriate threshold for positivity would depend on cost–benefit evaluations.

Petrelli *et al.*[25] evaluated a community screening programme in which kits containing Hemoccult II, HemoccultSENSA and HemeSelect were distributed to 39,000 people aged over 40 years. No dietary restriction or drug cessation was required. A total of 8933 kits were returned (23%) and positivity rates were 5.1, 9.4 and 4.9%, respectively. The positivity rate for at least one test was 13%. Of the 1165 positive individuals, physician-verified results were obtained for 631. In this group 20 cancers were found, of which the respective tests detected 13, 16 and 17. PPVs for cancer were slightly higher for HemeSelect, but the values were very similar for adenomas (Table 5.2).

Two studies have used both hydrated and non-hydrated Hemoccult tests. Mandel *et al.*[26] found that positivity for the test increased from 2.4 to 9.8% and sensitivity for cancer increased

Table 5.2. *Screening studies of occult blood tests**

Uncontrolled studies

Study	Year	No tested (%)	Diet	No. positive (%)	No. of cancers/ polyps	PPV: Cancer/ polyps	Comments
Greegor[60]	1969	278	Y	24 (8.6)	2/3	8/12	
Hastings[61]	1974	2625 (76)	Y	159 (6.1)	5/	3/	
Miller & Knight[62]	1977	2332	N/Y	11 (0.5)	1/3	9/33	Two stages/diet in 2nd stage
Goodman[63]	1977	1701 (68)	Y	9 (0.5)	0/	0/	Women only
Helfrich *et al.*[64]	1977	8930	N	157 (1.8)	3/2	2 /1	
Fruhmorgen & Demling[65]	1978	5016 (84)	Y	136 (2.7)	13/83	10/61	
Heeb & Ahlvin[66]	1978	3956 (69)	Y	79 (2.0)	515	6/6	
Elwood *et al.*[67]	1978	1690 (15)	Y	58 (3.4)	2/	3/	
Bralow & Kopel[68]	1979	3008 (79)	N/Y	180 (6.0)	7/11	4/6	Rehydrate/2 stages
Winchester *et al.*[69]	1980	14,074 (26)	Y	617 (4.4)	30/40	5/7	
Kurnick *et al.*[70]	1980	5420	N	120 (2.2)	9/	8/	
Gnauck & Thomas[71]	1980	16,100	–	531 (3.3)	75/106	14/20	
Schwartz *et al.*[72]	1980	3,480,000	–	38,030 (1.1)	–	–	
				4,262	322/	8/	Evaluable patients
Larkin[73]	1980	5565 (95)	Y	88 (1.6)	4/6	1/1	Unrehydrated/2 stages
Chambers & Morgan[74]	1980	1160 (46)		68 (5.9)	3/10	4/15	
Stuart *et al.*[75]	1981	4498 (68)	Y	150 (3.3)	13/31	9/21	
Farrands *et al.*[76]	1981	2439 (27)	N	124 (5.1)	4/8	3/6	
Million *et al.*[77]	1982	1646 (28)	N	37 (2.3)	2/5	5/16	
Sontag *et al.*[78]	1983	2964 (22)	Y	135 (4.6)	14/44	10/33	
Hardcastle *et al.*[79]	1983	3613 (37)	Y	77 (2.1)	12/27	16/35	
Habba & Doyle[80]	1983	1628 (76)	N	37 (2.3)	5/6	14/16	
Kapparis & Frommer[58]	1985	200	Y	10 (5.0)	1/3	10/30	Non-rehydrated
				21 (10.5)	1/5	5/24	Rehydrated
				15 (7.5)	2/4	13/27	Immunological

Table 5.2. *(Continued)*

Uncontrolled studies (with details on large adenomas)

Study	Year	No. tested (%)	Diet	No. positive (%)	No. cancers/large adenoma/polyps	PPV: cancer/ adenoma/polyps	Comments
Siba[81]	1983	3791	N	97 (2.6)	6/11/18	6/11/19	
Armitage *et al.*[82]	1985	1304 (44)	N	40 (3.1)	3/20/25	8/50/62	Hemoccult
				106 (8.1)	5/11/22	5/10/21	Immunological (Feca EIA)
Thomas *et al.*[83]	1990	10,176 (58)	Y	131 (1.3)	20/27/76	15/21/58	3-day test
		9461 (54)		160 (1.7)	24/35/83	15/22/52	6-day test
McGarrity *et al.*[84]	1990	46,014 (63)		1303 (2.8)	–	–	Follow-up only on subset
				799	67/ /174	8/ /22	
St. John *et al.*[23]	1993	1355	Y	68 (5.0)	1 /9/15	1/13/22	HemoccultSENSA
				41 (3.0)	1/10/10	2/24/24	HemeSelect
Caffarey *et al.*[85]	1993	5934 (79)	?	287 (4.8)	44/ /38	15/./13	High-risk population
Petrelli *et al.*[25]	1994	8933 (23)	N	456 (5.1)	13/18/44	5/7/18	Hemoccult
				849 (9.5)	16/24/85	4/5/19	HemoccultSENSA
				438 (4.9)	17/17/45	7/7/19	HemeSelect
Robinson *et al.*[86]	1994	1489 (38)		17 (1.1)	1/7/8	6/41/47	Hemoccult
				145 (9.7)	9/29/48	6/20/33	HemeSelect
Castiglione *et al.*[24]	1996	8008 (38)	Y	483 (6.0)	15/37/79	4/9/20	Rehydrated
				655 (8.2)	21/55/118	4/10/21	Low threshold – HemeSelect
				245 (3.1)	17/36/62	8/18/30	High threshold – HemeSelect

Controlled studies

Study	Year	No. tested (%)	Diet	No. positive (%)	No. cancers/large adenoma/polyps	PPV cancer/ adenoma/polyps	Comments
Kewenter *et al.*[27]	1991	16,711 (65)	Y	835 (5.0)	38/95/159	5/11/19	Most samples rehydrated
Mandel *et al.*[26]	1993			–			
	(annual)	14,051 (75)*	Y	–(9.6)	174/ /	2/ /28	Most samples rehydrated
	(biennial)	14,013 (78)*	Y		145/ /	3/ /29	
Kronberg *et al.*[30]	1996	20,672 (67)	Y	215 (1.0)	37/68/	17/32/	
Hardcastle *et al.*[29]	1996	40,214 (54)	Y	837 (2.1)	83/ /311	10/ /37	

* Incomplete entries reflect unavailable information.

from 80.8 to 92.2%, but the PPV fell from 5.6 to 2.2%. Kewenter *et al.*[27] found that the positivity rate increased from 1.9% for non-rehydrated kits to 6.1% (and subsequently as high as 14.3%) for rehydrated tests. In this study, the high rate of positivity in rehydrated tests led to a policy of retesting positives, which produced a positivity rate after the second test of 1.7–4.6%, depending on the cohort. Detection rates at the prevalent screening were 0.9/1000 for non-rehydrated tests and 2.7/1000 for rehydrated tests.

Rozen *et al.*[28] have compared Hemoccult II with flexible 60 cm sigmoidoscopy in 1176 previously unscreened asymptomatic individuals of mean age 52 years. About one-third of these patients had a first-degree relative with colorectal cancer, but otherwise they were at average risk. All abnormal results were followed by colonoscopy. FOBT detected only 16% (7/43) of the adenomas and 60% (3/5) of the cancers, compared with 95% (41/43) and 80% (4/5) respectively for sigmoidoscopy. Only two patients with cancers and five with an adenoma were positive by both tests, suggesting that FOBT might be a useful adjunct to sigmoidoscopy.

Mortality: follow-up studies

Three randomized clinical trials have thus far reported on the effect on mortality of occult blood testing (Table 5.4). Mandel *et al.*[26] reported on 46,501 individuals aged 50–80 years in Minnesota, USA, who were randomly allocated to one of three groups – control, annual FOBT or biennial FOBT by Hemoccult II. Rehydrated tests were mostly used and positivity rates were very high (9.6%) leading to a 38% colonoscopy rate in the group screened annually and a 28% rate in the biennial group. After 13 years of follow-up a 33% reduction (95% CI=18–50%) in mortality was observed in the group screened annually but thus far only a small and non-significant 6% decrease (95% CI 32% decrease to 31% increase) in mortality has been seen in the group randomized to biennial screening.

Hardcastle *et al.*[29] reported on 152,850 individuals aged 45–74 in Nottingham, UK, randomly allocated to control or biennial Hemoccult tests. Overall compliance was just under 60%. Samples were not rehydrated and positivity rates were 2.1%. After a median follow-up of 7–8 years, a significant (15%) reduction in mortality rate (95% CI=2–26%) has been found. A very similar trial of 61,933 Danes has given similar results:[30] after 10 years of follow-up the reduction in mortality rate was 18% (95% CI=1–34%).

A further trial in Gothenberg, Sweden, involving approximately 50,000 subjects and initiated in 1982, has not yet reported on effects on mortality, although a clear shift in stage distribution has been noted.[27]

A fourth trial has studied the value of adding FOBT to rigid sigmoidoscopy.[31] A total of 21,756 patients aged over 40 years were entered from 1975 to 1979, and were randomly allocated to annual screening by rigid sigmoidoscopy, either alone or in combination with Hemoccult. Initial compliance was high, but fell rapidly in follow-up visits. Follow-up was until 1984, at which time there were 199 cases of colorectal cancer (CRC) and 64 deaths from CRC. Randomization was not performed and patients were allocated to a treatment which alternated every year. A non-significant 26% reduction in CRC mortality was found.

These results have been generally supported by four published case–control studies (Table 5.4). Selby *et al.*[32] conducted a case–control study of FOBT using Hemoccult II in Northern California. Cases consisted of 485 persons who developed fatal CRC above the age of 50 years, and there were 727 age- and sex-matched controls. Overall, a 31% (95% CI=9–48%) reduction in CRC mortality was observed if at least one screening test had taken place in the past 5 years. Closer analysis indicated that the protection was confined to the 3 years following a screening test. The protection obtained was similar in men and women and unaffected by age. Cases had fewer periodic health checkups and sigmoidoscopies than controls, suggesting that the results may be at least partly due to a more healthy lifestyle in those screened. False-positive rates in controls were about 3%, in line with the clinical trials and series.

Wahrendorf *et al.*[33] conducted a case–control study based on a population screening programme in Saarland, Germany. Screening by FOBT became available under a government programme in 1977 and was offered to all men and women over the age of 45, but participation was low and based solely

Table 5.3. *Sensitivity of four occult blood tests. (Adapted from ref. 23.)*

Group	*n*	Hemoccult II	HemoccultSENSA	HemeSelect	HemoQuant (> 2 mg/g)
Colorectal cancer	107	88.8	93.5	97.2	71.0
Cancer proximal to splenic flexure	28	89.3	92.9	100.0	89.3
Cancer proximal to splenic flexure	79	88.6	93.7	96.2	64.6
Any adenoma	81	30.9	44.4	58.0	37.0
Adenoma > 1 cm	45	42.2	60.0	75.6	42.2
Adenoma < 1 cm	36	16.7	25.0	36.1	30.6

on the individual's wish to attend. The area studied had a population of 1.1 million and was covered by the Saarland cancer registry. Cases studied were those individuals who died of CRC between 1983 and 1986 and who were aged 55–75 at death, and for whom screening histories could be retrieved (163 male, 209 female). Age-matched controls were obtained from the GP files of the cases and also from gynaecologist's files for women. For men, 13% of cases and 14% of controls had at least one asymptomatic screen 6–36 months prior to diagnosis (OR = 0.92; 95% CI = 0.61–1.75), whereas for women, 16% of cases and 29% of controls had such a test (OR = 0.43; 95% CI = 0.27–0.68). Screening was more common in both male and female patients in the 6 months prior to diagnosis in each case, suggesting that some tests were performed because of symptoms. The benefit in women was ascribed to a higher participation rate; however, the low overall participation rate (15%), and the inability to separate symptomatic from asymptomatic cases reliably, limit the interpretations which can be drawn from this study.

Saito *et al.*[34] have reported a study of similar design from Aomori Prefecture, Japan, which has a population of 1.5 million. The main difference was that the FOBT test routinely used was an inmunochemical test for haemoglobin (HemeSelect). A total of 193 cases who died of CRC between 1986 and 1992 and who were diagnosed at ages 40–79 after the screening programme started in 1986 were considered. Three age-, sex- and location-matched controls were selected for each case and screening histories were abstracted for the 5 years prior to the date of diagnosis, in the case from a central screening registry for the area. In the 5 years prior to diagnosis 18.9% of cases and 22.8% of controls had been screened at least once (OR = 0.77; 95% CI = 0.34–1.74). The benefit was greatest in the first 2 years after screening and was no longer apparent after 4 years. The odds ratios for the first 5 years since the most recent screening test were 0.40, 0.39, 0.58, 0.90 and 1.20, respectively. Benefit did not differ by sex, age at diagnosis, or anatomical location of the cancer.

Lazovich *et al.*[35] conducted a case–control study based on a health-maintenance organization in western Washington state. Cases were individuals aged 40–84 who died of CRC between 1986 and 1991. A total of 248 eligible cases with available histories were matched on a two-to-one basis with 496 controls. Even though 'definitely symptomatic' tests were excluded, an increased amount of screening was found in cases in the first year before diagnosis (20 vs 17%), leading to an OR of 1.37 (95% CI = 0.92–2.03), suggesting that there was some misclassification in this regard. Mortality was reduced in subsequent intervals and there was a reduced mortality risk for 'ever' screening of 28% (95% CI = 49% benefit–2% harm) based on 50% of cases and 58% of controls having been screened at some time. The risk of fatal cancer was reduced by almost 50% in the second year following a test (6% of cases vs 11% of controls), and benefit appeared to be confined

Table 5.4. *Effect on mortality of faecal occult blood testing (FOBT)*

Clinical trials

Study	Year	Median FU* (years)	Frequency (months)	Screened CRC deaths/Pop	Controls CRC deaths/Pop	OR (95% CI)	Compliance (%)	Age (years)
Mandel *et al.*[26]	1993	13	12	82/15520	121 /15394	0.67 (0.50–0.82)	75	50–80
			24	117/15587	121/15394	0.94 (0.68–1.31)	78.4	50–80
Hardcastle *et al.*[29]	1996	7.8	24	360/76466	420/76384	0.85 (0.74–0.98)	59.6	45–74
Kronberg *et al.*[30]	1996	10	24	205/30967	249/30966	0.82 (0.68–0.99)	67	45–75
Winawer *et al.**[31]	1993	7	12	36/12974	28/8782	0.75 (0.45–1.21)	76 initially ~20 on FU	> 40

Case–control studies of FOBT

Study	Date	Cases/controls	Percentage screened in last 5 years (cases/controls)	Screened in last 5 years: OR (95% CI)	Screened in last 2 years: OR (95% CI)	Duration of effect
Selby *et al.*[32]	1993	485/727	31.5/42.6	0.69 (0.52–0.91)	0.76 (0.55–1.03)	2–3 years
Wahrendorf *et al.*[33]	1993	372/684	14.6/22.3	Male 0.92* (0.54–1.57)	Male 0.83† (0.42–1.64)	benefit only in years 1–3 after test
				Female 0.43* (0.27–0.68)	Female 0.30 (0.17–0.55)	
Saito *et al.*[34]	1995	193/577	18.9/22.8	0.77 (0.34–1.74)	0.41 (0.20–0.82)	2–3 years
Lazovich *et al.*[35]	1995	236/457	44/48	0.81 (0.62–1.19)	0.95 (0.66–1.35)	no trend

* 6–36 months asymptomatic tests.

† 12–24 months asymptomatic tests.

CI, confidence interval; CRC, colorectal cancer; FU, follow-up; OR, odds ratio; Pop, population;

to years 1–3 after a test. Benefit also appeared to be confined to patients aged under 75 at diagnosis, and to tests performed at home, compared with those performed in the doctor's office.

SIGMOIDOSCOPY

Randomized trials

At least two large randomized trials are evaluating the efficacy of screening by flexible sigmoidoscopy. In the United States, the PLCO trial is examining the role of 3-yearly screening in 37,000 men and 37,000 women aged 60–74. In the United Kingdom a trial of once-in-a-lifetime sigmoidoscopy for individuals aged 55–64 is underway. This trial will involve 200,000 individuals in 14 centres, of which 65,000 will be randomized for screening. It will be many years before either of these trials have definitive mortality results, but the UK trial has published baseline data for the first two centres.[12] A two-stage entry procedure is used in which randomization is performed only among those who express an interest for screening in a pre-randomization questionnaire. The positive response rate to this initial questionnaire has been 60%, and 75% of those invited to be screened have accepted, leading to screening being performed in 45% of the target population. In the first 1285 sigmoidoscopies there have been seven (0.5%) individuals with cancer, 76 (6%) with high-risk adenomas (>1 cm, villous, tubulo-villous, severely dysplastic or multiple), 120 (9%) with any adenoma, and a further 196 (15%) with metaplastic polyps only.

A pilot screening programme has been completed on 3500 asymptomatic subjects, aged 55–59, in Freemantle, Western Australia of which 2881 (86%) were estimated to be eligible.[36] Initial compliance was only 12%, with a 3.5% increase after a telephone follow-up. Among the 342 screened individuals, 35% had polyps of which just under half (16% of those screened) were adenomas. Nineteen (5.6%) individuals had an adenoma of 1 cm or more. The procedure was well tolerated and 99% of those screened agreed to be tested again, if necessary.

Hoff *et al.*[37] have published results of a pilot trial of flexible sigmoidoscopy screening in Telemark County, Norway: 400 men and women aged 50–59 were randomly allocated to screening, and there were 399 unscreened controls. If a polyp was found at screening, colonoscopy was performed initially and at 2- and 6-year follow-up examinations. Attendance for screening was high, at 81%. Polyps were found in 35% of the participants and adenomas greater than 5 mm were detected in 10%. After a 10-year follow-up, four cancers (one fatal) were found in the control group and one (fatal) cancer among the screened group, which was in a non-complier. These numbers are far too small to make any conclusions regarding efficacy; however, no significant pathology had occurred on the follow-up examinations, suggesting that follow-up could be much less frequent (or omitted altogether in some cases).

Observational studies

Most of the information on the efficacy of endoscopic screening comes from clinical or screening series and case–control studies (Table 5.5). A number of studies have examined CRC rates in patients offered repeated sigmoidoscopy or colonoscopy. In an early study, Gilbertson and Nelms[38] reported an 85% reduction in rectal cancer in 21,000 subjects who had annual rigid sigmoidoscopy, but others have suggested that the reduction may not have been as great. Friedman *et al.*[19] reported a 60% reduction in distal CRC in 10,000 patients randomly allocated to undergo sigmoidoscopy every 3 years, but subsequent analysis showed that the use of this procedure was similar in both arms of the study. However, a case–control study on the same population confirmed a 70% reduction in mortality associated with a single sigmoidoscopy which lasted up to 10 years.[39] This has also been confirmed in another, smaller, case–control study involving 66 cases and 196 controls, in which a 79% reduction in mortality was found following a single sigmoidoscopy.[40] A very large case–control study among American veterans has recently been reported.[41] After excluding patients with familial polyposis coli or inflammatory bowel disease, they examined the records of 4358 patients (98% males) who died from CRC between 1988 and 1992, and a set of 16,531 matched living controls and 16,199 matched dead controls. Overall, they found a 59% (95% CI = 50–67%) reduction in death associated with any prior colorectal procedure. The protection was 70% in the first year fol-

Table 5.5. *Efficacy of sigmoidoscopy*

Study	Year	Cases/no. of subjects	Percentage reduction in colorectal cancer incidence in region examined (95% CI)	Type of study
Gilbertson and Nelms[38]	1978	13/21,150	60–85	Prospective uncontrolled
Friedman *et al.*[19]	1986	110/10,713	60	Prospective randomized
Selby *et al.*[39]	1992	261/1129	70 (52–81)	Case–control
Newcomb *et al.*[40]	1992	66/290	79 (48–92)	Case–control
Atkin *et al.*[42]	1992	3**/1618	85	Retrospective cohort
Winawer *et al.**[30]	1993	5/1 418	90 (76–97)	Prospective cohort (colonoscopy)
Muller and Sonnenberg[41]	1995	4358/16,531	59* (50–67)	Case–control

* Any colorectal procedure.
** Excluding cancers arising in incompletely excised adenomas.

lowing the procedure but remained near 60% for the subsequent period of up to 10 years (Figure 5.2). Protection was most related to removal of tissue, suggesting a direct benefit of adenoma removal. In addition, some of the procedures examined only part of the bowel (sigmoidoscopy), suggesting a larger benefit in the specific regions investigated.

Two prospective studies have also shown a marked reduction of the anticipated cancer rates in patients who have had adenomas completely removed. Atkin *et al.*[42] followed up a cohort of 1618 patients in whom rectosigmoid adenomas had been removed during rigid rectosigmoidoscopy up to 14 years ago. Using the estimate of progression of large adenomas described by Stryker *et al.*,[43] a predicted 85% reduction of distal CRC was associated with complete adenoma removal. However, rectal cancer rates remained high among individuals who had an incomplete removal of their adenoma.

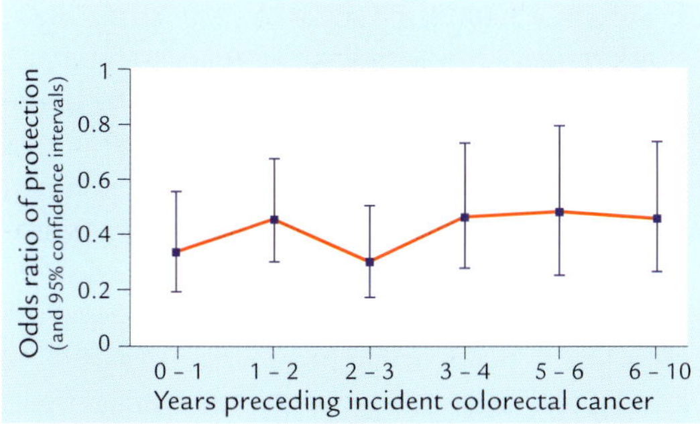

Figure 5.2. *Reduction in incidence of colorectal cancer following endoscopic surveillance.*

In the National Polyp Study, 1418 patients with one or more adenomas removed at complete colonoscopy were followed up by periodic colonoscopy for an average of 5.9 years.[30] A 76% (95% CI = 44–92%) reduction in CRC was observed, compared with the standard US population, and a 90% reduction was found if this was compared with other, similar, populations who did not receive follow-up surveillance. If the first 2 years of follow-up are omitted to adjust partially for a clear colon, the reductions were 66 and 85%, respectively.

A similar study from Australia,[44] of 645 patients followed up for a mean of 4.4 years found cancer rates similar to those for the general population (3 observed, 3.75 expected). The mean size of initial adenoma was 9 mm and 29% had a villous component; thus if one assumes a 2.5-fold increase in risk in this cohort compared with the general population, the cohort provides some evidence for a reduction of the order of 60–70%.

One observational study has shown a mortality benefit associated with colonoscopic surveillance of patients with ulcerative colitis.[45] The study consisted of 41 patients who developed carcinomas within a cohort of 2050 patients who had been seen for ulcerative colitis, 19 of whom were under colonoscopic surveillance. Although potentially subject to confounding and biases, both groups had longstanding ulcerative colitis before development of cancer (median 18 vs 15 years for surveillance vs no surveillance, respectively). An earlier stage distribution was associated with surveillance ($P = 0.04$) and survival was significantly better (4 vs 11 deaths, $P = 0.03$).

Safety and complications

The main complication of colorectal screening is perforation of the bowel. The risks are substantially greater for colonoscopy, than for sigmoidoscopy. For colonoscopy perforation rates are about 1–3/1000 and mortality approximately 1/10,000.[46,47] Complications occur more frequently after polypectomy, with a 2% incidence of haemorrhage, 0.3% incidence of perforation and a 0.1% mortality rate. Rates are much lower for sigmoidoscopy, where perforation rates are about 1–2/10,000 examinations,[48,49] although results of larger series with the 60 cm fibre-optic scopes have not yet been reported. Somewhat higher rates occur after biopsy or polypectomy, but as yet there are no mortality figures. Much lower perforation rates are reported for barium enema. A small risk of cardiac complication is associated with each of these procedures, relating possibly to the enema, sedation or anxiety about the test.

Endoscopic procedures are uncomfortable and colonoscopy usually requires sedation. However, the discomfort is short-lived, as sigmoidoscopy usually requires 6–10 minutes and colonoscopy 15–30 minutes. Wind and soiling are the most common complaints following these procedures.

Occult blood testing has virtually no direct complications, although many people find it an unacceptable procedure. However, because the test is performed frequently, the overall false-positivity rate is high, leading to a high proportion of those screened undergoing colonoscopy with its attendant complications.

References

1. Day NE. Estimating the sensitivity of a screening test. *J Epidemiol Community Health* 1985; 39: 364–366
2. Moss SM. Case–control studies of screening. *Int J Epidemiol* 1991; 20: 1–6
3. Simon JB. Occult blood screening for colorectal carcinoma: a critical review. *Gastroenterology* 1985; 88: 820–837
4. Lauridsen LH, Bohn L. Testing of feces for occult blood: a review. *Dan Med Bull* 1976; 23: 230–235
5. Irons GV, Kirsner JB. Routine chemical tests of the stool for occult blood: an evaluation. *Am J Med Sci* 1965; 249: 247–260
6. Greegor DH. Diagnosis of large-bowel cancer in the asymptomatic patient. *JAMA* 1967; 201: 943–945
7. Morris DW, Hansell JR, Ostrow JD, Lee CS. Reliability of chemical tests for fecal occult blood in hospitalized patients. *Am J Dig Dis* 1976; 21: 845–852
8. Wells HJ, Pagano JF. 'Hemoccult'(tm) test-reversal of false-negative results due to storage (abstr). *Gastroenterology* 1977; 72: 1148
9. Winawer SJ, Andrews M, Fleichinger B *et al.* Progress report on controlled trial of fecal occult blood testing for the detection of colorectal neoplasia. *Cancer* 1980; 45: 2959–2964
10. Kewenter J, Björk S, Haglind E *et al.* Screening and rescreening for colorectal cancer. A controlled trial of fecal occult blood testing in 27700 subjects. *Cancer* 1988; 62: 645–651
11. Atkin WS, Cuzick J, Northover JMA, Whynes DK. Prevention of colorectal cancer by once-only sigmoidoscopy. *Lancet* 1993; 341: 736–740
12. Atkin WS, Hart A, Edwards R *et al.* Uptake, yield of neoplasia and adverse effects of flexible sigmoidoscopy screening. *Gut* 1998; 42: 560–565

13. Eddy DM. Screening for colorectal cancer. *Ann Intern Med* 1990; 113: 373–384

14. Ott DJ, Scharling ES, Chen YM *et al.* Barium enema examination: sensitivity in detecting colonic polyps and carcinomas. *South Med J* 1989; 82: 197–200

15. Ott DJ. Role of the barium enema in colorectal carcinoma. *Radio Clin North Am* 1993; 31: 1293–1313

16. Stevenson GW. Radiology and endoscopy in the pretreatment diagnostic management of colorectal cancer. *Cancer* 1993; 71: 4198–4206

17. Lieberman D. Cost–effectiveness of colon cancer screening. *Am J Gastroenterol* 1991; 86: 1789–1794

18. Lieberman DA, Smith FW. Screening for colon malignancy with colonoscopy. *Am J Gastroenterol* 1991; 86: 946–951

19. Williams C. Electronic 3-dimensional imaging of intestinal endoscopy. *Lancet* 1993; 341: 724–725

20. Friedman GD, Collen MF, Fireman BH. Multiphasic health checkup evaluation: a 16-year follow-up. *J Chron Dis* 1986; 39: 453–463

21. Herrinton L, Selby JV, Friedman GD *et al.* A case–control study of digital-rectal screening in relation to mortality from cancer of the distal rectum. *Am J Epidemiol* 1995; 142: 961–964

22. Ahlquist DA, Wieand S, Moertel CG *et al.* Accuracy of fecal occult blood screening for colorectal neoplasia. *JAMA* 1993; 269: 1262–1267

23. St. John DJB, Young GP, Alexeyeff MA *et al.* Evaluation of new occult blood tests for detection of colorectal neoplasia. *Gastroenterology* 1993; 104: 1661–1668

24. Castiglione G, Zappa M, Grazzini G *et al.* Immunochemical vs guaiac faecal occult blood tests in a population-based screening programme for colorectal cancer. *Br J Cancer* 1996; 74: 141–144

25. Petrelli N, Michalek AM, Freedman A *et al.* Immunochemical versus guaiac occult blood stool tests: results of a community-based screening program. *Surg Oncol* 1994; 3: 27–36

26. Mandel JS, Bond JH, Church TR *et al.* Reducing mortality from colorectal cancer by screening for fecal occult blood. *N Engl J Med* 1993; 328: 1365–1371

27. Kewenter J, Asztely M, Engaras B *et al.* A randomised trial of faecal occult blood testing for early detection of colorectal cancer. In: Miller AB, Chamberlain J, Day NE *et al.* (eds.) *Cancer Screening. Results of Screening and Rescreening of 51325 Subjects.* Cambridge: Cambridge University Press, 1991, pp. 116–125

28. Rozen P, Ron E, Fireman Z *et al.* The relative value of fecal occult blood tests and flexible sigmoidoscopy in screening for large bowel neoplasia *Cancer* 1987; 60: 2553–2583

29. Hardcastle JD, Chamberlain JO, Robinson MHE *et al.* Randomised controlled trial of faecal-occult-blood screening for colorectal cancer. *Lancet* 1996; 348:1472–1477

30. Kronberg O, Fenger C, Olsen J, *et al.* Randomised study of screening for colorectal cancer with faecal-occult-blood test. Lancet 1996; 348: 1467–1471

31. Winawer SJ, Flehinger BJ, Schottenfeld D, Miller DG. Screening for colorectal cancer with fecal occult blood testing and sigmoidoscopy. *J Natl Cancer Inst* 1993; 85: 1311–1318

32. Selby JV, Friedman GD, Quesenberry CP, Weiss NS. Effect of fecal occult blood testing on mortality from colorectal cancer. A case-control study. *Ann Intern Med* 1993; 118: 1–6

33. Wahrendorf J, Robra BP, Wiebelt H *et al.* Effectiveness of colorectal cancer screening: results from a population-based case–control evaluation in Saarland, Germany. *Eur J Cancer Prev* 1993; 2: 221–227

34. Saito H, Soma Y, Koeda J *et al.* Reduction in risk of mortality from colorectal cancer by fecal occult blood screening with immunochemical hemagglutination test. A case–control study. *Int J Cancer* 1995; 61: 465–469

35. Lazovich DA, Weiss NS Stevens NG *et al.* A case-control study to evaluate efficacy of screening faecal occult blood. *J Med Screening* 1995, 2: 84–89

36. Olynyk JK, Aquilia S, Fletcher DR, Dickinson JA. Flexible sigmoidoscopy screening for colorectal cancer in average-risk subjects: a community-based pilot project. *Med J Aust* 1996: 165: 74–76

37. Hoff G, Sauar J, Vatn MH *et al.* Polypectomy of adenomas in the prevention of colorectal cancer: 10 years' follow-up of the Telemark Polyp Study I. *Scand J Gastroenterol* 1996; 31: 1006–1010

38. Gilbertson VA, Nelms JM. The prevention of invasive cancer of the rectum. *Cancer* 1978; 41: 1137–1139

39. Selby JV, Friedman GD, Quesenberry CP Jr, Weiss NS. A case–control study of screening sigmoidoscopy and mortality from colorectal cancer. *N Engl J Med* 1992; 326: 653–657

40. Newcomb PA, Norfleet RG, Storer BE, Surawicz TS, Marcus PM. Screening sigmoidoscopy and colorectal cancer mortality. *J Natl Cancer Inst* 1992; 84: 1572–1575

41. Muller AD, Sonnenberg A. Protection by endoscopy against death from colorectal cancer: a case–control study among veterans. *Arch Intern Med* 1983; 155: 1741–1748

42. Atkins WS. Morson BC. Cuzick J. Long-term risk of colorectal cancer after excision of rectosigmoid adenomas. *N Eng I J Med* 1992; 326: 658–662

43. Stryker SJ, Wolff BG, Culp CE *et al.* Natural history of untreated colonic polyps. *Gastroenterology* 1987; 93: 1009–1013

44. Meagher AP, Stuart M. Does colonoscopic polypectomy reduce the incidence of colorectal carcinoma? *Aust NZ J Surg* 1994; 64: 400–404

45. Choi PM, Nugent FW, Schoetz DJ *et al.* Colonoscopic surveillance reduces mortality from colorectal cancer in ulcerative colitis. *Gastroenterology* 1993; 105: 418–424

46. Macrae FA, Tan KG, Williams CB. Towards safer colonoscopy: a report on the complications of 5000 diagnostic or therapeutic colonoscopies. *Gut* 1983; 24: 376–383

47. Waye JD, Lewis BS, Yessayan S. Colonoscopy: a prospective report of complications. *J Clin Gastroenterol* 1992; 15: 347–351

48. Portes C, Majarakis JD. Proctosigmoidoscopy: incidence of polyps in 50,000 examinations. *JAMA* 1957; 163: 411–413

49. Winnan G, Berci G, Panish J *et al.* Superiority of the flexible to the rigid sigmoidoscope in routine proctosigmoidoscopy. *N Engl J Med* 1980; 302: 1011–1012

50. Griffith CDM, Turner DJ, Saunders JH. False negative results of Hemoccult test in colorectal screening. *Br Med J* 1981; 283: 472–473

51. Macrae FA, St. John DJ. Relationship between patterns of bleeding and Haemoccult sensitivity in patients with colorectal cancers or adenomas. *Gastroenterology* 1982; 82: 891–898

52. Doran J, Hardcastle JD. Bleeding patterns in colorectal cancer: the effect of aspirin and the implications for faecal occult blood testing. *Br J Surg* 1982; 69: 711–713

53. Farrands PA, Hardcastle JD. Accuracy of occult blood tests over a six-day period. *Clin Oncol* 1983; 9: 217–225

54. McDonald C, Goulston K. Colorectal test for occult blood. *Med J Aust* 1984; 140: 183

55. Ahlquist DA, McGill DB, Schwartz S *et al.* Faecal blood levels in health and disease. A study using HemoQuant. *N Engl J Med* 1985; 312: 1422–1428

56. Crowley ML, Freeman LD, Mottet MD *et al.* Sensitivity of guaiac-impregnated cards for the detection of colorectal neoplasia. *J Clin Gastroenterol* 1983; 5: 127–130

57. Songster CL, Barrows GH, Jarrett DD. Immunochemical detection of fecal occult blood – the fecal smear punch-disc test: a new non-invasive screening test for colorectal cancer. *Cancer* 1980; 45: 1099–1102

58. Kapparis A, Frommer D. Immunological detection of occult blood in bowel cancer patients. *Br J Cancer* 1985; 52: 857–861

59. Reilly JM, Ballantyne GH, Fleming FX *et al.* Evaluation of the occult blood test in screening for colorectal neoplasms. A prospective study using flexible endoscopy. *Am Surg* 1990; 56: 119–123

60. Greegor DH. Detection of silent colon cancer in routine examination. *CA Cancer J Clin* 1969; 19: 330–337

61. Hastings JB. Mass screening for colorectal cancer. *Am J Surg* 1974; 127: 228–233

62. Miller SF, Knight AR. The early detection of colorectal cancer. *Cancer* 1977; 40: 945–949

63. Goodman MJ. Mass screening for colorectal cancer – a negative report. *JAMA* 1977; 237: 2380

64. Helfrich GB, Petrucci P, Webb H. Mass screening for colorectal cancer. *JAMA* 1977; 238: 1502–1503

65. Fruhmorgen P, Demling L. Early detection of colorectal carcinoma with a modified guaiac test. A screening examination in 6000 humans. *Acta Gastroenterol Belg* 1978; 41: 682–687

66. Heeb MA, Ahlvin RC. Screening for colorectal carcinoma in a rural area. *Surgery* 1978; 83: 540–541

67. Elwood TW, Erickson A, Lieberman S. Comparative educational approaches to screening for colorectal cancer. *Am J Public Health* 1978; 68: 135–138

68. Bralow SP, Kopel J. Hemoccult screening for colorectal cancer. An impact study in Sarasota, Florida. *J Florida Med Assoc* 1979; 66: 915–919

69. Winchester DP, Shull JH, Scanlon EF *et al.* A mass screening program for colorectal cancer using chemical testing for occult blood in the stool. *Cancer* 1980; 45: 2955–2958

70. Kurnick JE, Walley LB, Jacob HH *et al.* Colorectal cancer detection in a community hospital screening program. *JAMA* 1980; 243: 2056–2057

71. Gnauck R, Thomas L. Haemoscreen in Vergleich mit Haemoccult als Suchtest auf kolorektalen Krebs. *Dtsch Med Wochenschr* 1980; 105: 1642–1646

72. Schwartz FW, Holstein H, Brecht JG. Preliminary report of fecal occult blood testing in Germany. In: Winawer SJ, Schottenfeld D, Sherlock P (eds.) *Colorectal Cancer: Prevention, Epidemiology, and Screening*, pp. 267–270 New York: Raven, 1980

73. Larkin KK. Mass screening in colorectal cancer. *Aust NZ J Surg* 1980; 50: 467–469

74. Chambers KJ, Morgan BP. Mass screening in colorectal cancer. *Aust NZ J Surg* 1980; 50: 467–469

75. Stuart M, Killingback MJ, Sakker S *et al.* Hemoccult II test. Routine screening procedure for colorectal neoplasm? *Med J Aust* 1981; 1: 629–631

76. Farrands PA, Griffiths RL, Britton DC. The Frome experiment – value of screening for colorectal cancer. *Lancet* 1981; i: 1231–1232

77. Million R, Howarth J, Turnberg E, Turnberg LA. Faecal occult blood testing for colorectal cancer in general practice. *Practitioner* 1982; 226: 659–663

78. Sontag SJ, Durczak C, Aranha GV *et al.* Faecal occult blood screening for colorectal cancer in a Veterans Administration hospital. *Am J Surg* 1983; 145: 89–93

79. Hardcastle JD, Farrands PA, Balfour TW *et al.* Controlled trial of faecal occult blood testing in the detection of colorectal cancer. *Lancet* 1983; 11: 1–4

80. Habba SF, Doyle JS. Colorectal cancer screening of asymptomatic patients in Ireland. *Ir J Med Sci* 1983; 152: 121–124

81. Siba S. Experience with Haemoccult screening in Hungary. A multicenter trial. *Hepatogastroenterol* 1983; 30: 27–29

82. Armitage N, Hardcastle JJ, Amar SS *et al.* A comparison of an immunological faecal occult blood test Fecatwin sensitive/FECA EIA with Haemoccult in population screening for colorectal cancer. *Br J Cancer* 1985; 51: 799–804

83. Thomas WM, Pye G, Hardcastle JD, Mangham CM. Faecal occult blood screening for colorectal neoplasia: a randomized trial of three days or six days of tests. *Br J Surg* 1990; 77: 277–279

84. McGarrity TJ, Long PA, Peiffer LP. Results of a repeat television-advertised mass screening program for colorectal cancer using fecal occult blood tests. *Am J Gastroenterol* 1990; 85: 266–270

85. Caffarey SM, Broughton CIM, Marks CG. Faecal occult blood screening for colorectal neoplasia in a targeted high-risk population. *Br J Surg* 1993; 80: 1399–1400

86. Robinson MHE, Marks CG, Farrands PA *et al.* Population screening for colorectal cancer: comparison between guaiac and immunological faecal occult blood tests. *Br J Surg* 1994; 81: 448–451

Chapter 6

CHEMOPREVENTION OF COLORECTAL CANCER

M.J.S. Langman and P. Boyle

Introduction

Any chemoprevention strategy, whether in patients at risk of cancer or in those with other disease, must be underpinned by the basic principle that the chosen agent must be safe enough to be administered to a group of individuals where significant proportions (usually the great majority) would not have developed the disease in question even if the preventive treatment had not been given. It would be unacceptable to exchange disease successfully prevented, for significant amounts of disease caused by the preventive agent. This principle is particularly important in the chemoprevention of cancer because treatment is likely to be given for very long periods, probably 5 years or much longer.

In applying the principle, account should be taken of the clinical circumstances. Thus, it might be acceptable to administer a modestly toxic treatment to patients with familial polyposis coli (where the cancer risk is universal) if the prospects of complete polyp remission were good, and therefore the chances of avoiding rectal excision high. By contrast it would be unwise to attempt any form of mass population prophylaxis in the absence of a high degree of confidence in safety, since in any one year the risk of colon cancer occurrence would be of the order of one in every 1000 people. Therefore 999 of those would be exposed to potentially toxic treatment, but without benefit.

The second important principle is of biological value in the given situation. It is possible that the required characteristics of an agent will differ in the primary prevention of adenomatous polyps, and in prevention of transformation from benign polyps to malignant disease.

Thirdly, any chemopreventive measure should be combinable with desirable lifestyle changes and, in those who have already developed malignant disease, should be compatible with any chemotherapeutic or other measures thought useful in disease management.

Chemotherapeutic regimes have obvious attractions compared with lifestyle changes in potentially being easy to apply and not being dependent upon major alterations in established behaviour patterns. Studies of cardiovascular disease have already shown that lifestyle changes can be extremely difficult to implement.

If chemopreventive agents work then it is to be expected that they will influence one or more of the steps in a multistage process in which genetic abnormalities – either of control mechanisms over cell multiplication or of suppressor mechanisms and repair processes – lead to unrestrained proliferation.

The adenoma–carcinoma sequence is now widely accepted as part of this process, and in animal studies an initial step would seem to be the development of aberrant crypt foci.

The molecular background includes the activation of various oncogenes and the loss or inactivation of tumour-suppressor genes. Identification of the APC *gene associated with the development of multiple adenomatous polyps in familial adenomatous polyposis coli has been associated with a greatly expanded understanding of the multistep process. However, it is clear that there is variation in the type and number of defects accumulated during carcinogenesis. Secondly, it is seldom clear at which stage of the process any putative chemotherapeutic agent acts, for how long that action lasts, and whether it necessarily prevents further stages in the process taking place.*

Potential treatments

Those treatments worthy of consideration either singly or together in chemotherapeutic regimens, include a range of vitamins, mineral supplements, anti-inflammatory drugs, histamine H_2 antagonists, bile acids, and other substances with properties such as those of antioxidants which have plausible biological bases. Evidence of value for any of these regimens is currently limited, and our understanding of their mechanisms of action is equally limited.

Candidate treatments have also been extensively studied (Table 6.1) in animal models – typically, rats treated with the colon carcinogen azoxymethane – and in isolated cell systems. Those compounds studied have included the non-steroidal anti-inflammatory drugs (NSAIDs) and also organoselenium compounds, alpha-difluoromethylornithine, flavonoids, retinoid-based agents, adrenocorticoids, trace metals and others.

Table 6.1. *Approaches to chemoprevention*

Agents	Postulated mechanism
Nutritional supplements	
Calcium	Reduced proliferation Enhanced differentiation Bile acid binding
Carotenoids	Reduced oxidation
Selenium	
Vitamin C	Reduced proliferation
Vitamin D	Reduced proliferation Enhanced differentiation
Vitamin E	Reduced proliferation
Anti-inflammatory agents	Selective or non-selective COX inhibition
Difluoromethylornithine	Inhibitor of ornithine decarboxylase
Retinoids	Induce cell differentiation
Oltipraz	Glutathione transferase enhanced (improved detoxication)

VITAMIN A

Distinctions have to be drawn between vitamin A as the pre-retinoid β-carotene, retinol, and a range of retinoids such as 9- or 13-*cis*-retinoic acid. The differences are important because retinoids such as 9-*cis*-retinoic acid are clearly mutagenic in their own right. This property raises potential therapeutic and practical difficulties: first, a mutagen could increase the frequency of cancer, if not at the site being considered for treatment then possibly elsewhere; secondly, precautions have to be taken to avoid such treatments in women who might become pregnant.

On the one hand, later liability to cancer, particularly of the lung and stomach, has been associated with low serum levels of β-carotene;[1] on the other hand, no influence on the later frequency of colon cancer has been detected, either here or in a review of available dietary studies.[2]

Direct intervention has also given mixed and unpromising results. A relatively small European study indicated that vitamin A, in combination with vitamins C and E, might prevent the recurrence of colonic adenomata;[3] elsewhere vitamin A or β-carotene, respectively in conjunction with vitamin C and with vitamin C and vitamin E, reduced epithelial cell proliferation in the colon.[4]

In contrast, a randomized controlled study of over 800 patients with colorectal adenomata suggested that vitamins A, C and E in combination did not decrease the frequency of recurrence of colorectal adenomatous polyps.[5] Although it is possible that the effects of vitamin A could be negated by the addition of vitamin C or vitamin E, it is noteworthy that three large and prolonged randomized trials of β-carotene have shown either no value, or significant and disturbing trends in influencing the risk of lung cancer in high-risk populations.[6–8]

Experimental evidence obtained in malignant cell lines has to be interpreted cautiously because such simple systems may be biologically far divorced from those in intact humans. However, in such systems, 9-*cis*-retinoic acid appeared capable of either inhibiting or enhancing the effects of vitamin D in reducing cell proliferation.[9]

Retinoids, of which there are large numbers of molecular variants, are not free from adverse effects. Thus, adverse effects of isotretinoin include drying of the skin, eyes and nasopharynx; headache; optic neuritis; and hepatitis; as well as teratogenicity.

VITAMIN D

Apart from its well-known role in modulating calcium transport, the activated vitamin (the dihydroxylated form) promotes cell differentiation in many tissues. Epidemiological evidence also suggests that high serum levels of vitamin D are associated with protection from colon cancer.[10] Furthermore, low intakes of vitamin D have been associated with raised risks.[11] Added plausibility is given by evidence that vitamin D-responsive receptors are demonstrable in the large bowel mucosa, and that these receptors are likely to be functional, as judged by inhibition of cell multiplication by low concentrations, of the order of 10^{-10} M in cancer cell lines maintained *in vitro*,[12] and from prevention of experimental animal tumours by vitamin D.[13,14]

Accessory evidence of value derives from studies of the effects of calcium salts taken by mouth upon indices of cell proliferation, where reductions have been detected by some, but not others. Whether positive effects are attributable to the actions of absorbed calcium on nuclear receptors, or to some other property, notably bile acid binding, is unclear. Two dietary studies using vitamin D also suggest that there are potential benefits.[15,16]

The limitations of vitamin D as therapy derive from the ease with which hypercalcaemia can be induced, particularly if in combination with calcium salts. However, if effects attributable to vitamin D can be detected epidemiologically, then this implies that enhancing intake while retaining levels within the physiological range would be likely to give significant benefit. A second way of avoiding hypercalcaemic adverse effects would be through using analogues that are non calcaemic. These are already available and in use for treating psoriasis where, despite quite widespread licensed use, the frequency of hypercalcaemia seems low. Experimental studies also indicate that non-calcaemic analogues are at least as effective as dihydroxy-vitamin D in reducing multiplication rates in intestinal cancer cell lines.[17]

VITAMINS C AND E

Vitamins C and E, together with vitamin A, have been aggregated in varying doses and combinations as part of antioxidant regimens in attempting to reduce the rate of recurrence of adenomatous polyps. Epidemiological evidence has suggested that diets high in fruit, vegetable and fibre content may be protective against colorectal cancer, and a reduced risk of colon cancer has been associated with vitamin C intake.

Combined vitamin A and C supplementation, and combined vitamin A, C and E supplementation, have been noted to reduce colonic crypt-cell proliferation rates.[1,18]

In contrast, of three polyp studies, one using vitamin C alone in familial adenomatous disease suggested protection,[19] whereas another employing vitamins C and E was negative, as was a third employing vitamins C and E in the prevention of simple polyps.[20,21]

A full antioxidant regimen employing vitamins A, C and E appeared to be highly protective in a study of 255 polyp patients (209 evaluable), recurrence rates being 5.7% on the vitamin regimen, 14.7% on lactulose, and 35.9% on placebo.[4] These findings differ from those obtained in an 864-patient study (751 completing), where there was no evidence of benefit from the combined treatment (relative risk 1.08, with 95% confidence intervals of 0.91–1.29).[5]

The disappointing results obtained, particularly in the last study, can be contrasted with the moderately strong evidence that vitamin E alone may have value. Combination of data from five independent studies indicated a reduced risk of developing colon cancer with an odds ratio (adjusted for serum cholesterol level) of 0.7 (0.4–1.1) comparing the highest and lowest quartiles.[22] The Iowa Women's Health Study[23] also suggested a strongly significant trend with colon cancer risk falling as serum levels of vitamin E rose.[23]

A coherent synthesis of all these findings is not easily achieved. Interference by one component of a regimen with the activity of another seems an unlikely basis, given that the same full regimen of vitamins A, C and E gave either no protection against polyp recurrence or apparently good protection. A second possibility is that there is a divergence between cancer prevention and adenoma prevention (i.e. the regimens retard progression). Again, there are no consistent patterns to suggest that this is plausible.

FOLATE

The epidemiological evidence of an inverse association between fruit and vegetable intake and the occurrence of colorectal cancer, has raised the possibility that the phenomenon is explained by dietary folate intake.[24] Supportive evidence is limited, and there appear to have been no direct intervention studies.

SEX HORMONES AND ADRENOCORTICOIDS

It has been known for many years that, when age-specific colorectal cancer incidence rates are compared in men and women, there is a progressive increase in the proportions of men with colonic or rectal cancer as age increases. The basis for this observation is unclear, but sex-steroid receptors are demonstrable in the large bowel epithelium, indicating that a direct sex-steroid action is possible.[25] Direct studies of the effect of oestrogen, in particular, on the multiplication of intestinal cancer cell lines, has not yielded particularly striking results; however, epidemiologically it has been consistently noted that the use of hormone replacement therapy in women is associated with about a one-third reduction in the risk of large bowel cancer.[26,27] Direct application of this finding has not been attempted. Although tamoxifen – an anti-oestrogen – has been explored as a treatment for established disease on the basis of a possible similarity between breast and bowel cancer, no evidence of material alterations in patterns of tumour behaviour have emerged.

Dehydroepiandrosterone (DHEA) has antiproliferative actions that may depend in some way on adrenocorticoid actions or possibly upon inhibition of glucose-1-phosphate dehydrogenase and the pentose phosphate pathway.[28]

ANTI-INFLAMMATORY DRUGS

It has been known for many years that, if experimental animals are treated with NSAIDs at the time that they are exposed to carcinogens such as azoxymethane, then there is a reduced yield of bowel tumours.[29] The possible clinical significance of these observations was not realized until epidemiological studies indicated that NSAID use appeared to be associated with a reduced risk of large bowel cancer, and that the same did not appear true for other drugs, such as sedatives.[30–32]

There have now been a large series of studies of experimental carcinogenesis in animals, as well as multiple case–cohort or case–control observational studies and explanatory molecular and biochemical investigations.

In general, the epidemiological studies have indicated that takers of NSAIDs appear to have reduced risks of colorectal cancer and of adenomatous polyps. These findings do not appear attributable to confounding factors and they seem to apply generally to aspirin and to other NSAIDs.

Observational studies are not entirely secure as bases for determining cause and effect. However, the support of animal studies showing inhibition of tumour induction and of clinical studies showing evidence of polyp regression in familial adenomatous polypsis coli strongly indicate causal influences.[33,34] These findings have prompted examination of the mechanistic bases, and attempts to decide on appropriate dosage of particular NSAIDs. The NSAIDs appear to increase the occurrence of programmed cell death (apoptosis).[35] The best-known property of these drugs is their inhibition of cyclo-oxygenase (COX), which is probably (but not certainly) responsible. It is now known that this is divisible into two broad types – one (COX-1) associated with cell restitution and the other (COX-2) with the facilitation of antiinflammatory responses. Examination of tissue COX activity indicates that COX-2 tends to be upregulated in colorectal tumours, suggesting that an agent selective for COX-2 might be of particular benefit.[36] Furthermore, avoidance of COX-1 inhibitors would seem likely to reduce the occurrence of the most important adverse effects of the non-selective inhibitors, e.g. upper gastrointestinal intolerance.

The classical NSAIDs (aspirin, indomethacin, piroxicam and others), first marketed some 20 years or more ago, are non-selective. Recently introcuced selective COX-2 inhibitors, celecoxib and rofecoxib, if proven to be nontoxic in prolonged use, are logical replacements. Interesting as these are, there is good clinical sense in considering the classical NSAIDs for chemoprophylaxis because their long-term therapeutic effects and adverse effects are well understood.

Considerations of dosage here become important. It seems unlikely that doses required would be materially lower than for ordinary treatment of musculoskeletal disease. Thus, the epidemiological studies, showing something of the order of one-third reductions of cancer frequency, imply a need for at least standard doses. Some epidemiological investigations would suggest that exposure must be substantial and prolonged.

MINERALS

Calcium salts

Reduced cellular proliferation has been demonstrated in colonic epithelial cells in animals but not in humans.[37,38] Whether benefits from taking calcium salts would be any different from those of vitamin D are unclear. One extra effect of potential value would be the binding of bile acids.

Selenium

Selenium has to be added as an essential mineral to parenteral feeds. Observational studies have indicated that those individuals with levels detected in the blood or tissues (typically the nails) that are relatively high but within the normal range, may be protected partially against colorectal cancer.[39] There is at least an equal body of evidence to indicate lack of effect.[40,41] Currently, there would seem to be insufficient basis for recommending selenium supplements in chemoprophylaxis.

OTHER SUBSTANCES

Bile salts

Although bile acids have come under suspicion as promoters of the occurrence of colorectal cancer, there could well be important differences between individual primary or secondary members of the series. Such differences are well understood in proneness or otherwise to cause hepatotoxicity.

Ursodeoxycholic acid, in particular, appears to reduce the frequency of experimental animal tumours.[42] It is an attractive candidate because long-term use has already been well studied in patients with gallstones or with primary biliary cirrhosis without evidence of important hazards emerging.

Histamine H_2 antagonists

Suggestions of beneficial immunological properties *inter alia* prompted interest in possible value in cancer prevention or modulation of disease occurrence. A single trial in gastric cancer suggested enhanced survival in treated disease, whether resectable or not, but confirmation of value has not been obtained.[43]

Difluoromethylornithine

Difluoromethylornithine, an ornithine decarboxylase inhibitor, reduces the occurrence of experimental animal colonic tumours.[44] Use in humans appears to be limited by ototoxicity.[45]

Oltipraz

Oltipraz, a glutathione transferase enhancing agent, appears to reduce the occurrence of experimental animal tumours by enhancing xenobiotic detoxication.[46]

Conclusions

Despite a wide range of candidate treatments, none can yet be recommended as being of proven efficiency. Novel agents have the drawback of requiring full safety testing, because most recipients of chemopreventive agents will never actually develop the disease in question if left untreated. Of the standard well-proven pharmaceuticals available, the NSAIDs show most promise. Non-selective agents have acceptable safety profiles, but these may be enhanced in time with the emergence of selective COX inhibitors. Amongst the vitamins, vitamin D and possibly retinoids as differentiating agents, are of particular interest.

References

1. Stahelin HB, Gey KF, Eicholzer M, Ludin E. Beta-carotene and cancer prevention: the Basel study. *Am J Clin Nutr* 1991; 53(Suppl 1): 265S–269S

2. Willett WC, Hunter DJ. Vitamin A and cancers of the breast, large bowel, and prostate: epidemiological evidence. *Nutr Rev* 1994; 52: S53–59

3. Roncucci L, Di-Donato P, Carati L *et al.* Antioxidant vitamins or lactulose for the prevention of the recurrence of colorectal adenomas. *Dis Colon Rectum* 1993; 36: 227–234

4. Paganelli GM, Biasco G, Brandi G *et al.* Effect of vitamin A, C and E supplementation on rectal cell proliferation in patients with colorectal adenomas. *J Natl Cancer Inst* 1992; 84: 47–51

5. Greenberg ER, Baron JA, Tosteson TD *et al.* for the Polyp Prevention Study Group. A clinical trial of antioxidant vitamins to prevent colorectal adenoma. *N Engl J Med* 1994; 331: 141–147

6. Omenn GS, Goodman G, Thornquist MD *et al.* Effects of combination of beta-carotene and vitamin A on lung cancer and cardiovascular disease. *N Engl J Med* 1996; 334: 1150–1155

7. Hennekens CH, Buring JE, Manson JE *et al.* Lack of effect of long-term supplementation with beta-carotene on the incidence of malignant neoplasms and cardiovascular disease. *N Engl J Med* 1996; 334: 1145–1149

8. The Alpha-Tocopherol, Beta-carotene Cancer Prevention Study Group (1994). The effect of vitamin E and beta-carotene on the incidence of lung cancer and other cancers in male smokers. *N Engl J Med* 1994; 330: 1029–1035

9. Kane KF, Langman MJS, Williams GR. Anti-proliferative responses of two human colon cancer cell lines to vitamin D3 are differentially modified by 9 cis retinoic acid. *Cancer Res* 1996; 56: 623–632

10. Garland CF, Comstock GW, Garland FC *et al.* Serum 25-hydroxyvitamin D and colon cancer: eight year prospective study. *Lancet* 1989; 2: 1176–1178

11. Garland CF, Shekelle RB, Barrett Connor E *et al.* Dietary vitamin D and calcium and risk of colorectal cancer: a 19-year prospective study in men. *Lancet* 1985; 1: 307–309

12. Kane KF, Langman MJS, Williams GR. 1,25-Dihydroxy vitamin D_3 and retinoid X receptor expression in human colorectal neoplasms. *Gut* 1995; 36: 255–258

13. Belleli A, Shany S, Levy J *et al.* A protective role of 1,25-dihydroxy vitamin D_3 in chemically induced rat colon carcinogenesis. *Carcinogenesis* 1992; 13: 2293

14. Sitrin MD, Halline AG, Abrahams C, Brasitus TA. Dietary calcium and vitamin D modulate 1,2 dimethylhydrazine-induced colonic carcinogenesis in the rat. *Cancer Res* 1991; 51: 5608–5613

15. Kampman E, Giovannucci E, van't Veer P *et al.* Calcium, vitamin D, dairy foods, and the occurrence of colorectal adenomas among men and women in two prospective studies. *Am J Epidemiol* 1994; 139: 16–29

16. Bostick RM, Potter JD, Sellers TA *et al.* Relation of calcium, vitamin D, and dairy food intake to incidence of colon cancer among older women. The Iowa Women's Health Study. *Am J Epidemiol* 1993; 137: 1302–1317

17. Binderup L, Bramme E. Effects of a novel vitamin D analogue MC903 on cell proliferation and differentiation *in vitro* and on calcium metabolism *in vivo*. *Biochem Pharmacol* 1988; 37: 889–895

18. Cahill RJ, O'Sullivan KR, Matthias PM *et al.* Effects of vitamin antioxidant supplementation on cell kinetics of patients with adenomatous polyps. *Gut* 1993; 34: 963–967

19. Bussey HJ, De Cosse JJ, Deschner EE. A randomised trial of ascorbic acid in polyposis coli. *Cancer* 1982; 50: 1434–1439

20. De Cosse JJ, Miller HH, Lesser ML. Effect of wheat fibre and vitamins C and E on rectal polyps in patients with familial adenomatous polyposis. *J Natl Cancer Inst* 1989; 81: 1290–1297

21. McKeown-Eyssen G, Holloway C, Jazmaji V *et al.* A randomised trial of Vitamins C and E in the prevention of recurrence of colorectal polyps. *Cancer Res* 1988; 48: 4701–4705

22. Longnecker MP, Martin-Moreno JM, Knekt P *et al.* Serum alphatocopherol concentration in relation to subsequent colorectal cancer: pooled data from five cohorts. *J Natl Cancer Inst* 1992; 84: 430–435

23. Bostick RM, Potter JD, McKenzie DR *et al.* Reduced risk of colon cancer with high intake of Vitamin E: the Iowa Women's Health Study. *Cancer Res* 1993; 53: 4230–4237

24. Little J. Is folic acid pluripotent? A review of the associations with congenital anomalies, cancer and other diseases. In: Ioannides C, Lewis DFV (eds) *Drugs, diet and disease. Vol. 1: Mechanistic approaches to cancer.* New York: Ellis Horwood, 1995.

25. Singh S, Sheppard MC, Langman MJS. Sex differences in the incidence of colorectal cancer: an exploration of oestrogen and progesterone receptors. *Gut* 1993; 34: 611–615

26. Calle EE, Miracle-McMahill HL, Thorn MJ, Heath CW Estrogen replacement therapy and risk of fatal colon cancer in a prospective cohort of post-menopausal women. *J Natl Cancer Inst* 1995; 87: 517–523

27. Newcomb PA, Storer BE. Post-menopausal hormone use and risk of large bowel cancer. *J Natl Cancer Inst* 1995; 87: 1067–1071

28. Schwartz AG, Pashko LL. Cancer chemoprevention with the adrenocortical steroid dehydroepiandrosterone and structural analogs. *Cell Biochem* 1993; Suppl 17G: 73–79

29. Reddy BS, Rao CV, Rivenson A, Kelloff G. Inhibitory effect of aspirin on azoxymethane-induced colon carcinogenesis in F 344 rats. *Carcinogenesis* 1993; 14: 1493–1497

30. Kune GA, Kune S, Watson JF. Colorectal cancer risk, chronic illnesses, operations and medications: case control results from the Melbourne Colorectal Cancer Study. *Cancer Res* 1988; 48: 4399–4404

31. Rosenberg L, Palmer JR, Zauber AG *et al.* A hypothesis: non-steroidal anti-inflammatory drugs reduce the incidence of large bowel cancer. *J Natl Cancer Inst* 1991; 83: 355–358

32. Peleg I, Maibach HT, Brown SH, Wilcox CM. Aspirin and non-steroidal anti-inflammatory drug use and the risk of subsequent colorectal cancer. *Arch Intern Med* 1994; 154: 394–399

33. Labayle D, Fischer D, Vielh P *et al.* Sulindac causes regression of rectal polyps in familial adenomatous polyposis. *Gastroenterology* 1991; 101: 635–639

34. Giardiello FM, Hamilton SR, Krush AJ *et al.* Treatment of colonic and rectal adenomas with sulindac in familial adenomatous polyposis. *N Engl J Med* 1993; 328: 1313–1316

35. Piazza GA, Kulchak Rahm AL, Krutzysch M *et al.* Anti neoplastic drugs sulindac sulfide and sulfone inhibit cell growth by inducing apoptosis. *Cancer Res* 1995; 55: 3110–3116

36. Eberhart CE, Coffey RJ, Radhika A *et al.* Upregulation of cyclo-oxygenase 2 gene expression in human colorectal adenomas and adenocarcinomas. *Gastroenterology* 1994; 1183–1188

37. Reshef R, Rozen P, Fireman Z *et al.* Effect of a calcium enriched diet on the colonic epithelial hyperproliferation induced by N-methyl-N-nitro-N-nitrosoguanidine in rats on a low calcium and fat diet. *Cancer Res* 1990; 50: 1764–1767

38. Bostick RM, Potter JD, Fosdick L *et al.* Calcium and colorectal epithelial proliferation – a preliminary randomised double-blinded placebo-controlled clinical trial. *J Natl Cancer Inst* 1993; 85: 132–141

39. Clark LC, Hixson LJ, Combs GF Jr *et al.* Plasma selenium concentration predicts the prevalence of colorectal adenomatous polyps. *Cancer Epidemiol, Biomark Prevent* 1993; 2: 41–46

40. Vanden Brandt PA, Goldbohm RA, van't Veer P *et al.* A prospective cohort study on toenail selenium levels and risk of gastrointestinal cancer. *J Natl Cancer Inst* 1993; 85: 224–229

41. Garland M, Morris JS, Stampfer MJ *et al.* Prospective study of toenail selenium levels and cancer among women. *J Natl Cancer Inst* 1995; 87: 497

42. Ernest DL, Holubec H, Wali RK *et al.* Chemoprevention of azoxymethane-induced colonic carcinogenesis by supplemental dietary ursodeoxycholic acid. *Cancer Res* 1994; 54: 5071–5074

43. Tonneson H, Knigge U, Bulow S *et al.* Effect of cimetidine on survival after gastric cancer. *Lancet* 1988; ii: 990–992

44. Rao CV, Rivenson A, Katiwalla M *et al.* Chempreventive effect of oltipraz during different stages of experimental colon carcinogenesis induced by azoxymethane in male F344 rats. *Cancer Res* 1993; 53: 2502–2506

45. Love RR, Carbone PP, Verma AK *et al.* Randomised phase 1 chemoprevention dose-seeking study of alpha-difluoromethylornithine. *J Natl Cancer Inst* 1993; 85: 732–737

46. O'Dwyer PJ, Szarka CE, Yao KS *et al.* Modulation of gene expression in subjects at risk for colorectal cancer by the chemopreventative dithiolethione oltipraz. *J Clin Invest* 1996; 98: 1210–1217

Chapter 7

ELECTIVE SURGERY FOR COLORECTAL CANCER

S. Dorudi and N.S. Williams

Introduction

This chapter discusses the central issues in colorectal cancer surgery performed on an elective basis. Surgery for complications of colorectal cancer (obstruction and perforation), which is covered elsewhere, has been specifically excluded. In addition, any discussion of laparoscopic surgery for colorectal cancer has been avoided, as the author is of the opinion that this technique should be employed only in the context of a clinical trial examining its oncological safety versus that of open surgery. Following the diagnosis of colorectal cancer, it is necessary to decide on the optimal management of the patient. Surgery remains the primary treatment modality for cure, whether performed as a major colorectal resection at laparotomy or as a transanal excision in selected rectal cancers.

Preoperative evaluation

EVALUATION OF THE PATIENT

A thorough history and examination of the patient will often give valuable information as to their suitability for a general anaesthetic and major surgery. Any correctable co-morbidity (especially cardiorespiratory) must be treated – or, certainly, stabilized – prior to surgery. Old age does not necessarily preclude any patient from a potentially curative resection: elderly patients have to be assessed individually and the risk–benefit ratio of any proposed surgery carefully examined in the context of their current quality of life and future life expectancy. However, surgery for colorectal cancer is inadvisable if the risks of the operation are deemed to be greater than the potential benefits. Preoperative full blood count and renal function should be assessed, as these indices can be adversely affected by the patient's colorectal cancer.

FAMILY HISTORY

The importance of obtaining a detailed family history for colorectal cancer and, indeed, other malignancies is now well recognized.[1] Approximately 80% of colorectal cancers are sporadic or occur in individuals with no known predisposition to the disease. The remainder arise in patients with a family history of colorectal cancer or polyps, previous colorectal cancer, or a predisposing condition such as inflammatory bowel disease. Patients with a family history of colorectal cancer in one or more first-degree relatives (parent, sibling or offspring), but with no defined genetic syndrome, may account for 10–15% of patients with colorectal cancer; 5–8% of all colorectal adenocarcinomas can be attributed to patients with hereditary non-polyposis colorectal cancer (HNPCC), while familial adenomatous polyposis accounts for the remaining 1% (see Chapter 3). These observations underscore the importance of taking a detailed family history for malignancies. In our own unit, a standardized cancer family history questionnaire is completed by all patients with colorectal cancer.

EVALUATION OF THE TUMOUR

The site, multiplicity, size, local extent and regional/distant spread of the tumour need to be evaluated carefully before surgery can be planned.

Site

The site of the tumour will dictate the proposed resection. In rectal cancers a careful digital examination, together with rigid sigmoidoscopy, will determine accurately the lowest level of the tumour from the anal verge.

Multiplicity

Synchronous cancers are reported in 1.5–7.5% of cases, whereas synchronous polyps occur more frequently (between 25 and 40% of cases)[2]. These lesions will be detected either by careful and complete preoperative colonoscopy or by high quality double contrast radiology. The reliability of an air-contrast barium enema approaches that of endoscopy for significant lesions, but small lesions (up to 1 cm) will be detected more accurately by colonoscopy. The advantages of colonoscopy are that a histological diagnosis can usually be established, if appropriate, polypectomy can be performed. The preoperative detection of significant lesions will lead to a change of the planned surgical procedure in approximately 10% of patients. A preoperative colonoscopy is thus ideal, provided that the tumour can be intubated and the rest of the colon visualized. If this is not possible, a double-contrast barium enema will suffice.

Size and local extent

Although tumour size is rarely problematic in colon cancer surgery, large rectal cancers may benefit from adjuvant preoperative chemo- and/or radiotherapy, as these tumours are often advanced and locally invasive. Patients found to have large rectal cancers should be carefully assessed by an examination under sedation or a general anaesthetic, together with local imaging to determine local tumour extent (see below). Digital examination of a rectal tumour will establish its circumferential extent and its mobility or fixation, providing information on the suitability of local excision. On the other hand, detection of submucosal tumour extension and extrarectal involvement do not augur well for a curative procedure, if the lesion can be resected at all. Such findings will support the use of adjunctive preoperative therapy.

The local extent of a colonic tumour rarely alters the surgical approach that is undertaken. Generally, adjacent organ involvement is uncommon but its presence and local surgical resectability will dicate the precise surgical approach. However, some pivotal management decisons will have to be considered as a result of accurate local regional staging of rectal cancers, particularly those in the lower two-thirds. Three questions need to be addressed: (1) what is the depth of intramural penetration, (2) is there extramural invasion, and (3) are lymph node metastases present? Thus, the discussion below concerns the staging of rectal cancer.

Digital examination remains important in the assessment of the extent of distal rectal tumours (see above). When performed by an experienced clinician, rectal examination can predict the local extent of a tumour in 80% of patients,[3] but mesorectal lymph node involvement is often difficult to detect unless such nodes are enlarged and indurated. The accuracy of clinical examination is highest for advanced lesions and lowest for early cancers, limiting its use in the selection of tumours amenable to local treatment. Complete local regional staging requires cross-sectional imaging with computed tomography (CT), endorectal ultrasound (ERUS) or magnetic resonance imaging (MRI).

CT does not allow accurate assessment of

the depth of penetration of a rectal cancer, as this imaging modality cannot discriminate between the layers comprising the gut wall. Its greatest advantage lies in the detection of extrarectal spread; thus, it should be employed in all patients deemed to have a locally advanced tumour on clinical examination. The assessment of nodal involvement within the mesorectum and pelvis is also inaccurate using CT, as it is dependent upon the detection of enlarged lymph nodes. However, lymph nodes less than 1.5 cm in diameter often contain micrometastases. Not surprisingly, CT staging has been found to have a poor correlation with subsequent pathological staging, but it is reasonably accurate in identifying extrarectal extension, especially in the presence of adjacent organ involvement.[4] The knowledge that there is extrarectal organ involvement may well alter the surgical approach and should alert the surgeon of potential technical difficulties during the surgery. Thus, its primary use in the management of patients with rectal cancer lies in assisting the selection of patients with advanced tumours who may benefit from adjuvant preoperative radiotherapy. Additionally, CT does have a well-established role in the detection of distant metastatic disease, which is discussed below.

ERUS is currently undisputed as the technique of choice in accurately assessing the depth of transmural invasion of a rectal cancer.[5] Using a circumferential 7.0 mHz transducer, the rectal wall is imaged as a five-layered structure through which the extent of tumour penetration can be assessed. The layers are alternatively echogenic and echo poor. There are three echogenic (white) lines and two echo-poor (black) lines (see Figure 7.1). The middle echogenic submucosa is extremely important, as breach of this tissue defines an invasive cancer. In the presence of this finding, the muscularis propria is carefully evaluated throughout the length of the tumour, as invasion beyond this layer denotes tumour extension into the perirectal fat. ERUS is user dependent and the accuracy of published series has varied. However, in experienced hands the overall correlation of ERUS staging with pathological stage (for transmural tumour penetration) ranges between 87 and 94%, with up to 10% either over- or under-staged.[6] As with CT, ERUS accuracy improves with advanced tumour stage and is thus very reliable in determining whether a cancer is confined to the rectal wall or has extended beyond. The reported accuracy of identifying lymph node metastases varies between 60 and 80%.[6] Large nodal size does not necessarily imply the presence of tumour metastases, but involved nodes are generally more than 5 mm in diameter; moreover, they do possess some specific morphological features that aid their diagnosis.[7] The use of ERUS-guided fine-needle aspiration, or even needle biopsy, will undoubtedly increase the accuracy for detecting lymph node spread. ERUS cannot be performed in patients with stenotic lesions or in lesions beyond 12 cm from the anal verge, as the entire length of the tumour needs to be examined to establish the local stage accurately.

MRI suffers from the same limitations as CT in staging rectal cancer because it does not allow discrimination between layers of the bowel wall and, again, relies on the presence of nodal enlargement to identify lymph node metastases. The technique has not been widely adopted in rectal cancer staging, other than in

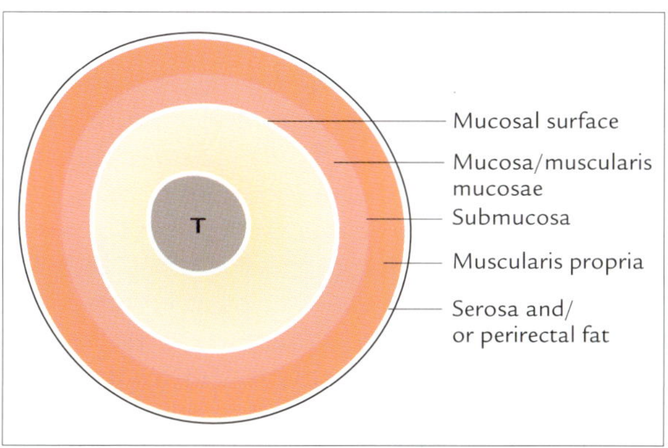

Figure 7.1. *Endoanal ultrasound appearance of the rectal wall.*

a research setting. However, the recent advent of endoluminal coils with enhanced resolution may improve the accuracy of MRI staging in rectal neoplasms.

Preoperative assessment of the local regional extent of rectal cancer should identify four groups of patients: (1) those who are suitable for a potentially curative resection without any further therapy; (2) those who require adjuvant radiotherapy prior to surgery; (3) those whose tumours may be amenable to local excision; and, finally (4), patients whose tumours will necessitate extended regional resections to achieve cure, or at least adequate local control.

Distant spread

Establishing the presence or absence of distant metastatic disease should be the ideal aim in all patients. At present there is no evidence that such assessment alters the final prognosis. Chest radiography and liver imaging – either by ultrasound or, preferably, by CT scan – should be performed. Liver metastases, detected preoperatively, are present in 15–20% of patients.[8] Even in their presence, the majority of patients with locally operable tumours will benefit from resection of the primary. However, the extent and number of liver metastases, pulmonary spread and the age of the patient are all important factors in reaching a final decision (see below in the section on palliative surgery; pp. 125). Intra-operative ultrasound of the liver is also employed to assess liver metastases, but it is usually performed in the context of planning a liver resection (see Chapter 8).

Preparation of the patient

Before a patient can undergo colorectal cancer surgery, some specific preoperative issues must be addressed.

INFORMED CONSENT

All patients will need to give informed consent prior to their surgery; however, precisely what factors constitute such consent have only recently come under scrutiny. In our opinion, it is mandatory to inform the patient of the following issues that are germane to their surgery. The possibility of stoma formation will always need to be discussed, irrespective of the resection planned. However, it is the authors' practice to ensure that all patients undergoing anterior resection (not just low anterior resection) are seen and prepared for a stoma by appropriate specialist nurses. The risks of autonomic nerve dysfunction, with the likelihood of developing urinary and sexual problems (particularly impotence in male patients), also should always be discussed in patients undergoing rectal surgery. All patients undergoing any colorectal resection should be warned of postoperative stool frequency, and the poor functional results after low anterior resection will need to be explained and emphasized in some depth. Finally, in the authors' opinion, patients undergoing anterior resection of the rectum must be informed of the possibility of anastomotic failure and its sequelae.

BOWEL PREPARATION

Mechanical bowel preparation is still regarded as necessary in patients undergoing elective colorectal cancer surgery. There have been recent successful challenges to this long-held doctrine,[9,10] but reducing the total faecal mass is still generally considered as desirable. However, osmotic-based cathartics can cause significant preoperative fluid shifts, resulting in dehydration; it is, therefore, the author's practice to ensure that patients receive appropriate intravenous fluids on the evening before surgery. Elderly patients, in particular, will need longer periods of intravenous hydration, as they are often not able to tolerate the large volumes of oral fluids that need to be taken during bowel preparation.

THROMBOEMBOLISM PROPHYLAXIS

Thromboembolism prophylaxis is mandatory for all patients undergoing colorectal resection unless there is a specific contraindication. The incidence of deep vein thrombosis, pulmonary emboli and fatal pulmonary emboli can all be reduced in general surgical patients with the use of subcutaneous heparin administered peri- and postoperatively.[11] This can be supplemented with intermittent calf compression during surgery and the use of graduated compression stockings in the postoperative period.

Surgery for colorectal cancer

The abdomen is explored through a midline incision, although other incisions are commonly used. A thorough laparotomy is performed, with special reference to the primary tumour, other colonic pathology (e.g. severe diverticulosis, synchronous cancers) and the presence/absence of peritoneal or distant metastatic disease in the liver. Assessment of the primary cancer should ascertain the size of the tumour and whether the malignancy has infiltrated local peritoneum or adjacent structures. At this stage it is usually possible to decide whether surgery is being undertaken with curative or with palliative intent.

Curative surgery: colon cancer

GENERAL PRINCIPLES

The standard surgical treatment for colon cancer is a hemicolectomy and regional lymphadenectomy. The precise resection depends upon the location of the tumour and its arterial supply, which in turn will dictate the extent of the regional lymph node dissection. A 'no-touch technique' now seems unnecessary as there is no convincing evidence that Turnbull's original concept of initial vascular ligation bestows a significant survival advantage.[12] Similarly, extended regional lymphadenectomy (i.e. beyond the regional blood supply of the colonic segment to include para-aortic lymph nodes) does not appear to confer any consistent survival advantage and increases the morbidity of the procedure.[13] The most compelling reason to perform an adequate regional lymphadenectomy is the emerging evidence that patients with lymph node-positive cancers benefit from adjuvant chemotherapy;[14] it is, therefore, necessary to remove sufficient lymph nodes to allow accurate staging.

The surgery should be performed by careful sharp dissection along anatomical planes with identification and preservation of important structures. Extensive malignant infiltration of the local peritoneum and contiguous organ involvement are both uncommon but their management can be problematic and may preclude curative surgery. However, the ultimate aim in this situation is achievement of a tumour-free resection margin. Infiltrated peritoneum should be circumcised with the tumour along a macroscopically normal margin. If possible, attached adjacent organs, whether such attachment is due to direct tumour penetration or to an inflammatory process, should be removed *en bloc* with the primary lesion. This may involve resection of small bowel or a segment of bladder wall, or cholecystectomy. The area of invasion should be marked with metal surgical clips, and postoperative radiotherapy should be considered once the final histopathology report is available.

The outcome of restoration of intestinal continuity following the resection of a colonic tumour is as important to the patient as the outcome of the cancer resection itself. Anastomotic failure is associated with high morbidity and not insignificant mortality. Irrespective of the precise technique used (i.e. sutured vs stapled, one layer vs two layers), it is necessary to heed some fundamental principles of surgical technique to ensure success. An anastomosis must be performed between well-perfused bowel ends, in the absence of tension and significant sepsis. It is useful to cut the marginal artery of the colon prior to its ligation to observe pulsatile arterial flow before constructing an anastomosis.

SPECIFIC MANAGEMENT ISSUES

There are a number of specific management issues in a subset of patients with colon cancer that deserve particular discussion.

Patients with synchronous tumours

The true incidence of synchronous carcinoma can be assessed only by rigorous preoperative colonoscopy in all patients with colorectal cancer, or at least early endoscopy following surgery (certainly within 6 months). However, pooled data from several series indicate an incidence of approximately 6%.[2] A cancer discovered on early postoperative colonoscopy most probably represents a synchronous lesion rather than a true metachronous tumour. Every effort should be made to perform a complete examination of the colon once a colorectal cancer is diagnosed. In patients with stenotic lesions this is not always possible and some authors have suggested intra-operative colonoscopy to examine the mucosa proximal to the constricting cancer.[15] Certainly, careful intra-operative assessment is required in all patients undergoing surgery for synchronous cancers. Before the surgical strategy for such patients is formulated, the characteristics and biology of these tumours need to be considered, as does the patient's age. Patients with more than one cancer have an extremely high incidence of both synchronous and metachronous adenomas[16] (50% of patients develop metachronous polyps), but do not appear to exhibit a consistent predisposition towards developing metachronous cancers. Synchronous cancers are widely distributed throughout the colon and there is no evidence to suggest clustering within the same bowel segment.

The primary consideration is an adequate cancer resection, but subtotal colectomy (with ileorectal or ileosigmoid anastomosis) should be strongly considered for many patients with synchronous carcinomas. The indication for this procedure is particularly strong in young patients in whom a curative resection can be performed, and also in the presence of synchronous adenomas. The surgery removes the bulk of the mucosa at risk and facilitates endoscopic follow-up. In the elderly, subtotal colectomy can lead to poor functional results with disabling bowel frequency, although this complication is generally avoided if a short segment of the sigmoid colon is retained. Discontinuous colonic resections for synchronous cancers can be performed in patients who will attend lifelong colonoscopic surveillance. This strategy may well be appropriate when one of the tumours is located in the upper rectum. Alternatively, partial colectomy (i.e. a single resection) is an appropriate option if an early cancer in a polyp can be removed endoscopically prior to surgery. Interestingly, subtotal colectomy does not appear to result in any survival advantage over segmental resection in patients with synchronous cancers.[2]

Patients with HNPCC (Lynch syndromes)

Patients with HNPCC can be distinguished from those with sporadic colorectal cancer by a series of quite stringent diagnostic criteria used originally to identify family kindreds for genetic analysis. However, the fundamental features of the condition are young age, proximal location of cancers and synchronous and metachronous colonic lesions. A patient with HNPCC who develops colon cancer should undergo subtotal colectomy with an ileorectal anastomosis. Excision of all of the colonic mucosa is justified because of the high incidence of synchronous and metachronous colonic cancers. Removal of the rectum and its attendant morbidity should be avoided, as the majority of the cancers (>80%) are proximal to the rectum in patients with HNPCC. Regular sigmoidoscopy is required, as the risk of developing a metachronous rectal cancer is currently unknown after subtotal colectomy in patients with HNPCC. If HNPCC is subsequently diagnosed in a patient who has already undergone a segmental resection, a strong case can be made for a completion colectomy as there is a 45% risk of developing a metachronous cancer in the residual colon in the ensuing 10 years.[17] Interestingly, Lynch himself has recently proposed that patients with proven HNPCC germline genetic lesions should be offered prophylactic subtotal colectomy before a cancer develops.[17]

Patients with ulcerative colitis

In the context of malignant disease there are two indications for surgery in patients with ulcerative colitis: First, a minority develop a carcinoma; secondly, surgery is performed following the detection of dysplasia on colonoscopic surveillance. Clearly, these conditions are not mutually exclusive in patients with ulcerative colitis. The risk of cancer in ulcerative colitis is increased by both the extent of the disease and its duration and not by the disease severity. Colitis-associated carcinoma can be difficult to diagnose and often presents at an advanced stage, but cancer development is often associated with dysplastic changes within the colon. Surveillance programmmes have been instituted to screen for this change and encourage prophylactic colectomy in such patients. There are a number of problems with this approach as dysplasia can be difficult to diagnose with confidence in the presence of mucosal inflammation. Furthermore, cancers can occur in the absence of dysplasia; conversely, frequent dysplasia screening fails to detect some carcinomas.

There is no place for segmental resections in patients with ulcerative colitis who develop an adenocarcinoma and four options should be considered:[18] these include total proctocolectomy with end ileostomy; total proctocolectomy and Kock continent ileostomy; subtotal colectomy and ileorectal anastomosis; and, finally, restorative proctocolectomy with formation of an ileo-anal pouch. The Kock continent ileostomy provides a flush ileostomy with a continent inverted nipple valve. The technique is complex and prone to complications and is now rarely performed in the UK. Total proctocolectomy with an end (Brooke) ileostomy is a tried and tested procedure and should be regarded as the standard against which all other options are compared. It may be an appropriate option in the elderly patient, as the entire mucosa at risk is removed in one familiar operation. The potential morbidity of the pelvic and perineal dissections and the prospect of a permanent ileostomy should not be dismissed lightly and will prove unacceptable to many younger patients. These problems are obviated by subtotal colectomy and the formation of an ileorectal anastomosis but the residual rectum, if diseased, can cause troublesome symptoms and may develop a cancer. This procedure is a good option in young patients with relative rectal sparing and a proximal cancer, particularly, as it obviates the risk of pelvic nerve dysfunction. Lifelong endoscopic surveillance of the residual mucosa is mandatory and completion proctectomy with ileostomy or restorative proctectomy may be necessary at a later date. Restorative proctocolectomy goes some distance in achieving many of the objectives of the 'ideal' operation in this situation. The procedure is technically demanding and generally requires two stages. Moreover, there is a comparatively high early and late (pouchitis) complication rate, and final pouch function can be very variable. Complete mucosectomy should be performed in patients with cancer as, if the rectum is transected at the pelvic floor, the risk of developing dysplasia in the remaining columnar cuff above the anal transition zone is high in such cases.[19] Indeed, some surgeons are reluctant to perform restorative surgery after proctocolectomy in patients with ulcerative colitis who develop a cancer.

Curative surgery: rectal cancer

LOCAL EXCISION

It is important to distinguish between local excision of a rectal cancer with curative intent and local excision performed as a compromise in treatment of a very elderly or unfit patient or alternatively as a palliative procedure. Inevitably, the boundary between these groups of patients becomes indistinct. Nevertheless, the discussion below addresses the issues involved in the selection of appropriate patients for curative local excision and the techniques currently in practice. Pathological studies have revealed that some early stage rectal cancers have a very low propensity for lymph node metastasis.[20] It is now recognized that in these patients no additional benefit will be accrued by a procedure that does any more than remove the primary cancer. One of the future areas of intensive study in this field will be the development of greater precision in determining which patients can undergo only local excision and which need a standard radical excision with regional lymphadenectomy.

Selection of patients for local excision

Favourable rectal cancers should be less than 3 cm in diameter and preoperative biopsies should not reveal any adverse pathological features. There is significant discrepancy between tumour grade, assessed on biopsy, and the final differentiation status of the excised specimen. Nevertheless, a tumour biopsy revealing poor differentiation or the presence of vascular or lymphatic invasion should be regarded as contraindications to local excision of a rectal cancer for cure. Several biopsies should be taken both to confirm an adenocarcinoma and to maximize the amount of pathological information obtained. Patients with moderately or well-differentiated cancers and no other adverse pathological features should undergo preoperative staging with ERUS. Clear uT1 lesions with no discernible lymph node metastases can be treated by local excision. Tumours should be located in the lower rectum and, certainly, the upper margin of the tumour should be within reach of the palpating finger. However, endoscopic techniques now allow cancers of the upper rectum, with favourable pathology and stage, to be excised locally as well.

Local excision techniques

There are four surgical approaches – transanal, trans-sacral, trans-sphincteric and transanal endoscopic microsurgery (see ref. 21 for review). The two open dorsal approaches (trans-sacral and trans-sphincteric) are now seldom performed.

Transanal excision

The patient is positioned to maximize access to the tumour. Thus, patients with anterior cancers should be placed prone in the jack-knife position, whereas posterior lesions are best approached in the lithotomy position. Excision of carcinomas must be full thickness down to the perirectal fat with an appropriate clearance margin. The authors perform the excision with diathermy dissection, sequentially excising and placing sutures so that good control of the tumour and rectal wall wound can be maintained throughout the procedure. A large defect in the rectal wall following excision must be repaired in a transverse axis to obviate narrowing of the lumen. Double-action needle holders are very useful in this surgery as they provide excellent grasping power, while being long enough not to obliterate the view.

Dorsal approaches

The trans-sacral approach was first described by Kraske in 1885 for high or mid-rectal tumours.[22] The rectum is accessed through a posterior midline incision from the tip of the coccyx to just short of the anus and external sphincter. This is deepened through the layers of the levator ani to the retrorectal fat and posterior rectal wall. A trans-sphincteric approach can be be employed for distal rectal tumours closer to the anal sphincters. Initially described by Bevan in 1917,[23] the technique was reintroduced into practice by York Mason in 1970.[24] This procedure is particularly suitable for lesions that span more than a quarter of the circumference of the anterior rectum but do not extend onto the posterior rectal wall. Such cancers can be difficult to excise using a transanal approach. The technique involves a parasacral incision that is extended to the anal verge and deepened in the midline to the anal sphincter. This muscle complex is divided and all ends tagged precisely with marking sutures for subsequent reconstruction. Problems with wound healing and sepsis were common to both of these dorsal approaches and they are now rarely used.

Transanal endoscopic microsurgery (TEM)

The transanal approach to mid-rectal tumours can be problematic and is compounded further by hindrance due to the anal retractors necessary for luminal access. Because of this, and the relative invasiveness of dorsal approaches, Buess has developed a transanal endoscopic microsurgical technique.[21] TEM is a complex technique that requires substantial training. The technology for TEM has now evolved since its first clinical application in 1983. The rectum is distended with a closed system using a 40 mm diameter rectoscope and the surgery performed with endoscopic instruments, while the operative field is viewed with a binocular stereoscope. Using TEM, tumours amenable to full-thickness excision should be confined to the extraperitoneal rectum. Thus, the maximum distance from the anal verge on the anterior rectal wall will be at 12 cm, laterally at 15 cm, while extending no more than 20 cm posteriorly.

Results of local excision

Cure rates comparable to those obtained with radical surgery can be achieved in appropriately selected patients with local excision alone. An analysis of over 400 patients accrued from 10 series revealed a collective cancer-specific survival of 94% with a 19% local recurrence rate for T1 and T2 lesions.[25] Even if series without 5-year follow-up are excluded, the figures for cancer-specific survival and local recurrence rate are still 89 and 24%, respectively. Moreover, nearly half of the patients with local treatment failure were considered to be cured by subsequent radical salvage surgery. Buess and his group have recently reported that only two of 64 patients undergoing TEM for T1 rectal cancers developed local recurrence,[26] and curative salvage surgery was possible in both of these cases.

It should be emphasized that only in a very few patients with rectal cancer (T1 lesions with no adverse pathology) is a local excision technique appropriate. Such surgery should at no time compromise the curative intent of conventional cancer surgery. Perhaps, with the advent of more accurate prognostic indices of tumour biology, more patients with rectal cancer (for instance, T2 lesions) can be treated regularly by local excision.

RADICAL SURGERY

Radical surgery is the primary treatment modality for the vast majority of patients with non-disseminated rectal cancer but the choice of surgeon is now recognized as an important determinant of patient outcome.[27] Presumably, this is due to variations in surgical technique. When performing radical surgery for rectal cancer a surgeon should have five major aims in mind: (1) cure; (2) avoidance of locoregional recurrence; (3) sphincter-saving reconstruction; (4) adequate anorectal function and, finally, (5) avoidance of autonomic nerve dysfunction. The presence of distant metastases will almost certainly preclude a cure, irrespective of the quality of the pelvic surgery. Notwithstanding the pathological stage of the tumour, local disease control and the avoidance of autonomic nerve damage are intimately related to the technique of pelvic dissection.

Avoidance of locoregional recurrence

There is considerable variation in the incidence of local recurrence among surgeons performing rectal cancer surgery: the published figures vary from between less than 3% to more than 30%.[28] Surgical technique appears to be a vital factor in accounting for this wide variability. There are three potential sources of local recurrence in the pelvis that need to be addressed in the surgical treatment of rectal cancer – lateral/circumferential spread, the presence of mesorectal tumour beyond the distal margin of the intraluminal cancer and, finally, the contribution of the distal resection margin. The lowest incidences for locoregional treatment failure are reported by surgeons who perform complete mesorectal excision. The role of lateral pelvic lymphadenectomy also needs to be addressed, although, this is not widely practised by Western surgeons.

Circumferential tumour clearance

Unsuspected microscopic tumour involvement of the lateral margins of the resection represents a major cause of local treatment failure. Quirke and colleagues[29] demonstrated that, when present, such microscopic disease almost invariably leads to a macroscopic recurrence if left untreated. Previously, tumour specimens were not carefully examined with this circumferential tumour spread in mind. This group has recently demonstrated that, even when a curative resection is thought to have been performed, some 25% of specimens had positive circumferential margins.[30] Positive lateral margins are due to inadequate clearance of the entire mesorectum from the lateral pelvic walls. This will be obviated by careful sharp dissection rather than a blunt or 'push' technique that causes trauma to the tumour/mesorectum package. Sharp dissection with scissors or diathermy allows careful and haemostatic excision of the rectum and mesorectum along the parietal pelvic fascia.

Mesorectal excision

Complete excision of the mesorectum is undoubtedly associated with a low incidence of local treatment failure.[31] Distal tumour spread within the mesorectum can occur beyond intramural tumour extension from the luminal surface. Scott and colleagues[32] have reported this distal mesorectal tumour spread in four of 20 patients who underwent complete mesorectal excision. In this study, the presence of mesorectal disease was associated with poor outcome (both local recurrence and distant metastasis). This pattern of tumour extension may be a marker of an aggressive tumour phenotype rather than a mechanism of local recurrence in itself. These findings do provide a rational oncological basis for total mesorectal excision, but the case numbers are insufficient to draw general conclusions about the frequency and biological significance of distal mesorectal tumour spread. It remains unclear as to whether such tumour spread occurs even in high rectal cancers or is limited to more distal carcinomas. Complete mesorectal excision commits the surgeon to performing a very low anastomosis with the probability of temporary faecal diversion. Subsequent anorectal function may well be less than satisfactory when intestinal continuity is subsequently restored. Total mesorectal excision does facilitate precise dissection of the mesorectal/tumour package within its visceral pelvic fascial sling. This in itself may well be of benefit to the patient with rectal cancer. For a cancer at or below the peritoneal reflection, we would recommend total mesorectal excision. In patients with high rectal cancers or rectosigmoid tumours the authors do not perform total mesorectal excision but, nevertheless, undertake extensive circumferential rectal mobilization and resect the tumour with a distal margin of at least 5 cm. In this way, the distal clearance margins of both rectal and mesorectal resections are not compromised by 'coning' down during the dissection (see below).

Distal resection margin

Williams and co-workers[33] have demonstrated that distal intramural tumour spread beyond the lowest level of the intraluminal lesion, when present, rarely exceeds 2 cm. In the absence of an intra-operative problem, a positive distal resection margin is invariably associated with aggressive pathological characteristics such as high tumour grade. Indeed, with a moderately or well-differentiated tumour, a distal resection margin of 2 cm does not adversely affect the incidence of pelvic recurrence.[34] These data taken together with increasing experience in circular stapling and, latterly, the 'staple on staple' technique, has led to widespread adoption of sphincter-saving procedures for low rectal cancers. Determination of the precise length of the distal resection margin can be difficult during surgery for a low rectal cancer, especially in a male with a narrow pelvis or after radiotherapy. It is vital to assess the extent of this clearance accurately and to mark the level at which the rectum is to be transected. This can be achieved only after full circumferential rectal mobilization down to the pelvic floor. This obviates 'coning down' to the site of the rectal resection, which may compromise both mesorectal and lateral tumour clearance. Thus, the issue of the distal resection margin should not be confused with the distal extent of the dissection, as the latter level will be lower than the former.

Pelvic lymphadenectomy

The biological significance and incidence of lateral spread to involve internal iliac artery lymph nodes has been the subject of some debate. The precise frequency of such tumour spread is not accurately known. Meticulous histopathological studies by Japanese surgeons indicate that this occurs in as many as 30% of patients undergoing rectal cancer surgery.[35] Whether lateral internal iliac lymph node spread is a primary feature in some patients with rectal cancer, or only an anomalous finding in the presence of occluded lymphatic pathways in the mesorectum, again is not known. Japanese surgeons performing extended pelvic lymphadenectomy report local recurrence rates of 5%,[36] but this is achieved at a significant cost in terms of morbidity from postoperative urinary and sexual dysfunction. The Japanese data do not provide a comparison between conventional rectal cancer surgery and extended pelvic lymphadenectomy, and the technique is not practised by Western surgeons.

Sphincter-saving reconstruction

As already discussed above, the frequency of sphincter-saving surgery for rectal cancer has increased markedly over the last two decades. Even if the top of the anal canal cannot be stapled and transected at the pelvic floor, a transanal hand-sewn colo-anal anastomosis can be performed as long as the distal margin of the tumour has been adequately cleared. There are tumours that are just too low for such surgery and there are patients, particularly men with a narrow pelvis, in whom it is technically not possible to extend the dissection safely below the tumour. In such instances, abdominoperineal excision of the anorectum needs to be performed to ensure tumour clearance. Notwithstanding the discussion above, a minimum distance of 6 cm between the anal verge and distal edge of the tumour is probably required to permit a sphincter-saving reconstruction. However, it should be stressed that the distal clearance of a low rectal tumour can be determined only after full mobilization of the rectum down to the pelvic floor.

Anorectal function

Total mesorectal excision for low rectal cancer necessitates total resection of the rectum. Bowel function after a straight colo-anal reconstruction can be very unsatisfactory, particularly in the first postoperative year. The technique of colon J pouch–anal reconstruction is well established, with reported improved function over a straight anastomosis,[37] but has not gained widespread acceptance outside specialist units. However, a recent prospective randomized trial has demonstrated that a colon pouch–anal anastomosis afforded superior function over a straight colo-anal anastomosis, and that this improvement was maintained even after 12 months.[38] Some key technical points have emerged and are important to consider in order to optimize function and avoid poor pouch evacuation. The pouch should be short – a maximum of 7–8 cm – as this reduces the emptying difficulties associated with pouches constructed with longer limbs. Additionally, sigmoid colon should be excised and not used for pouch construction. This segment of colon is often narrowed with diverticular disease and a pouched left colon is preferred. The decreased stool frequency observed with a colon pouch is not associated with increased reservoir capacity or compliance; rather, this functional advantage is probably sustained through the negative propulsive activity exerted by the short reversed limb of the pouch. Colon pouch reconstruction can be undertaken even in patients who are likely to require postoperative radiotherapy.

Autonomic nerve dysfunction

Sexual and urinary dysfunction occur after rectal excision for cancer. It is difficult to estimate the incidence of these complications as there is a paucity of good studies in the literature examining the problem; however, the incidence of impotence can be as high as 40% after radical surgery for rectal cancer. Sexual dysfunction in women undergoing rectal excision has been studied even less and the components of this morbidity are not clear. Cadaveric dissections have provided detailed information about the anatomy of the pelvic autonomic nerves[39,40] but, surprisingly, there has been little application of this knowledge to clinical surgery of the rectum. Injury to the hypogastric (sympathetic) nerves occurs most commonly on entry into the true pelvis at the commencement of the rectal mobilization. The pelvic parasympathetics are most commonly damaged by traction injuries due to blunt dissection or during division of the lateral ligaments.

This distressing morbidity can be largely obviated by using sharp dissection performed under direct vision with good haemostasis. The true pelvis should not be entered unless the hypogastric nerve trunks are identified medial to the ureters above the pelvic brim (see Figure 7.2). This will then ensure entry into the pelvis anterior to the nerves and within the pelvic parietal fascia. The trunks can then be followed during extension of the dissection inferiorly and laterally. Enker has developed a formal autonomic nerve-preserving pelvic side-wall dissection and has reported excellent results, with a low incidence of impotence in men undergoing low anterior resection for rectal cancer.[41]

TOTAL ANORECTAL RECONSTRUCTION (TAR)

Despite the improvements in the design of stapling instruments and their wider use, there remain patients whose low rectal tumours can be removed only by abdominoperineal excision. Many patients with a permanent colostomy are able to return to a full and active life, but a significant number experience severe social and psychological problems and seek an alternative. For such patients one of the authors has developed a technique to restore both gastrointestinal continuity and acceptable anorectal function. Various methods of reconstruction have been described (see ref. 42 for review). All techniques employ a perineal colostomy, while neo-anal sphincters have been fashioned from either smooth muscle or transposed striated muscle pedicles.

As a result of extensive experience with the use of the electrically stimulated anal neosphincter[43] for incontinent patients with an intact anorectum, the author has moved on to use this technique as part of total anorectal reconstruction.[44] TAR is performed both in patients at the time of abdominoperineal excision of the rectum for rectal cancer and in those individuals who have previously undergone their cancer surgery. In both groups of patients it was considered that their cancer surgery was curative. The author's standard technique of TAR now comprises three stages. The first stage of the operation consists of a coloperineal pull-through to create the perineal stoma at the site of the original anus. Complete mobilization of the remnant left colon, splenic flexure and transverse colon is necessary to achieve this without tension. A loop ileostomy is raised at this time. During this procedure, a continent colonic conduit is fashioned,

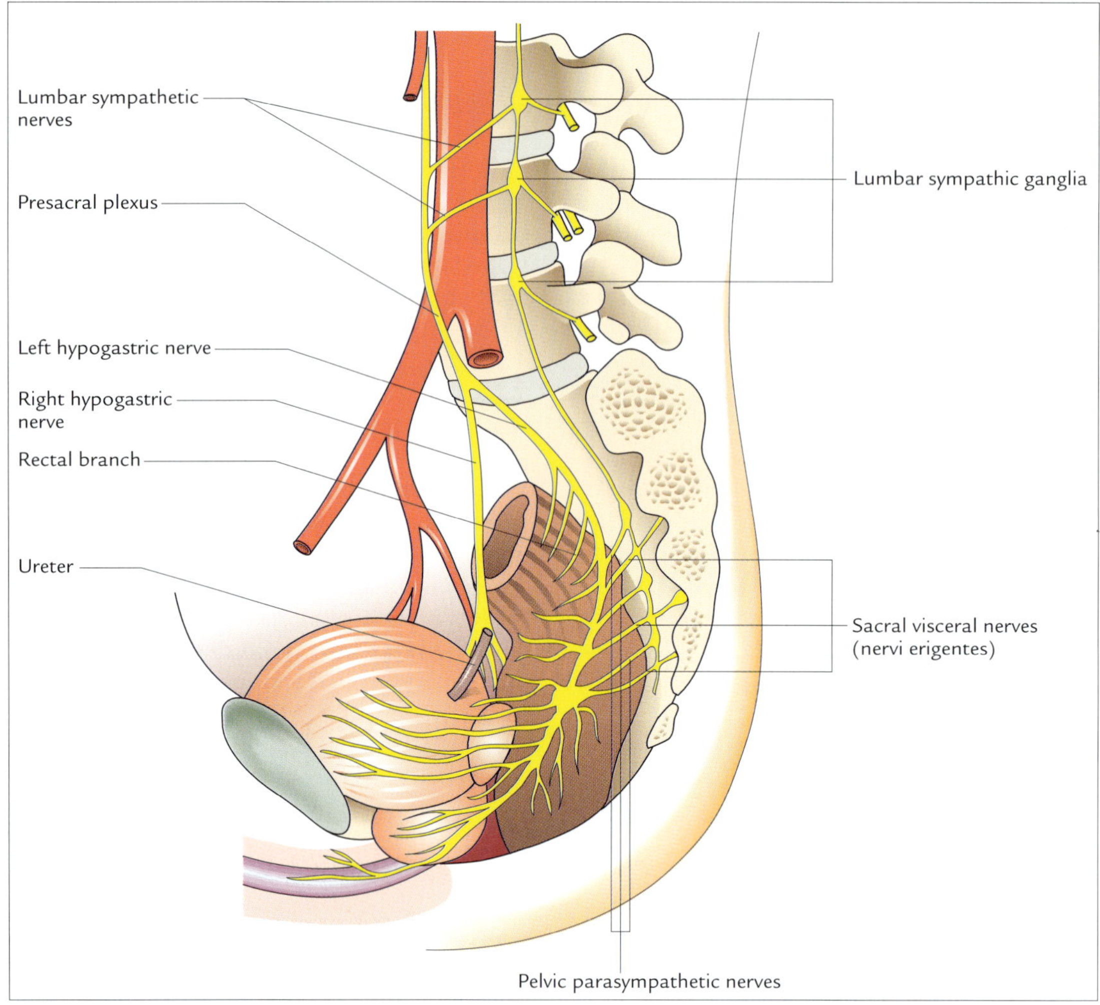

Figure 7.2. *The hypogastric nerves: the true pelvis should not be entered until these have been identified above the pelvic brim.*

consisting of a segment of colon incorporating a stabilized intussusception to act as a non-return valve. The colonic conduit has been developed from the author's work with patients with severe idiopathic constipation, with either slow transit in the left colon or a rectal evacuation disorder.[45] The conduit has been added for antegrade irrigation, as most patients who have had their continence restored after TAR experience problems with evacuation of the neorectum. Patients seem to accept the irrigation readily in preference to a permanent colostomy.

About 6–8 weeks later, the gracilis muscle is transposed from the thigh and is wrapped around the neo-anus in a gamma configuration, and the tendon of the muscle is sutured to the contralateral ischial tuberosity (see Figure 7.3). An electrode is carefully sutured over the main nerve to the muscle and its lead connected to an implantable generator positioned in a subcutaneous pocket in the left upper quadrant of the abdomen. The muscle is intermittently stimulated with incremental increases to a continuous stimulus until conversion has taken place from fast-twitch to slow-twitch muscle. The ileostomy is closed as the final stage of the surgery.

It should be emphasized that this technique for TAR is still evolving. However, this procedure has proved to be feasible and successful in a small number of patients who have

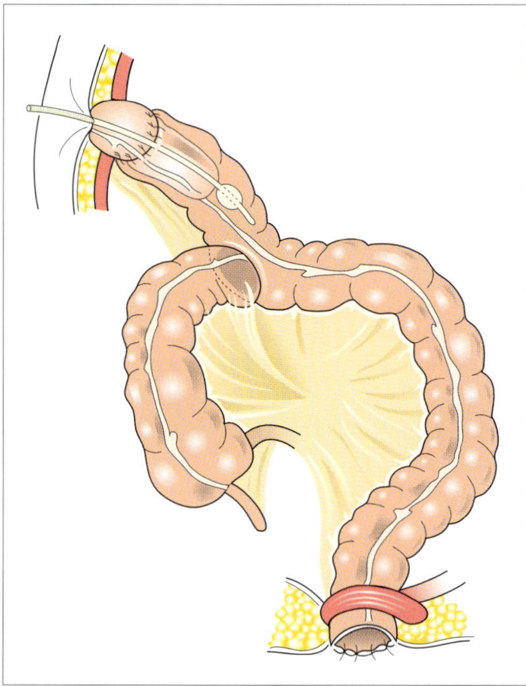

Figure 7.3. *Total anorectal reconstruction. Coloperineal anastomosis, electrically stimulated neosphincter and transverse colonic conduit. The neosphincter maintains continence, while antegrade irrigation via the conduit achieves evacuation.*

rejected the prospect of a permanent colostomy. Currently, TAR is being prospectively evaluated by an independent investigator who is assessing anorectal function and quality of life following the procedure.

Palliative surgery

Synchronous hepatic metastases are present in up to 25% of patients presenting with colorectal cancer.[8] A minority of such patients will have hepatic disease that is amenable to liver resection; however, for the remainder, a decision has to be made on the indications for surgery of the primary carcinoma. Resection of the primary lesion is generally advisable if the cancer is stenotic and causing obstructive symptoms. Bleeding and pain are also strong indications for palliative resection. Palliative procedures are particularly appropriate in patients with a relatively small burden of incurable hepatic disease, whose survival is likely to be sufficiently prolonged to accrue the benefits of surgery. Frail or elderly patients, and those with a high percentage of hepatic replacement, probably should not be offered palliative surgery. However, each patient will need to be assessed on an individual basis with potential operative morbidity and quality of life in mind.

Operable rectal cancer or advanced rectal lesions, both in the presence of incurable liver disease, need special consideration. For instance, it is difficult to justify abdominoperineal excision of the anorectum for a low rectal cancer in the majority of patients with diffuse hepatic metastases. If the anal sphincters can be preserved, then an extended Hartmann's operation (where the rectum is transected and stapled at the pelvic floor) should be considered as an alternative to very low colo-anal reconstruction with its attendant distressing bowel dysfunction. This procedure is especially useful in fit elderly patients with poor anal sphincter function.

In addition to laser treatment and palliative radiotherapy of colorectal cancers, the use of stent endoprostheses to obviate bowel obstruction in stenotic cancers should also be considered.[46] These expanding metallic stents can be used either to provide long-term palliation in patients in whom surgery is not appropriate or, alternatively, as an interval procedure before definitive resection. The author's initial experience of this approach as palliation for stenotic rectosigmoid cancers has been promising.

References

1. Cunningham C, Dunlop MG. Molecular genetic basis of colorectal cancer susceptibility. *Br J Surg* 1996; 83: 321–329

2. Davison AJ, Stern HS. Additional specific management problems. In: Cohen AM, Winawer SJ, Friedman GD, Gunderson (eds) *Cancer of the Colon, Rectum and Anus*. New York: McGraw Hill, 1995, pp. 477–489.

3. Nicholls RJ, York Mason A, Morson BC *et al*. The clinical staging of rectal cancer. *Br J Surg* 1982; 69: 404–409

4. Adalsteinsson B, Glimelius B, Graffman S *et al.* Computed tomography in staging of rectal cancer. *Acta Radiol Diagn* 1985; 26: 45–55

5. Wong WD, Orrom WJ, Jensen LL. Preoperative staging of rectal cancer with endorectal ultrasonography. *Perspect Colon Rectal Surg* 1990; 3: 315–334

6. Rothenberger DA, Buie WD. Local regional staging of rectal cancer. In: Cohen AM, Winawer SJ, Friedman GD, Gunderson (eds) *Cancer of the Colon, Rectum and Anus.* New York: McGraw Hill, 1995, pp. 521–531

7. Katsura Y, Yamada K, Ishizawa T *et al.* Endorectal ultrasonagraphy for the assessment of wall invasion and lymph node metastasis in rectal cancer. *Dis Colon Rectum* 1992; 35: 362–368

8. Taylor I. Liver metastases from colorectal cancer: lessons from past and present studies. *Br J Surg* 1996; 83: 456–460

9. Irving AD, Scrimgeour D. Mechanical bowel preparation for colon resection and anastomosis. *Br J Surg* 1987; 74: 580–581

10. Burke P, Mealy K, Gillen P *et al.* Requirement for bowel preparation in colorectal surgery. *Br J Surg* 1994; 81: 907–910

11. Collins R, Scrimgeour A, Yusuf S, Peto R. Reduction in fatal pulmonary embolism and venous thrombosis by perioperative administration of subcutaneous heparin. *N Engl J Med* 1988; 1: 593–595

12. Wiggers T, Jeekel J, Arends JW *et al.* No-touch isolation technique in colon cancer: a controlled prospective trial. *Br J Surg* 1988; 75: 409–415

13. Sugarbaker PH, Corlew S. Influence of surgical techniques on survival in patients with colorectal cancer: a review. *Dis Colon Rectum* 1982; 25: 545–557

14. IMPACT (International multicentre pooled analysis of colon cancer trials) investigators. *Lancet* 1995; 345: 939–944

15. Finan P, Ritchie JK, Hawley PR. Synchronous and 'early' metachronous carcinomas of the colon and rectum. *Br J Surg* 1987; 74: 945–947

16. Evers BM, Mullins RJ, Matthews TH *et al.* Multiple adenocarcinomas of the colon and rectum: an analysis of incidence and current trends. *Dis Colon Rectum* 1988; 31: 518–522

17. Lynch TL. Is there a role for prophylactic subtotal colectomy among hereditary nonpolyposis colorectal cancer germline mutation carriers? *Dis Colon Rectum* 1996; 39: 109–110

18. Madoff RD, Goldberg SM. Operative approaches to patients with inflammatory bowel disease. In: Cohen AM, Winawer SJ, Friedman GD, Gunderson LL (eds) *Cancer of the Colon, Rectum and Anus.* New York: McGraw Hill, 1995, pp. 379–390.

19. Thompson-Fawcett MW, Mortensen NJMcC. Anal transitional zone and columnar cuff in restorative proctocolectomy. *Br J Surg* 1996; 83: 1047–1055

20. Lockhart-Mummery HE, Dukes CE. The surgical treatment of malignant rectal polyps. *Lancet* 1952; ii: 751–755

21. Banerjee AK, Jehle EC, Shorthouse AJ, Buess G. Local excision of rectal tumours. *Br J Surg* 1995; 82: 1165–1173

22. Hargrove WCIII, Gertner MH, Fitts WT Jr. The Kraske operation for carcinoma of the rectum. *Surg Gynecol Obstet* 1979; 148: 931–933

23. Bevan AD. Carcinoma of the rectum – treatment by local excision. *Surg Clin Chicago* 1917; 1: 233–239

24. York-Mason A. Rectal cancer: the spectrum of selective surgery. *Proc R Soc Med* 1976; 69: 237–244

25. Graham RA, Garnsey L, Jessup JM. Local excision of rectal carcinoma. *Am J Surg* 1990; 160: 306–312

26. Mentges B, Buess G, Effinger G *et al.* Indications and results of local treatment of rectal cancer. *Br J Surg* 1997; 84: 348–351

27. McArdle CS, Hole D. Impact of variability among surgeons on postoperative morbidity and mortality and ultimate survival. *Br Med J* 1991; 302: 1501–1505

28. Expert advisory group of The Royal College of Surgeons of England and Association of Coloproctology of Great Britain and Ireland. In: *Guidelines for the management of colorectal cancer*, June 1996; 14–37

29. Quirke P, Durdey P, Dixon MF, Williams NS. Local recurrence of rectal adenocarcinoma due to inadequate surgical resection: histopathological study of lateral tumour spread and surgical excision. *Lancet* 1986; ii: 996–999

30. Adam IJ, Mohamdee MO, Martin IG *et al.* Role of circumferential margin involovement in the local recurrence of rectal cancer. *Lancet* 1994; 344: 707–711

31. Heald RJ, Ryall RDH. Recurrence and survival after total mesorectal excision for rectal cancer. *Lancet* 1986; i: 1479–1482

32. Scott N, Jackson P, al-Jaberi T *et al.* Total mesorectal excision and local recurrence: a study of tumour spread in the mesorectum distal to rectal cancer. *Br J Surg* 1995; 82: 1031–1033

33. Williams NS, Dixon MF, Johnston D. Reappraisal of the 5 centimetre rule of distal excision for carcinoma: a study of distal intramural spread and of patient survival. *Br J Surg* 1983; 70: 150–154

34. Vernava AM, Moran M, Rothenberger DA *et al.* A prospective evaluation of distal margins in carcinoma of the rectum. *Surg Gynecol Obstet* 1992; 175: 333–336

35. Hojo K, Koyama Y, Moriya Y. Lymphatic spread and its prognostic value in patients with rectal cancer. *Am J Surg* 1982; 144: 350–354

36. Moriya Y, Hojo K, Sawada T, Koyama Y. Significance of lateral node dissection for advanced rectal carcinoma at or below the peritoneal reflection. *Dis Colon Rectum* 1989; 32: 307–315

37. Seow-Choen F. Colonic pouches in the treatment of low rectal cancer. *Br J Surg* 1996; 83: 881–882

38. Ho YH, Tan M, Seow-Choen F. Prospective randomised controlled study of clinical function and anorectal physiology after low anterior resection: comparison of straight and colonic J pouch anastomoses. *Br J Surg* 1996; 83: 978–980

39. Lee JF, Maurer VM, Block GE. Anatomic relations of pelvic autonomic nerves to pelvic operations. *Arch Surg* 1973; 107: 324–328

40. Havenga K, DeRuiter MC, Enker WE, Welvaart K. Anatomical basis of autonomic nerve-preserving total mesorectal excision for rectal cancer. *Br J Surg* 1996; 83: 384–388

41. Enker WE. Potency, cure and local control in the operative treatment of rectal cancer. *Arch Surg* 1992; 127: 1396–1402

42. Abercrombie JE, Williams NS. Total anorectal reconstruction. *Br J Surg* 1995; 82: 438–442

43. Abercrombie JF, Williams NS. Development of an electrically-stimulated skeletal muscle neoanal sphincter. *Baillières Clin Neurol* 1995; 4: 21–34

44. Mander BJ, Abercrombie JF, George BD, Williams NS. The electrically stimulated gracilis neosphincter incorporated as part of total anorectal reconstruction after abdominoperineal excision of the rectum. *Ann Surg* 1996; 224: 702–711

45. Hughes SF, Williams NS. Continent colonic conduit for the treatment of faecal incontinence associated with disordered evacuation. *Br J Surg 1995;* 82: 1318–1320

46. Mainar A, Tejero E, Maynar M *et al.* Colorectal obstruction: treatment with metallic stents. *Radiology* 1996; 198: 761–764

Chapter 8

TREATMENT OF COLORECTAL CANCER THAT HAS SPREAD TO THE LIVER

J.L.A. Bastos, S. Bramhall and P. McMaster

Introduction

Colorectal cancer is one of the most common malignancies in developed countries, with 20,000–30,000 new cases per year in England and Wales[1] and 130,000–150,000 in the US.[2,3]

The liver is the commonest site of distant metastases from colorectal cancer; it is estimated that approximately 50% of patients with colorectal cancer will develop liver metastases during the course of their disease, and they may or may not be associated with local recurrence.[4,5] About 20–25% of those patients already have synchronous liver metastases by the time of initial laparotomy for colorectal resection.[6–8] In over 90% of all other patients, liver metastases will be diagnosed within the first 3 years after colonic resection, after this, the development of liver metastases seems to be uncommon.[8] In about 20% of patients the metastases are confined to the liver.[9]

The spread of malignant cells from primary colorectal cancer into the liver occurs mainly via portal venous drainage and there is evidence to suggest that in the majority of (if not all) patients with primary colorectal cancer, micrometastases already exist in the liver in a dormant state. It seems likely, however, that only a proportion of these metastases develop into clinically overt disease.[5]

Approximately 5–10% of patients with liver metastases from colorectal cancer could become candidates for curative surgical resection.[9,10] Considering the incidence of colorectal cancer,[1] it would be expected that a median of 750–2500 patients per year would be suitable for resection of hepatic metastases from colorectal cancer in England and Wales. If they are left untreated, hepatic colorectal metastases carry a dismal prognosis, with a median survival of 10.6 (range 3–24) months, and a 5-year survival of less than 1%.[2–8,11–13]

Currently, hepatic resection is the only potential curative treatment available for colorectal metastases. The 5-year survival in resected patients is between 16 and 35%,[2,7,12,14–18] in a highly selected group of patients, this survival rate can be higher than 40%.[11,19,20] In experienced hands, this surgery can be done safely, with 30-day mortality rates ranging from 0 to 10%, and with specific postoperative morbidity in approximately 25% of patients.[17,18,20]

Screening

There is no definite protocol for screening of liver metastases from colorectal cancer but, because metastases are common and easily detectable,[1,4,5,8] it is the authors' opinion that every patient presenting with a primary colorectal cancer should specifically be screened for liver metastases. This should be performed both synchronously with the diagnosis of the primary tumour and metachronously during the follow-up of patients with colorectal cancer.

PREOPERATIVE SCREENING: SYNCHRONOUS METASTASES

Approximately 25% of patients with liver metastases from colorectal cancer already have synchronous hepatic lesions by the time of initial laparotomy for colorectal resection.[6–8] The screening for synchronous hepatic metastases from colorectal cancer should be performed during the diagnostic work-up for the primary colorectal cancer, because preoperative detection of these metastases in the liver or elsewhere may influence the general therapeutic planning for the primary lesion. The screening for synchronous liver metastases should be performed using abdominal ultrasound scan (USS); this may be complemented by other more sophisticated imaging methods, such as computed tomography (CT), magnetic resonance imaging (MRI) and intraoperative ultrasound (IOUS). Figure 8.1 is an algorithm of diagnostic screening and treatment pathways that could be applied to synchronous liver metastases from colorectal cancer.

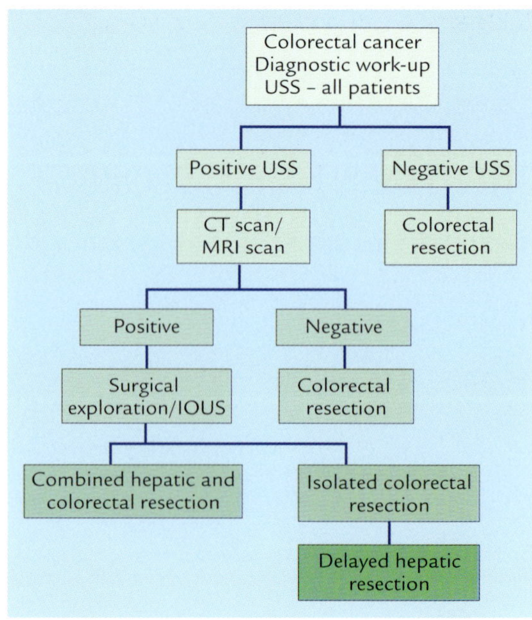

Figure 8.1 *Screening for synchronous liver metastases from colorectal cancer. USS, ultrasound scan; IOUS, intraoperative ultrasound; CT, computed tomography; MRI, magnetic resonance imaging.*

Imaging methods

Ultrasound scan (USS)

Transabdominal ultrasound is the screening investigation of choice for the detection of liver tumours, because of its sensitivity, ease of use and cost-effectiveness. Preoperative USS is reported to have a sensitivity of up to 94% in lesions greater than 20 mm and up to 59% for smaller lesions.[21,22]

Using technical refinements, such as high-resolution machines or duplex ultrasonography, sensitivity has been improved with the evaluation of hepatic arterial and portal blood flow. Using this technology, it is possible to determine the Doppler perfusion index, which is higher in patients with liver metastases than in normal controls. The use of this index is reported to improve sensitivity to 100% in patients with liver metastases, with a specificity of 70%, giving a positive predictive value of 62% and a negative predictive value of 100%.[21,23,24] Table 8.1 shows the efficacy of USS and IOUS in diagnosing liver tumours.

Computed tomography (CT)

CT scanning is rarely used as a primary screening tool in patients with colorectal cancer but is often used when the USS is positive or equivocal. CT scanning is considered to be the 'gold standard' imaging method for the detection of liver metastases, but availability and cost usually reduce its use in screening. Sensitivity and specificity can, however, vary widely, depending on the equipment, contrast enhancement techniques and the size of the hepatic lesion. Four techniques are currently in use, as described below.

Table 8.1. *Comparison of preoperative (USS) and intraoperative ultrasound (IOUS) in diagnosing liver tumours*

Author/year	Number of patients	Technique	Sensitivity (%)	Specificity (%)	Positive predictive value
Sheu *et al.* 1984[21]	Review	USS	94	/	/
Tanaka *et al.* 1986[22]	Review	USS	59	99	99
Olsen *et al.* 1990[25]	213	USS	66	/	/
		IOUS	98	/	/
Charnley *et al.* 1991[26]	99	USS	34	100	/
		IOUS	92	96	/
Machi *et al.* 1991[27]	189	USS	41	97	90
		IOUS	93	95	92
Machi & Siegel 1996[36]	Review	USS	41	96	87
		IOUS	94	94	92

Bolus contrast dynamic computed tomography (BCDCT)

The BCDCT is the most widely used CT technique for the delineation of liver lesions. In this method, an immediate CT scan is performed after intravenous infusion of a bolus of a water-soluble contrast agent. Using BCDCT, liver metastases from colorectal carcinoma can be detected in up to 93% of patients. The sensitivity for nodules greater than 20 mm is almost 100% and for those smaller than 10 mm the sensitivity is between 50 and 70%.[28–30] The BCDCT can be extended to cover other anatomical regions (e.g. the thorax and lower abdomen), and is more effective in detecting disease in these sites than an USS.[28,29]

Delayed scanning computed tomography (DSCT)

In DSCT, CT scanning is carried out 4–6 hours after intravenous infusion of a water-soluble contrast agent in order to give better definition of hepatic metastases, but the technique is no more sensitive or specific than BCDCT. DSCT is a useful technique for instruments with a slow image acquisition rate, but has the disadvantage of using higher doses of iodine contrast than BCDCT.[29,31,32]

Computed tomographic arteriography (CTA) and computed tomographic arterial portography (CTAP)

CTA and CTAP involve performing a CT scan after infusion of the contrast media directly into the hepatic or mesenteric artery. It is a widely held belief that CTA and CTAP are the most sensitive imaging methods for detecting metastases from colorectal cancer.[33,34] The high sensitivity of these techniques allows the detection of lesions less than 10 mm in diameter and definition of the relationship between the lesions and vascular structures. Both techniques are, however, expensive and invasive, and may have a high rate of false-positive results.[29,32] They should be used after USS and BCDCT in cases where there is doubt and when more information is required to assess the resectability of lesions.[33] Table 8.2 shows the results of different computed tomographic techniques in diagnosing liver tumours.

Magnetic resonance imaging (MRI)

T1-weighted MRI is as sensitive as CTAP without the disadvantage of a high rate of false-positive results. With the development of specific hepatobiliary contrast agents, such as those that are gadolinium based, T1-weighted MRI will be the imaging method of choice in preoperative assessment of liver metastases from colorectal cancer as soon as it becomes widely available.[8,35]

INTRA-OPERATIVE ASSESSMENT

Intra-operative ultrasound (IOUS)

Once synchronous liver metastases from colorectal cancer have been detected and staged during the preoperative screening, they should be assessed again with IOUS. This is particularly

Table 8.2. *Comparison of different CT imaging methods in diagnosing liver tumours*

Author/year	Number of patients	Technique	Sensitivity (%)	Specificity (%)	Positive predictive value
Miller *et al.* 1987 [32]	15	CTAP	77	/	63
		DSCT	83	/	90
		EOECT	82	/	81
Chezmar *et al.* 1988 [28]	59	BCDCT	92	/	81
		DSCT	82	/	/
Heiken *et al.* 1989 [33]	42	CATP	100	/	91
		DSCT	100	/	71
		BCDCT	92	/	88
Soyer *et al.* 1992 [34]	28	CTAP	93	100	/
		BCDCT	71	100	/
Knoll *et al.* 1993 [30]	51	DSCT	54	72	/
		BCDCT	50	72	/
Machi *et al.* 1996 [36]	Review	BCDCT	49	94	86

CTAP, computed tomography arterial portography; DSCT, delayed scanning computed tomography; BCDCT, bolus contrast dynamic computed tomography; EOECT, ethiodized oil emulsion computed tomography.

important if a combined colorectal and hepatic resection is planned.

IOUS in conjunction with palpation has a higher sensitivity and specificity than other preoperative imaging methods.[25–27,30,36] It has been shown that IOUS can demonstrate synchronous liver metastases in about 10% of patients in whom lesions were otherwise unrecognized at the time of colorectal resection.[26,27,30,36] In a lesion-by-lesion analysis, it was demonstrated that IOUS can detect up to 30% more tumours than preoperative diagnostic methods.[25,36] Besides its value as an efficient diagnostic tool, IOUS is essential in evaluating the feasibility of surgical resection of liver lesions.[36] Tables 8.1 and 8.3 show the sensitivity of IOUS in diagnosing liver tumours, compared with other imaging techniques.

POSTOPERATIVE ASSESSMENT: METACHRONOUS METASTASES

About 25–30% of patients with liver metastases from colorectal cancer will develop the disease as a metachronous lesion. Of these patients, 90% will develop the metastases during the first 3 years after colorectal resection and, of these, 20–25% will have disease limited to the liver.

Early detection of these lesions, when they are small in size and few in number, is associated with an increased rate of curative resection and therefore survival.[8,9] There has never been a prospective study to determine which is the most appropriate method of screening for metachronous metastases from colorectal cancer. Biochemical tests are often inadequate for screening. Some prospective studies however, have shown that measurements of alkaline phosphatase, γ-glutamyl transpeptidase, lactate dehydrogenase, aspartate aminotransferase and carcinoembryonic antigen (CEA) are worthwhile as screening tests if they are simultaneously and significantly elevated. In cases of small metastases, however, these tests can be entirely normal. In general, serial estimations of CEA seem to be the most useful biochemical test for screening metachronous liver metastases.[15,37–41] Table 8.4 shows the sensitivity and specificity of biochemical tests as screening methods in diagnosing hepatic metastases from colorectal cancer.

The results of immunoscintigraphy with radiolabelled monoclonal antibodies against tumoral antigens are inconsistent and are not superior to those obtained with USS and CT.

Abdominal USS and serial determinations of CEA performed at 4- or 6-month intervals during the first 2–3 years after colorectal resection is probably the most appropriate method of screening because of its sensitivity, wide availability and ease of use. A CT or a MRI scan should then be done if a lesion is detected on

Table 8.3. *Comparison between different computed tomography techniques and ultrasonography in diagnosing liver tumours*

Author/year	Number of patients	Technique	Sensitivity (%)	Specificity (%)	Positive predictive value
Sheu *et al.* 1984[21]	Review	USS	94	/	/
		BCDCT	84	/	/
Charnley *et al.* 1991[26]	99	USS	34	100	/
		BCDCT	69	96	/
		IOUS	92	96	/
Soyer *et al.* 1992[34]	28	USS	66	100	/
		BCDCT	71	100	/
		CTAP	93	100	/
Machi *et al.* 1991[27]	189	USS	41	97	90
		BCDCT	47	94	84
		IOUS	93	95	92
Machi *et al.* 1996[36]	Review	USS	41	96	87
		BCDCT	49	94	86
		IOUS	94	94	92

USS, preoperative ultrasound scan; BCDCT, bolus contrast dynamic computed tomography; CTAP, computed tomography arterial portography.

Table 8.4. *Sensitivity and specificity of biochemical tests as a screening method in diagnosing hepatic metastases from colorectal cancer*

Author/year	Number of patients	Test	Sensitivity (%)	Specificity (%)
Tartter *et al.* 1981[37]	327	CEA	81	57
		ALKp	77	43
Kemeny *et al.* 1982 [38]	80	CEA	86	60
		ALKp	50	30
		LDH	55	28
Minton *et al.* 1985 [39]	Review	CEA	81	/
Kemeny, 1986 [40]	100	CEA	86	/
		ALKp	63	/
		IDH	61	/

CEA, carcinoembryonic antigen; ALKp, alkaline phosphatase; LDH, lactate dehydrogenase.

USS or if the CEA is persistently elevated. Colonoscopic surveillance and imaging to detect local recurrence should be performed in conjunction with screening for liver metastases.

The number of patients presenting with metachronous metastases from colorectal cancer is substantial, and hepatic resection can be potentially curative with low rates of morbidity and mortality. Therefore, an aggressive follow-up policy for all patients who have undergone colorectal resection is justified, but individual judgement on the suitability of each patient for resection is important and the diagnostic screen should be done only when there are no contraindications for hepatic resection. These may include residual primary disease, extensive hepatic involvement, co-morbid disease or other relative contraindications to hepatic surgery such as advanced age and a poor general clinical condition.[7,10,11,20] As approximately 90% of metachronous hepatic metastases will develop during the first 3 years after colorectal resection, this period needs more intensive screening whatever method of follow-up is used.[8] Figure 8.2 shows an algorithm for screening and treatment pathways which could be applied to metachronous liver metastases from colorectal cancer.

POSTOPERATIVE ASSESSMENT: RECURRENT METACHRONOUS METASTASES

After hepatic resection for colorectal metastases, the disease will relapse in 65–85% of patients and tumour recurrence is the main cause of death after resection. The liver will be the primary site of recurrence in 70%, and in 20–48% of the patients it will be the only site of recurrence.[18,41] More than 50% of these recurrences will be detected within 2 years after the first hepatic resection, but only 10–30% of these will be amenable to further resection,[18,41] this represents only 5–15% of the total number of patients who have undergone resection of colorectal metastases.[3,17,18,41] As these numbers are significant, in the authors' opinion the same follow-up policy should be used for patients presenting with recurrence of hepatic metastases from colorectal cancer. Figure 8.3 shows an algorithm for screening and treatments pathways that could be applied to recurrent liver metastases from colorectal cancer.

Treatment

SURGICAL RESECTION

Surgical resection is the treatment of choice in patients with hepatic colorectal metastases, but this potentially curative treatment is indicated in only 10–20% of all patients who develop metastases.[42] Long-term survival rates and long-term disease-free survival are reported to be 35 and 25%, respectively, and higher survival rates (46%) have been reported in carefully selected patients.[19] Table 8.5 shows the morbidity, operative mortality and survival rates after hepatic resection of colorectal cancer metastases. There is a general agreement, however, that hepatic resection should be attempted only if all macroscopic malignant tissue can be removed and if enough viable liver tissue can be left in place.

There are some parameters that may affect the outcome of the surgery and should be

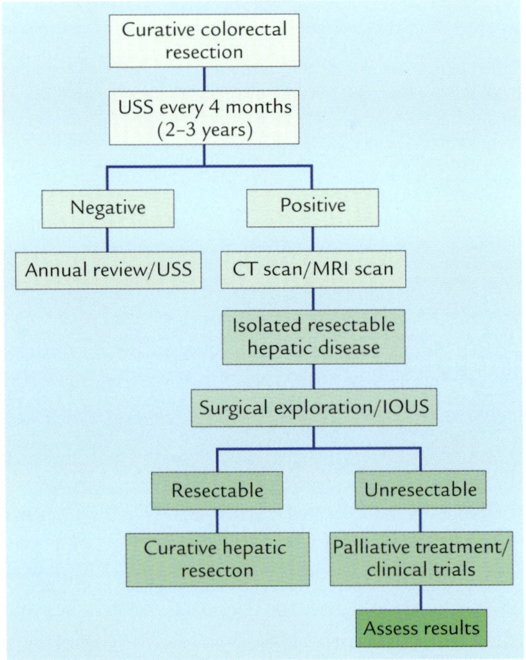

Figure 8.2 *Screening for metachronous liver metastases from colorectal cancer. USS, ultrasound scan; IOUS, intraoperative ultrasound; CT, computed tomography; MRI, magnetic resonance imaging.*

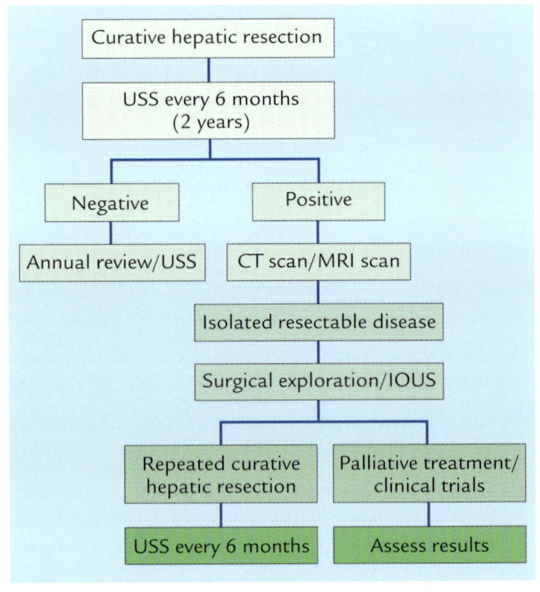

Figure 8.3 *Screening for recurrent liver metastases from colorectal cancer. USS, ultrasound scan; IOUS, intraoperative ultrasound; CT, computed tomography; MRI, magnetic resonance imaging*

Table 8.5. *Morbidity, operative mortality and survival rates after hepatic resection for colorectal cancer metastases*

Author/year	Number of patients	Morbidity (%)	Operative mortality (%)	Survival			
				Disease free (months)	MST (months)	3 year (percentage)	5 year (percentage)
Bradpiece *et al.* 1987[1]	48	12.5	4	17	30	44	/
Registry of hepatic metastases, 1988[14]	748	/	/	/	30	/	32
Hughes *et al.* 1989[15]	125	/	/	/	30	/	32
Scheele *et al.* 1990[11]	183	/	5	32	50	41	32
Scheele *et al.* 1991[20]	219	22	5.5	32	40	50	39
Savage & Malt 1992[12]	104	/	/	/	25	36	18
Gayowski *et al.* 1994[16]	204	0	1	17	33	43	32
Pinson *et al.* 1996[17]	95	/	0	16	34	43	32
Adam *et al.* 1997[43]	243	16	0	/	39	54	33

MST, median survival time.

Table 8.6. *Hepatic resection for colorectal cancer metastases: prognostic factors*

- Liver volume replaced by tumour
- Clear resection margins
- Lymph node involvement/extrahepatic disease
- Clearance of the primary tumour
- Number of metastases
- Disease-free interval (timing of surgery)
- Staging of primary colorectal tumour
- Anatomical limitations
- Preoperative carcinoembryonic antigen
- Size of metastases
- Site of hepatic metastases

analysed in the decision-making process of whether to resect hepatic metastases from colorectal cancer. Table 8.6 shows the prognostic factors related to hepatic resection of colorectal cancer metastases.

Clearance of the primary tumour

Before hepatic resection is considered, it should be established that all of the primary colorectal tumour has been removed completely and that there is no evidence of either anastomotic or local recurrence. If synchronous surgery is being considered, it must be established that the primary tumour is suitable for total clearance.[42]

Lymph node involvement/extrahepatic disease

It has been shown that metastatic spread from colorectal cancer to hilar or coeliac lymph nodes carries a poor prognosis. The 5-year survival rate for patients with involved lymph nodes at hepatic resection is less than 5%.[12,15,20,42] Some groups, however, advocate a more radical approach by resecting all of the lymph nodes from the hilum and coeliac region and have reported 5-year survival rates of approximately 15%.[8] Stangl *et al.*[42] reported a survival rate of only 16–24 months in patients with positive lymph nodes, even though this selected group of patients had less than 25% of liver volume replaced by tumour, no other extrahepatic disease and a well-differentiated primary tumour.

Patients having resection of extrahepatic metastases (e.g. in the lungs, adrenal gland and peritoneum) simultaneously with hepatic resection are reported to have a 20% 5-year survival, the 5-year disease-free survival, however, was only 4%. Some authors advocate this radical approach in patients who are a very good surgical risk.[15,43] Extrahepatic disease, however, is associated with a very poor outcome in terms of survival, whether it consists of a primary residual colorectal tumour or metastases in the other organs, and irrespective of whether a more aggressive treatment strategy is adopted. This approach is indicated only in cases of isolated disease in the organ, and in the absence of a better therapeutic option.[3,42] An exception may be made for certain types of endocrine tumours, such as carcinoid.[7,12,15,20]

Number of metastases

The best results are reported after resection of single hepatic metastases from colorectal cancer, and the 5-year survival rate is reported to be approximately 35%, with higher survival rates being reported in carefully selected cases.[7,11,14,15,20] The current consensus is that liver resection should be the treatment of choice for patients with up to three lesions, but it is important that tumour-free resection margins are obtained and an adequate amount of normal liver tissue is left in place to avoid the development of hepatic failure after resection. The 5-year survival for patients with up to three lesions can be similar to that observed in cases of resection for single lesions.[10,11,14,15,41] Patients with more than four metastases may have a worse prognosis.[7,11,16] The limit of three hepatic metastases, however, has been contested as a prognostic factor by some authors who argue that, provided that clear resection margins can be obtained and that there is no extrahepatic disease, it is reasonable to perform resection for four or more metastases and that in such cases there is a chance of long-term benefit.[15,20]

Clear resection margins

The resection of hepatic metastases from colorectal cancer is justified only when it is potentially curative; therefore, clear resection margins are considered to be a crucial factor for long-term survival.[7,12,14] If resection margins greater than 10 mm cannot be obtained, the prognosis is poor, and median survival (in cases where there are residual liver metastases after resection) ranges from 13 to 26 months.[7,12,15,16] Patients with positive resection margins after hepatic resection had survival rates similar to those who were left untreated.[11,12]

Disease-free interval

The time interval between the colorectal resection and hepatic resection seems to have a positive impact on long-term survival. Patients with metachronous liver metastases resected more than a year after colorectal resection had a 5-year survival rate of approximately 40%.[14,15] In cases of either synchronous or metachronous metastases detected less than a year after colorectal resection, the 5-year survival rate was approximately 28%.[14,15] It is possible that patients with a longer disease-free interval have slower-growing tumours, but synchronous disease or a short disease-free interval should not be a contraindication to hepatic resection.[14,15,20,42]

Site of hepatic metastases

There was no difference in long-term survival rate or long-term disease-free survival rates among patients with multiple unilobar metastases when compared with patients presenting with multiple bilobar metastases.[14,15,20,42]

Liver volume replaced by tumour (LVRT)

The extent of liver involvement at the time of diagnosis has an important effect on the long-term survival and is probably the single most important prognostic factor after liver resection for colorectal metastases. The 3-year survival rate in patients with more than 25% of LVRT was 0%.[7, 42]

Size of metastases

The size of solitary hepatic metastases does not seem to have a prognostic impact if analysed as an isolated factor. The 5-year survival rate for patients with lesions of 5.0 cm or more was similar to that observed in patients with smaller lesions.[14,15,20,42]

Staging of primary colorectal tumour

Both the grade and stage of the primary colorectal tumour are also important prognostic factors after resection of hepatic metastases. Poorly differentiated tumours have a worse prognosis than tumours that are well or moderately differentiated.[7,11,12,42] Patients with Dukes' classification A or B tumours have a significantly better survival and disease-free interval (47 and 28%, respectively) than those with Dukes' C tumours (18–23%).[14,15]

Preoperative carcinoembryonic antigen (CEA)

Low preoperative levels of CEA are associated with an improved prognosis:[42] patients with CEA levels below 5.0 ng/ml had a 5-year survival rate of 45%, whereas CEA levels higher than 5.0 ng/ml were associated with a 5-year survival of 30%.[14,15]

Timing of surgery

Better results could be obtained by improving the diagnosis of otherwise occult disease in order to obtain a true picture of the extent of the disease. Improved diagnostic accuracy would mean that a considerable proportion of patients could be spared an unnecessary operation.

Some specialized centres perform combined resection of the primary colorectal tumour and liver metastases with low rates of morbidity and mortality, however, this has no effect on 5-year survival rates.[11,12,19,20] Combined resection has a higher morbidity and mortality than sequential resection, which is mainly due to septic complications, and the indication for combined resection should be highly selective.[20] Preoperative screening can be helpful in this process because patients with small isolated lesions which are suitable for wedge resection may be detected. Patients with larger metastases in the left lateral lobe, which could be resected during an uncomplicated colonic resection, can be properly assessed. Generally, however, surgical enthusiasm should be restrained until the biological behaviour of the hepatic metastases can be properly assessed.[10] It would seem more appropriate to resect the primary colorectal tumour and to assess accurately the extension of liver involvement as well as the extrahepatic disease or metachronous lesions, and aim for a delayed hepatic resection.[7,10,13]

Anatomical limitations

Surgical resection is undoubtedly the treatment of choice for liver metastases from colorectal cancer; however, clear resection margins and the preservation of an adequate amount of normal liver parenchyma after resection should always be the aim. The balance between these two aims needs to be judged in each individual case and therefore surgical resection may be difficult and sometimes contraindicated. Surgical contraindications may include involvement of the portal vein bifurcation, hepatic vein confluence, inferior vena cava and Couinand's liver segment I. In these situations it may be impossible either to obtain a clear resection margin or to preserve enough liver parenchyma. Definitive information on these features can be obtained using IOUS; the adoption of ultrasound-guided oriented techniques to recognize vessels and bile ducts, and to assess resection margins, is now an essential component of the operative assessment.[8,10,44]

Two different groups of patients can be identified, using the above criteria. The first group comprises patients whose primary colorectal tumour has been completely removed with no evidence of extrahepatic disease and in whom the liver volume replaced is less than 25%, up to three hepatic metastases have been detected and all of these lesions are likely to be resected with a 10 mm excision margin. For these patients a hepatic resection is clearly indicated and carries a good prognosis. The second group comprises patients presenting with either advanced primary colorectal cancer or tumours with lymph node metastases; the volume of liver replaced by tumour is usually more than 25%, and there are often more than four hepatic lesions. The prognosis in these patients is very poor and the feasibility of hepatic resection should be considered carefully.[45] It is unclear however, whether the selection process outlined above is really worthwhile, because the exact impact of surgery is unlikely ever to be known as no surgeon will consider randomizing patients to resection or not in the presence of potentially resectable disease.[46]

Repeated hepatic resection

The indications for repeated hepatectomy for recurrent colorectal metastases are still unclear, however, initially, the same criteria as those used to select patients for the first hepatectomy should be adopted. Special attention, however, should be given to the clinical condition of the patient.[13,18] Recently, some centres have indicated re-resection for patients with synchronous extrahepatic disease, but the results of this approach are still under scrutiny.[43]

The 5-year survival rates reported after repeated hepatectomy are between 23 and 40%, with a median survival of 30 months, which are similar to those reported after the first resection.[3,17,41,43,47] At least one multicentre randomized trial, however, did not report a 5-year survival for patients undergoing repeated hepatectomy. The explanations for these differences are unclear, but may relate to the criteria adopted for hepatic resection or to differences in the biological behaviour of the tumours.[43] The use of adjuvant therapy did not seem to improve the results after a second liver resection.[47]

The mortality and morbidity rates after first hepatectomy are low – 0–10% and 8–40%, respectively,[3] but second hepatectomy is technically more difficult and is more time consuming, and the risk of bleeding is higher. Other complicating factors are perihepatic adhesions (making exposure of the liver difficult), modification of the intrahepatic anatomy due to regeneration, soft consistency of the remaining hepatic tissue secondary to regeneration and chemotherapy, and decreased resistance to ischaemia after clamping of the porta hepatis. The extent of the first surgery is, however, not an absolute contraindication to repeat surgery.

Because of these factors, re-resection after a relapse of hepatic disease from colorectal carcinoma should be considered a specialized procedure, and should be confined to specialized centres.[3,17,43,48]

Recurrence after a second hepatic resection is around 60%, with half of these confined to the liver.[3] These recurrences may occur when adequate resection margins could not be achieved during the resection, and may also be due to occult disease undetectable at the time of the operation.[3,43,48]

In carefully selected patients, repeated liver resection for relapsed colorectal cancer may be worthwhile: it may offer the chance of prolonged survival similar to that achieved after first hepatectomy, provided that the results of surgery are optimal. It would seem prudent, however, to delay re-resection for some months after the diagnosis of disease relapse, and this policy should allow the full spectrum of the recurrence in a given patient to become apparent.[43] The question of whether repeated hepa-

Table 8.7. *Therapeutic options for hepatic metastases from colorectal cancer*

Curative		
• Surgical resection		
Palliative		
• Palliative resection		
• Cryotherapy		
• Ethanol injection		
• Regional chemotherapy (intra-arterial)		
• Tumour ischaemia:	hepatic artery ligation	
	microsphere embolisation	
• Hyperthermia:	electromagnetic radiation	
	ultrasound	
	laser	
• Adjuvant systemic chemotherapy		
• Combined treatment		
• Clinical trials		

tectomy is warranted in patients with extra-hepatic relapse of colorectal cancer, however, is still unclear and further information is required.

ADJUVANT THERAPY

Adjuvant treatment of hepatic metastases from colorectal carcinoma requires a multidisciplinary approach and includes local and systemic treatment, such as cryotherapy, ethanol injection, regional chemotherapy and arterial embolization/chemoembolization. Other less common therapeutic modalities include tumour ischaemia, immunotherapy and adjuvant systemic chemotherapy. Table 8.7 shows the therapeutic options for hepatic metastases from colorectal cancer.

Cryotherapy

When curative hepatectomy cannot be performed, palliative resection alone is of no benefit in the treatment of hepatic metastases from colorectal cancer; however, cryotherapy has been proposed as an alternative therapeutic approach in such patients.[7,10,11,49,50]

Cryotherapy is a technique in which tumours can be destroyed by freezing and thawing cycles. One or more metallic probes (8–12 mm in diameter) are guided by IOUS and implanted through the hepatic tissue into the lesion. Freezing is obtained using two or three cycles of circulating liquid nitrogen at −169°C through the probe tip. The frozen tumour volume assumes an ice-ball shape around the probe. An adequate margin of 10 mm of frozen hepatic tissue should be achieved beyond the frozen tumour to assure completeness of cryoablation. The use of IOUS is essential to direct the probe and to control the amount of frozen tissue.[7,11,49,50]

Cryotherapy can be used alone, in conjunction with preoperative chemotherapy or with palliative resection; however, whatever the indication, complete tumour clearance should be the aim.[10,49,50]

Cryotherapy is normally indicated in patients with isolated hepatic metastases from colorectal cancer which are not amenable to curative surgical resection. The commonest indication is for bilateral metastases which would require extensive hepatic resection in which an adequate amount of liver parenchyma could not be preserved. In this situation, a combined approach has been advocated, the main lesion being removed by surgical resection and the remainder treated by cryotherapy.[7,10,46,49,50] Cryoablation may also be used in patients who have undergone attempted curative resection, but in whom a clear margin of resection has not been achieved. In such cases, the freezing of the cut edge of the remaining parenchyma can be performed using flat probes for cycles of 3–5 minutes.[49]

Cryosurgery is not indicated in the treatment of lesions adjacent to major vessels such as the vena cava or main hepatic veins, because the thermal dilution caused by rapid blood flow prevents adequate freezing of the tumour tissue.[46] Lesions close to the hepatic hilum should not be treated because of the risk of damage to the bile ducts, and tumours larger than 6.0 cm in diameter cannot be completely destroyed by cryotherapy because this exceeds the limits of the freezing process.

The reported mortality rate from cryotherapy is low, ranging from 0 to 4%, with an overall morbidity of approximately 8%. The reported complications include transient postoperative fever, leucocytosis, thrombocytopenia, disseminated intravascular coagulation, subphrenic or subhepatic fluid collections, pleural effusions and bile leak.[46,49,50,51]

The results of cryotherapy are very difficult to analyse because it has been used alone in very few patients, the follow-up period has been very short and the studies are not randomized. The ideal patient for cryotherapy is also likely to be an ideal candidate for surgical resection; therefore, cryotherapy should be used as complementary to, rather than as an alternative to, surgical resection.

Ethanol injection

The intratumoral injection of absolute alcohol guided by USS causes necrosis of malignant tissue and this technique has been used in the treatment of small hepatocellular carcinomas in patients with cirrhosis.[8,52] Alcohol injection has also been used in some selected patients with a few small (≤3.0 cm) and easily accessible hepatic metastases from colorectal cancer. Percutaneous injection of ethanol is cheap, is easy to perform requiring only local anaesthesia, can be repeated several times, and is well tolerated. The extent of alcohol-induced necrosis can be evaluated using USS or dynamic CT 24–72 hours after the procedure. The results of alcohol injection used to treat hepatic metastases from colorectal cancer, however, are inconclusive; because this technique may be ineffective for treating this type of metastasis, it should not be used as a first line of treatment.[52]

Regional chemotherapy

Regional hepatic artery chemotherapy is performed by placing a catheter in the gastroduodenal artery, connected to a subcutaneous reservoir or Infusaid pump. The adequacy of the hepatic perfusion is assessed by injecting methylene blue or fluorescein through the catheter at the time of its placement. Slightly different surgical approaches may be required in cases of arterial anatomical variations, and attempts should be made to identify these preoperatively by hepatic arteriography.[8,53] Intra-arterial chemotherapy is indicated in patients with unresectable hepatic metastases from colorectal cancer when extrahepatic disease is minimal or absent. Massive liver replacement by tumour, symptomatic extrahepatic disease and involvement of the central nervous system are to be considered contraindications for this treatment. Morbidity rates after the procedure for insertion of the catheter are high: the main complication is arterial thrombosis, with 50% occluding in the first 6 months of treatment. Other complications include drug-induced hepatitis, sclerosing cholangitis, gastroduodenitis, gastroduodenal ulcerations and reservoir or pump pocket infection.[53] In the authors' unit, 26 (39%) of 66 patients in whom hepatic artery chemotherapy was considered had abnormal arterial anatomy detected by a preoperative hepatic arteriogram. The morbidity rate following catheter placement in the authors' hands was 24% and there were no deaths related to the technique. Catheter blockage occurred in 16.6% of all patients and inadequate liver perfusion was more common in patients with arterial abnormalities (author, unpublished data).

There are several different regimens of regional chemotherapy which are reported as being effective in controlling hepatic disease in up to 80% of patients.[8] These results are considered to be two to three times superior to those obtained with conventional systemic chemotherapy; however, most of the reports have demonstrated a better control of local disease, rather than a real increase in the survival rates.[54] Only a small number of prospective studies have demonstrated a prolonged survival with regional chemotherapy and further studies are required to confirm these results.[53] The main disadvantage of this method is that it does not prevent the recurrence or development of extrahepatic disease, which occurs in up to 70% of patients.[8,53,54,55]

The combination of regional and systemic chemotherapy seems more likely to improve the overall survival, but the studies supporting this approach have had only preliminary reports.[8,54–56]

Tumour ischaemia

Tumour ischaemia is obtained either by hepatic artery ligation or hepatic artery embolization with starch or albumin microspheres. In spite of the related improvements in pain control, however, tumour ischaemia has not been shown to have a positive effect on the survival rates of patients with hepatic metastases from colorectal cancer.[8] The microspheres have also been used as vector for chemotherapeutic agents and lipiodol is also used as a vector for antitumour drugs because it can be selectively retained within the tumour. The use of either of these techniques, however, offers no apparent survival benefits.[54]

Hyperthermia

Attempts have been made to destroy hepatic tumours through heat produced by electromagnetic radiation, ultrasound waves and laser. Of these techniques, interstitial laser photocoagulation (ILP) seems to be the most effective. This therapeutic modality, however, has very little practical applicability because it has a number of technical problems which have yet to be solved; furthermore, it has not been shown to have a positive effect on survival rates.[8,52]

Conclusions

The high incidence of liver metastases from colon cancer justifies the adoption of aggressive diagnostic screening to detect metastases at an early stage and to offer surgical resection when appropriate, as this is currently the only treatment that can offer a prolonged survival or hope of a cure. Patients presenting with low levels of CEA, no extrahepatic disease, less than four hepatic metastases, lesions smaller than 5.0 cm and less than 25% of liver tissue replaced by tumour, with a well-differentiated primary colorectal cancer and more than a year's delay between the resection of the primary tumour and the diagnosis of liver metastases, have the best prognosis after hepatic resection. Patients with unresectable liver metastases can be offered an array of palliative treatments to improve their quality of life and, sometimes, their survival. Perhaps the most helpful of these are cryotherapy and hepatic artery chemotherapy, although the results of randomized trials are awaited.

In conclusion, with increasing patient awareness and further specialization by surgeons and oncologists, the management of patients with hepatic metastases from colorectal cancer will increasingly become the domain of highly specialized multimodality units. Such units will be able to offer the whole gamut of investigative tools and treatment modalities which will enable the evidence-directed and controlled application of the treatments discussed in this chapter.

References

1. Bradpiece HA, Benjamin IS, Halevy A *et al.* Major hepatic resections for colorectal liver metastases. *Br J Surg* 1987; 74: 324–326

2. Vauthey JN, Marsh RW, Cendan JC *et al.* Arterial therapy of hepatic colorectal metastases. *Br J Surg* 1996; 83: 447–455

3. Wanebo HJ, Chu QD, Avradopoulus KA *et al.* Current perspectives on repeated hepatic resection for colorectal carcinoma; a review. *Surgery* 1996; 119: 361–371

4. Cedermark BJ, Blumenson LE, Pickren JW *et al.* The significance of metastases to the adrenal glands in adenocarcinoma of the colon and rectum. *Surg Gynecol Obstet* 1977; 114: 537–546

5. Taylor, I. Liver metastases from colorectal cancer: Lessons from the past and present clinical studies *Br J Surg* 1996; 83: 456–460

6. Kemeny N, Niedzwiecki D, Shurgot B *et al.* Prognostic variables in patients with hepatic metastases from colorectal cancer. *Cancer* 1989; 63: 742–747

7. Ballantyne GH, Quin J. Surgical treatment of liver metastases in patients with colorectal cancer. *Cancer* 1993; 71: 4252–4256

8. Launois B, Landen S, Heaunit F. Colorectal metastatic liver tumour. In: Terblanche J (ed) *Hepatobiliary Malignancy. Its Multidisciplinary Management.* London: Edward Arnold, 1994, pp. 272–300

9. Bengmark S, Hafstrom L. The natural history of primary and secondary malignant tumors of the liver. I. The prognosis with hepatic metastases from colonic and rectal carcinoma by laparotomy. *Cancer* 1969; 23: 198–202

10. Scheele J. Hepatectomy for liver metastases. *Br J Surg* 1993; 80: 274–276

11. Scheele J, Stangl R, Altendorf-Hoffmann A. Hepatic metastases from colorectal carcinoma: impact of surgical resection on the natural history. *Br J Surg* 1990; 77: 1241–1246

12. Savage AP, Malt RA. Survival after hepatic resection for malignant tumours. *Br J Surg* 1992; 79: 1095–1101

13. Doci R, Gennari L, Bignami P *et al.* Morbidity and mortality after hepatic resection of metastases from colorectal cancer. *Br J Surg* 1995; 82: 377–381

14. Registry of hepatic metastases. Resection of the liver for colorectal carcinoma metastases: a multi-institutional study of indications for resections. *Surgery* 1988; 103: 278–288

15. Hughes K, Scheele J, Sugarbaker PH. Surgery for colorectal cancer metastatic to the liver. Optimizing the results of treatment. *Surg Clin North Am* 1989; 69: 339–359

16. Gayowski TJ, Iwatsuki S, Madriaga J *et al.* Experience in hepatic resection for metastatic colorectal cancer: analysis of clinical and pathologic risk factors. *Surgery* 1994; 116: 703–711

17. Pinson CW, Wright JK, Chapman WC *et al.* Repeated hepatic surgery for colorectal cancer metastases to the liver. *Ann Surg* 1996; 223: 765–779

18. Bines SD, Doolas A, Jenkins L *et al.* Survival after repeated hepatic resection for recurrent colorectal hepatic metastases *Surgery* 1996; 120: 541–596

19. Iwatsuki S, Esquivel CO, Gordon RD *et al.* Liver resection for metastatic colorectal cancer. *Surgery* 1986; 100: 804–810

20. Scheele J, Stangl R, Altendorf-Hoffmann A *et al.* Indicators of prognosis after hepatic resection for colorectal secondaries *Surgery* 1991; 110: 13–29

21. Sheu JC, Sung JL, Chen DS *et al.* Ultra-sonography of small hepatic tumours using high-resolution linear-array real-time instruments. *Radiology* 1984; 150: 797–802

22. Tanaka S, Kitamura T, Ohshima A *et al.* Diagnostic accuracy of ultrasonography for hepatocellular carcinoma. *Cancer* 1986; 58: 344–347

23. Leen E, Goldberg JA, Robertson J *et al.* Early detection of occult colorectal hepatic metastases using Duplex Colour Doppler Sonography. *Br J Surg* 1993; 80: 1249–1251

24. Leen E, Angerson WJ, Wotherspoon H *et al.* Comparison of the Doppler Perfusion Index and Intraoperative Ultrasonography in diagnosing colorectal liver metastases – evaluation with postoperative follow-up results. *Ann Surg* 1994; 220: 663–667

25. Olsen AK. Intraoperative ultrasonography and the detection of liver metastases in patients with colorectal cancer. *Br J Surg* 1990; 77: 998–999

26. Charnley RM, Morris DL, Dennison AR *et al.* Detection of colorectal liver metastases using intraoperative ultrasonography. *Br J Surg* 1991; 78: 45–48

27. Machi J, Isomoto H, Kurohiji T *et al.* Accuracy of intraoperative ultrasonography in diagnosing liver metastasis from colorectal cancer: evaluation with postoperative follow-up results. *World J Surg* 1991; 15: 551–557

28. Chezmar JL, Rumancik WM, Megibow AL *et al.* Liver abdominal screening in patients with cancer: CT versus MR imaging. *Radiology* 1988; 168: 43–47

29. Ward BA, Miller DL, Frank JA *et al.* Prospective evaluation of hepatic imaging studies in detection of colorectal metastases: correlation with surgical findings. *Surgery* 1989; 105: 180–187

30. Knoll JA, Marn CS, Francis IR *et al.* Comparisons of dynamic infusion and delayed computed tomography, intraoperative ultrasound and palpation in the diagnosis of liver metastases. *Am J Surg* 1993; 165: 81–88

31. Bernardino ME, Eerwin DC, Steinberg HV *et al.* Delayed hepatic CT scanning: increased confidence and improved detection of hepatic metastasis. *Radiology* 1986; 159: 71–74

32. Miller DL, Simmons JT, Chang R *et al.* Hepatic metastases detection: comparison of three CT contrast enhancement methods. *Radiology* 1987; 165: 785–790

33. Heiken JP, Weyman PJ, Lee JKT *et al*. Detection of local hepatic masses: prospective evaluation with CT, delayed CT, CT during arterial portography and MR imaging. *Radiology* 1989; 171: 47–51

34. Soyer P, Levesque M, Elias D *et al*. Prospective assessment of resectability of hepatic metastases from colonic carcinoma: CT portography vs sonography and dynamic CT. *Am J Radiol* 1992; 159: 741–744

35. Semelka RC, Shenut JP, Kroeker MA *et al*. Focal liver disease: comparison of dynamic contrast enhanced CT and T2-weighted fat-suppressed, FLASH, and dynamic gadolinium-enhanced MR imaging at 1,5 T. *Radiology* 1992; 184: 687–694

36. Machi J, Siegel B. Operative ultrasound in general surgery. *Am J Surg* 1996; 172: 15–20

37. Tartter PI, Slater G, Gelernt I *et al*. Screening for liver metastases from colorectal cancer with carcinoembryonic antigen and alkaline phosphatase. *Ann Surg* 1981; 193: 357–360

38. Kemeny MM, Sugarbaker PH, Smith TJ *et al*. A prospective analysis of laboratory tests and imaging studies to detect hepatic lesions. *Ann Surg* 1982; 195: 163–167

39. Minton JP, Hoen JI, Gerber DM *et al*. Results of a 400-patient carcinoembryonic antigen second-look colorectal cancer study. *Cancer* 1985; 55: 1284–1290

40. Kemeny M, Hogan JM, Ganteaume L *et al*. Preoperative staging with computorized axial tomography and biochemical laboratory tests in patients with hepatic metastases. *Ann Surg* 1986; 203: 169–172

41. Fernandez-Trigo V, Shamsa F, Sugarbaker PH. Repeated liver resections from colorectal metastasis. *Surg* 1995; 117: 296–304

42. Stangl R, Altendorf-Hoffmann A, Charnley RM *et al*. Factors influencing the natural history of colorectal liver metastases. *Lancet* 1994; 343: 1405–1410

43. Adam R, Bismuth H, Castaing D *et al*. Repeated hepatectomy for colorectal liver metastases. *Ann Surg* 1997; 225: 51–62

44. Bismuth H. Surgical anatomy and anatomical surgery of the liver. *World J Surg* 1982; 6: 3–9

45. Adson MA. Resection of liver metastases – when is it worthwhile? *World J Surg* 1987; 11: 511–520

46. Steele G, Ravikumar IS, Benotti PN. New surgical treatments for recurrent colorectal cancer. *Cancer* 1990; 65: 723–730

47. Neeleman N, Anderson R. Repeated liver resection for recurrent liver cancer. *Br J Surg* 1996; 83: 893–901

48. Elias D, Lasser JM, Hoang J *et al*. Repeated hepatectomy for cancer. *Br J Surg* 1993; 80: 1557–1562

49. Adam R, Akpinar E, Johann M *et al*. Place of cryosurgery in the treatment of malignant liver tumours, *Ann Surg* 1997; 225: 39–50

50. Korpan N. Hepatic cryosurgery for liver metastases. Long term follow-up. *Ann Surg* 1997; 225: 193–201

51. Ravikumar T, Kane R, Cady B *et al*. A 5-year study of cryosurgery in the treatment of liver tumours. *Arch Surg* 1991; 126: 1520–1524

52. Amin Z, Bown SG, Lees WR. Local treatment of colorectal liver metastases: a combination of interstitial laser photocoagulation (ILP) and percutaneous alcohol injection. *Clin Radiol* 1993; 48: 166–171

53. Allen-Mersh TG, Earla S, Fordy C *et al*. Quality of life and survival with continuous hepatic-artery floxuridine infusion for colorectal liver metastases. *Lancet* 1994; 344: 1255–1260

54. Hunt TM, Flowerdew ADS, Birch SJ *et al*. Prospective randomised controlled trial on hepatic arterial embolisation or infusion chemotherapy with 5-fluorouracil and degradable starch microspheres for colorectal liver metastases. *Br J Surg* 1990; 77: 779–782

55. Rougier P, Laplanche A, Huguier M *et al.* Hepatic artery infusion of floxuridine in patients with liver metastases from colorectal carcinoma: long-term results of a prospective randomised trial. *J Clin Oncol* 1992; 10: 1112–1118.

56. Kerr DJ, Lederman JA, McArdle CS *et al.* Phase I clinical trial and pharmacokinetic study of leucovorin and infusional hepatic arterial fluorouracil. *J Clin Oncol* 1995; 13: 2968–2972

Chapter 9

COLORECTAL CANCER AS A SURGICAL EMERGENCY

R.A. Audisio, W.E. Longo and F. Uggeri

Introduction

Colorectal cancer (CRC) remains one of the major causes of cancer morbidity and mortality in the Western world: 137,000 new cases affecting EC members are recorded every year, and this number is likely to increase by the year 2000. Regardless, the mortality from CRC remains high, often because many patients presenting with advanced disease at the time of diagnosis.

Surgery is currently considered to be the first therapeutic option for CRC under elective conditions: nevertheless, a number of patients with CRC present as a surgical emergency. This proportion varies widely according to geographical, cultural and economical factors. In the 1950s, Goligher[1] reported that one in five patients with CRC will present with a complete colon obstruction or perforation. This figure is in keeping with most recent reports, demonstrating an overall rate of 20–25% emergency surgical procedures for CRC today (range 6.1–48.1%).[2–10] It is difficult to know why such a percentage of patients currently exists. Patients who present with obstruction or perforation not only have a poor prognosis due to the presence of neoplastic disease, but also have a higher operative morbidity and mortality.

Surgery is being undertaken in an increasing number of elderly patients, and the proportion of this surgery undertaken as an emergency escalates with increasing age. The most common surgical emergencies seen in this age group are intestinal obstructions and perforations.[11] Regarding location, there is a significantly increased number of right-sided colonic tumours in the elderly, whereas rectal tumours present less often as a surgical emergency[2] There appears to be an increased prevalence for women.[12] No significant difference in stage distribution was recorded by Waldron et al.[2] *between the two age groups, but more aged subjects presented as an emergency.*

Age is the first risk factor for most solid tumours,[13] including CRC. If 5-year survival is worse for younger subjects under elective conditions,[14] it has been extensively reported that short-term prognosis of CRC elderly patients presenting as an emergency continues to be poor, with a clinical lethality of 50%, which compares with a 10% operative mortality for the same age group under elective conditions.[15,16] *Also, a higher co-morbidity or physiological derangement is expected for this age group. Treatment efforts are aimed at defining a therapeutic strategy that would represent a combination of an aggressive approach to the tumour and the lowest possible lethality.*[17] *An extensive overview of this topic has been presented by Koperna* et al.[17] *on a series of 110 subjects over 70 years old (obstruction: 74 patients; tumour perforation: 10 patients; colonic perforation due to obstructing CRC: 15 patients). The prevalence of co-morbidities and their clinical significance is reported in Table 9.1. These authors conclude that a pre-operative estimation of the operative risk, based on previous illnesses, is a useful tool. Similarly, the Acute Physiology and Chronic Health Evaluation (APACHE) II score might document physiological changes in the acute situation.*

Clinical data were also analysed by Wolters et al.[18] *who retrospectively compared the two age groups from a series of 411 CRC patients. The prevalence of postoperative cardiac complications, anastomotic leakage and pneumonia were significantly increased in the elderly group operated under emergency conditions, whereas none of these was more prevalent amongst elective cases. This resulted in a fivefold morbidity rate for the urgent elderly cases. Interestingly, the length of history before referral to the hospital does not seem to be affected by patient's age.*[2] *Finally, it is worth mentioning that the poor 5-year survival rate has been shown to be much more correlated with metastatic cancer and advanced disease than with advanced age, using logistic regression analysis.*[19]

In the elective setting, in over 90% of CRC patients the CRC is potentially resectable, of which 70% can effectively be treated for cure, while 13% receive a palliative procedure.[4,8] *In the emergency situation, results are not as favourable: the overall resection rate in the case of emergency surgery for CRC is usually inferior to that under elective conditions (77 vs 85% for elective series), and the resection-for-cure rate, including primary and staged resections in the emergency resections, is usually around 60%.*[4] *Thus, the primary objective of the surgical approach, in this case, is palliation of symptoms.*

Table 9.1. *Co-morbidities and their clinical significance for elderly emergency CRC patients*

Organ system or disease	Co-morbidity			Percentage mortality for patients affected
	None	Moderate	Severe	
Lungs	66	32	1	69.7
Heart	42	53	4	63.2
Kidneys	87	11	1	83.3
Liver	9	0	2	100.0
Blood	84	13	2	46.7
Intestine	97	2	0	50.0
CNS	54	40	3	58.1
Diabetes	88	0	11	90.9

After ref. 17.

Pathophysiological features

An early report by Gatch and Culbertson[20] showed that the intra-intestinal pressure increases and mesenteric venous flow decreases progressively, to stop entirely when the intra-intestinal pressure reaches the systolic pressure.[20] When this occurs, the blood flow to the mucosa is more severely affected than the flow to the muscularis or serosa. Besides oedema of the bowel wall, causing transudation of fluid, other mechanisms of circulatory changes take place and affect the remaining part of the large bowel. Often these mechanisms are mediated by circulating humoral agents or the effect of toxins.[21] Intra-intestinal fluids, which are normally absorbed in the unobstructed gut, become sequestered in the obstructed intestine so that dehydration occurs. If the ileocaecal valve is incompetent, faeculent vomiting may ensue, causing further fluid and electrolyte loss.[21]

The bowel just proximal to a left-sided large bowel occlusion has been shown to undergo initial increase in peristaltic activity, in a mini-pig model, together with decreased activity at the caecum; while the occlusive condition progresses, the peristaltic activity of the left colon will eventually decrease.[22]

Prospective clinical studies have shownhow patients with large bowel obstruction undergo changes in the intestinal flora, and are more likely to have micro-organisms translocating into the mesenteric nodes.[23] The number of anaerobic and aerobic organisms are also significantly increased in the occluded intestine,[24] and 39% of patients with occlusive disease have positive cultures from mesenteric lymph nodes.[25] Septic complications are more frequent, and occur in 43% of patients with obstruction and positive mesenteric cultures, and it was shown that the same organism was responsible for postoperative septic complication. Wound infection is doubled when surgery in performed as an emergency (25.6 vs 11.8%),[26] requiring drainage, frequent dressing and antibiotics. The risk of death from sepsis is markedly higher in patients who undergo emergency surgery.[4,17] Sepsis, peritonitis and septicaemia are responsible for the largest proportion of operative deaths in elderly patients (29% of all deaths).[11] This is caused by perforation as well as by absence of intestinal preparation and poor resistance to infection, resulting in a higher rate of persistent peritonitis.[4]

Symptoms and signs

Symptoms may vary widely, depending on the primary cause – either stricture, perforation, bleeding, or their combination. The symptoms and clinical course are also dependent on other factors such as the site of the stricture; the time between the onset of symptoms and presentation, and the patient's co-morbidities, nutritional status and age. Interestingly, the majority of patients presenting as emergencies have a relevant history of less than 3 months' duration, whereas most of the patients admitted electively have longer-lasting symptoms.[2] This might be explained by a different biological behaviour of the tumour.

The symptoms of large bowel obstruction include abdominal pain and distention, constipation and, finally, vomiting. Complete obstruction of the colon may show a dramatic onset, particularly when the patient has been experiencing increasing difficulty with bowel movements for weeks or even months, as in the case of the 'acute on chronic variety'. In this case the patient is not responding to purgatives, as was the case previously. Increasing abdominal discomfort may develop over a few days up to a week, while the subject is not experiencing nausea and vomiting, and often is eating. In other cases a more dramatic condition manifests itself with acute colicky pain, particularly when the stricture lies at the ascending colon.

CRC is reported to be responsible for approximately 50% of symptoms of large bowel obstruction, while volvulus, diverticular disease, hernia, faecal impaction and others produce the same condition in the remaining 50% of cases.[27] When a closed loop is present or the ileocaecal valve is competent, colonic distention is greater, increasing the risk of ischaemia and perforation, while an incompetent ileocaecal valve permits colonic decompression into the small bowel.

The patient with untreated large bowel obstruction may present signs of dehydration, septicaemia, abnormal bowel sounds and massive abdominal distension or shock. Hyperactive peristalsis may become evident, which may progress to a quiet abdomen, and occasionally an abdominal mass is present as well as signs of peritonism. Digital rectal examination is helpful in appreciating the 'ballooning' of the rectum, frequently elicited when the obstruction lies in the sigmoid or upper rectum. A rectal neoplasm can sometimes be palpated, although more commonly the growth is beyond the reach of the finger. Another relevant sign is the presence of blood or mucus on the examining finger. The physical examination of the obstructed patient should always include inspection of the hernial orifices, to exclude a strangulated external hernia.

A minority of patients with CRC will present with perforation and consequent peritonitis. The site of perforation can be at the site of the stricture as well as at the caecum, which becomes distended. The perforation may result into generalized faecal peritonitis, or a localized peritonitis and abscess. The former is more frequently observed when the stricture is at the left colon, and the latter in the case of growths affecting the right colon. For this reason, operative mortality is further increased in the case of perforation (Table 9.2). The presence of abdominal pain, poor performance status, tenesmus and vomiting were found by Scott *et al.*[7] to be statistically more frequent in the case of CRC presenting as an emergency. The majority (70%) of patients presenting as emergencies have a relevant history of less than 3 months, whereas 75% of patients with CRC admitted electively may report symptoms for longer than 3 months, regardless of the age group.[2]

Table 9.2. *Mortality rates (%) for obstructing and perforating CRC surgically treated as an emergency*

First author and ref. no.	Year	No. of patients	Operative deaths*
Obstructing CRC			
Glenn[28]	1971	204	27 (13)
Peloquin[29]	1975	127	27 (21)
Kronborg[30]	1975	97	14 (14)
Dutton[31]	1976	103	16 (16)
Irvin[32]	1977	66	25 (38)
Annest[33]	1979	34	6 (18)
Raftery[34]	1980	101	22 (22)
Kelley[35]	1981	156	28 (18)
Turunen[36]	1983	91	14 (15)
Umpleby[37]	1984	103	32 (31)
Hermaneck[38]	1985	173	43 (25)
Phillips[39]	1985	713	164 (23)
Waldron[40]	1986	238	78 (33)
Beuchter[41]	1988	99	23 (23)
Runkel[4]	1991	57	12 (21)
Viale[42]	1991	66	15 (23)
Tobaruela[43]	1997	34	3 (9)
Perforating CRC			
Glenn[28]	1971	99	15 (15)
Peloquin[29]	1975	59	24 (41)
Raftery[34]	1980	27	7 (26)
Kelley[35]	1981	27	8 (30)
Michowitz[44]	1982	42	16 (38)
Hermaneck[38]	1985	71	22 (31)
Runkel[4]	1991	20	6 (30)
Viale[42]	1991	38	6 (16)
Tobaruela[43]	1997	17	4 (23)

* Percentages in parentheses.

Investigations and diagnosis

In the patient who presents with CRC as a surgical emergency, few investigations are necessary to establish the diagnosis. Although physical examination can address diagnosis, one often relies on blood tests, abdominal radiographs and proctosigmoidoscopy to confirm the diagnosis.

A marked leucocytosis suggests ischaemia or perforation, while low haemoglobin levels obviously imply the presence of bleeding. These data should be interpreted cautiously, since the patient tends to show increased values of haemoglobin, platelets and white cells as a consequence of dehydration. An abdominal radiograph can confirm the clinical diagnosis, but the nature of the obstruction is not always obvious. Mechanical obstructions must be differentiated from pseudo-obstruction, the latter condition not always necessitating surgery.

In the setting of a suspected large bowel obstruction, a water-soluble contrast enema should be the initial test of choice. This may be completed with colonoscopy, especially when the aetiology is uncertain. In the setting of an incomplete obstruction, a computed tomography (CT) scan may be performed which obviously gives more anatomical information. In a number of instances the diagnosis is made only in the operating room.

Colonic haemorrhage is present less frequently than obstruction. When CRC presents as an emergency, following resuscitation and identification of underlying clotting disorders, rectal inspection can easily detect the obvious presence of fresh blood, thus requiring endoscopy. At times, nuclear scanning or angiography may be warranted.

Resuscitation

Physical status is the principal determinant of outcome after emergency admission, given the poor general condition of emergency patients.[3] Large bowel occlusion causes volume depletion and requires rehydration. The rate and type of crystalloid fluids required is defined on the basis of serum electrolyte analysis and clinical assessment. Complete blood count helps the clinician in deciding if and when blood transfusion is required. Blood transfusion has been suspected to be an independent prognosticator for both emergency and elective patients;[45] it has also been argued that the adverse impact of transfusion on cancer patient survival may be the result of unevaluated tumour variables and underlying illness.[46]

Urinary output is measured with a urinary catheter; a central venous system might be helpful for rapid fluid administration and central venous pressure assessment. Forced ventilation is infrequently required, since it is only at a late phase that the patient shows respiratory compromise, due to diaphragm compression. Ultimately, these patients should require resuscitation in an intensive care unit.

Perioperative antibiotics with a good anaerobic and Gram-negative spectrum, deep vein thrombosis prophylaxis, and preoperative stoma marking are advisable. Antibiotics should be continued for at least 5 days in the case of peritonitis.

Patients with perforation, or who are clinically suspected to have perforation or ischaemia require urgent laparotomy, as well as those who do not improve after resuscitation or if the caecal distenstion increases during 12–24 hours. Darby *et al.*[47] have suggested that, in such cases, surgery should be delayed until resuscitation is complete, thus reducing the number of unprepared patients being operated on during less than optimal operative hours. This view has also been supported by Lopez-Kostner,[21] who suggested that laparotomy is best performed during daylight hours by the regular surgical team and under the supervision of a senior anaesthetist, if the clinical condition allows it: however, other authors appear to support a contrary view. A prospective study by Kingston *et al.*[3] analysed the outcome of treating three groups of CRC patients – those operated upon within 24 hours after admission (urgent; 8.5% of cases), those whose operation was delayed for more than 24 hours (delayed; 20.5% of cases), and those who had elective surgery (71% of cases). Patients in both emergency groups were of a poorer performance status when admitted, compared with the elective group ($P < 0.0001$). Delayed surgery to allow complete resuscitation did not improve the operative mortality rate, nor did it affect the 5-year survival. Moreover, the operative mortality rate for the urgent group (15.9%) was not higher than that reported for the delayed one (15.2%), despite a greater proportion being operated on by junior staff.

Surgical options and techniques

The operative treatment of acutely obstructed left colon cancer is still a matter of debate. All efforts should be made to resect the tumour at the initial operation. Traditionally, a staged approach has been the rule, despite a relevant mortality affecting up to almost one-third of patients.[48] The advisability of postponing the resection of the tumour has been hampered by the poor 5-year survival (10–16%).[49–51] The rationale for a staged resection is based on the association with a high dehiscence rate (up to 50%), with consequent high mortality.[52] The Paul–Mikulicz tumour resection without primary anastomosis and the Hartmann's procedure have been suggested to avoid the delay of tumour resection and the high mortality and morbidity rates related to tumour staged surgery.[53] Nevertheless, temporary colostomy is reported to become definitive in 29% of patients presenting with acutely obstructed left colon cancers.[54] Colostomy closure itself carries a relevant morbidity (ranging from 11.6 to 49%) and mortality (ranging from 0.2 to 2.8%).[55]

More recently, there has been a trend towards definitive surgery with immediate resection and anastomosis, under certain conditions.[56] The presence of peritonitis, particularly when associated with purulent or faeculent peritonitis[57,58] (Table 9.3), is frequently regarded as a contraindication to primary resection and immediate anastomosis, although there is some clinical and experimental evidence to refute this view.[56,59,60] Two points are worthy of mention: first, in the preoperative setting, a metallic wall stent can be placed through the nearly obstructed colon, allowing for the patient to be adequately resuscitated and bowel 'prepped', and subsequently a one-stage procedure can be performed; secondly, in the case of immediate resection and anastomosis, often a subtotal colectomy with ileorectal anastomosis is warranted. The status of the remaining large bowel proximal to the tumour (second cancer) is unknown. Those who fear anastomotic dehiscence can perform a temporary loop ileostomy proximal to the anastomosis where a second-stage procedure does not require a full laparotomy.

Table 9.3. *Pathological grade of peritonitis according to the Hughes method,[57] modified by Krukowski[58]*

Grade	Definition
A	Acute inflammation
B1	Localized abscess
B2	Localized peritonitis
C1	Generalized purulent peritonitis
C2	Generalized faecal peritonitis

Current choices of operation have been enquired into by sending a questionnaire to 218 consultant surgeons in the UK, with a reply rate of 92%.[61] It transpired that Hartmann's procedure, with or without mucus fistula, was the most popular operation, while sigmoid colectomy with primary anastomosis was performed by 40% of surgeons, mainly for obstructing carcinomas. On-table lavage is apparently rarely used, and the majority of anastomoses were not protected by a proximal stoma. Subtotal colectomy was also unpopular, except when caecal perforation resulted from an obstructing left sided carcinoma. Standards in everyday practice show a relevant variation according to geographical distribution and surgeon's preference.

Operatively, the patient is placed in the modified lithotomy position so that the anus and the abdomen are accessible (for introducing a stapling device when required). The abdomen is opened with a midline incision and the peritoneal cavity is entered. The small bowel, when distended, can be deflated by 'milking' its content into the stomach. These procedures usually allow a better handling of the intestinal loops, although they increase the risk of contamination and mechanical injury of the ischaemic tract. The complex decision of resecting or not, the extent of the resection, and the option of a primary anastomosis or a staged procedure are discussed below.

ONE-STAGE, TWO-STAGE AND THREE-STAGE PROCEDURES

There are advocates for all these surgical approaches. Caecostomy was the principal diverting procedure until the first decades of the twentieth century,[62], but currently opinion is divided as to whether initial decompression followed by staged resection or immediate resection with or without primary anastomosis should be conducted.

Immediate resection for left-sided obstructing CRC was first introduced by Wangesteen in 1949.[63] Mealy *et al.*,[56] from Brigham and Women's Hospital, Boston, USA, have supported a one-stage resection. In their large series, which included both inflammatory conditions and CRC patients, 87.3% of subjects underwent immediate resection and two-thirds of these had primary anastomosis with no colostomy. Overall mortality was 14.3% (12.7% in the immediate resection group; 9.6% in those with primary anastomosis with no colostomy; 5.2% in the group with peritonitis undergoing resection and anastomosis and no colostomy; and 25% in those having non-resectional surgery). Their complication rate was 10.3% for infection and 7.2% for anastomotic dehiscence. A longer hospital stay for the colostomy group, especially when the colostomy was closed, was also reported. It was concluded that resection and primary anastomosis can be performed, with acceptable mortality and morbidity, in the largest proportion of cases of emergency large bowel conditions, irrespective of site of disease and presence of peritonitis.

Similarly, a retrospective analysis of 115 patients with complete neoplastic obstruction of the colon reported by Sjodahl *et al.*,[64] suggests that large bowel obstruction should be treated with primary resection, whenever possible: these authors recorded no difference between primary and staged resection when operative mortality is considered (10 vs 15%, respectively); the median hospital stay was 18 days vs 45 days for each group, with 5-year survival rates of 38 vs 29% (*P* not significant). These results are confirmed by Anderson *et al.* [65] who showed how a preliminary defunctioning stoma did not improve the survival of emergency patients compared with those undergoing primary resection (29 vs 20% 5-year survival).

Poor clinical results after primary resection and immediate colo-colonic anastomosis have been reported by Clark (27% operative mortality), [48] and Irvin (34% operative mortality).[32] A clinical trial was also conducted, to compare the two-stage procedure with the three-stage procedure. This study involved 138 patients with a left colonic or rectal stricture.[66] The two-stage procedure was conducted as follows: resection of the affected segment; colostomy on the left colon; and anastomosis of the descending loop at 1–2 months interval from primary resection. The three-stage procedure consisted of loop colostomy at the transverse colon, planned resection with anastomosis 2–3 weeks later, and transverse colostomy closure 2–3 months after resection. Complications after the two-stage procedure tended to be more frequent, but no statistical significance was recorded, whereas wound infections were statistically more frequent. Postoperative deaths were equally frequent (eight subjects in the two-stage and seven patients in the three-stage approach), and the overall recurrence rates and survival rates were also similar in the two groups. The duration of hospital stay was significantly reduced in the two-stage group, but the risk of a permanent colostomy was less in the three-stage group. This was explained by the surgeon's reluctance to perform a second operation in the presence of severe co-morbidities. High mortality figures are also reported from staged resection series, varying from 20–22% in the series of Umpleby[37] to 31% in that of Clark *et al.* [48] where the creation of a diverting colostomy and its closure is in part responsible for these high mortality rates.

At present, resection without anastomosis is a good option for patients with risk factors that preclude a primary anastomosis, such as severe nutritional impairment, immunosuppression, advanced (locally or metastatic) neoplastic disease, perforated left colon carcinoma and extreme cardiopulmonary risk. A staged procedure might also be considered for elderly subjects with increased number of co-morbidities. However, more emergency patients are given stomas than those operated on under elective conditions (56 vs 35%, $P<0.0001$).[7]

SUBTOTAL/TOTAL COLECTOMY

Hughes[67] reported emergency subtotal colectomy with ileosigmoid anastomosis (Figure 9.1) in 1970; the procedure was conducted on 17 patients with no operative mortality.[67] Several series have subsequently reported on its use in a number of patients.[5,68–72] The rationale for this procedure is based on the fact that the terminal ileum has a rich blood supply.[53] It is also supported by the fact that synchronous CRCs may hamper the efficacy of a segmental resection: there were 6.8% synchronous CRCs at the time of acute presentation in the series reported by Arnaud.[53]

Subtotal colectomy achieves relief of bowel obstruction and tumour resection. It has also been reported to ensure restoration of gut continuity by encompassing a massively distended and faeces-laden colon with ischaemic lesions and serosal tears on the caecum,[53] although the prevalence of these last pathological lesions has not been documented. Subtotal colectomy was previously thought of as a major undertaking requiring the intervention of an experienced surgeon.[73] Mean operative time averages 3 hours[5] and mean postoperative hospital stay is rather long (mean 26 days; range 8–31 days).[5,69,74,75] An extensive review of the literature was written by Arnaud *et al.*[53] summarizing an 8.2% rate of overall mortality and 0.4% rate of anastomotic mortality (Table 9.4). Notably, only 44 cases from his personal series of 118 subjects presenting with intestinal obstruction, were selected for such a procedure.

Although functional results have been questioned,[85] today this procedure is fairly routine.

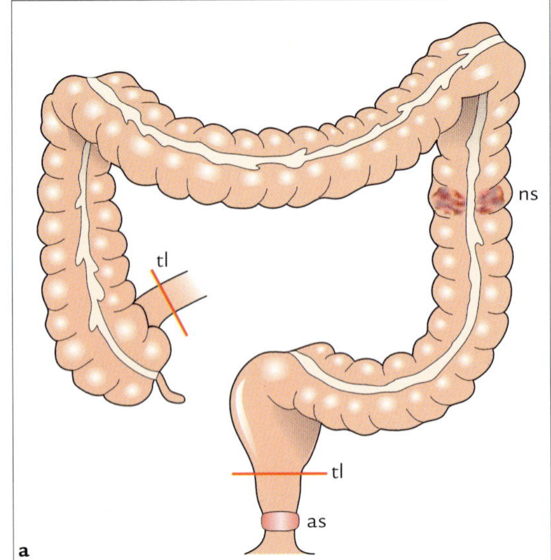

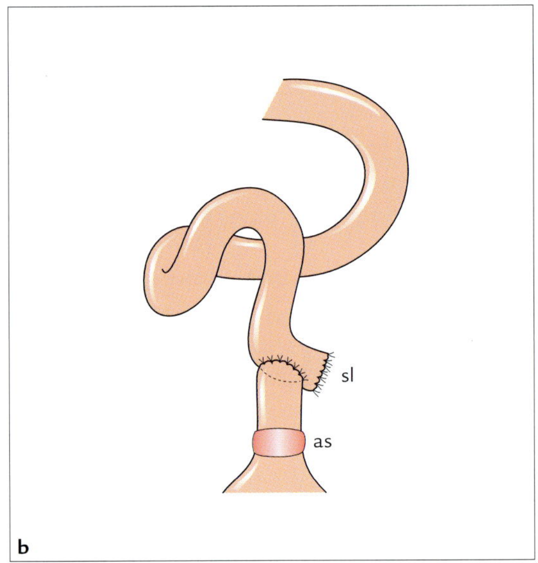

Figure 9.1: *Total/subtotal colectomy: the terminal ileal loop (a) is sutured to the rectal stump (b). as, anal sphincter; ns, neoplastic stricture; sl, suture line; tl, transection line.*

RIGHT HEMICOLECTOMY

Although CRC more frequently affects the left colon and rectum, 25% of patients will present with a right-sided colon cancer, and one-quarter of these will require emergency right hemicolectomy[72]. This procedure is defined as the resection of a portion of the terminal ileum, the whole of the ascending colon, and variable amounts of the transverse colon (Figure 9.2). This operative procedure is most frequently performed as an emergency for obstructing tumour (83%), and occasionally for perforated cancers (10%) especially caecal perforation, secondary to a left-sited obstruction (7%).[72]

A large series of right emergency hemicolectomies was reported by Smithers *et al.*[72] These authors recorded an average age of 68 years at presentation and complications were more common among patients whose age was over 70 years. The operative mortality did not differ statistically between emergency and

Table 9.4. *Total/subtotal colectomy for obstructing CRC*

First author and ref. no.	Year	No. of patients	Operative deaths*
Hughes[67]	1970	17	0 (0)
Valerio[68]	1978	5	1 (20)
Terry[76]	1981	5	1 (20)
Klatt[74]	1981	5	0 (0)
Deutsch[75]	1983	14	1 (7)
Brief[77]	1983	15	0 (0)
Glass[70]	1983	7	1 (14)
Weddel[78]	1983	12	1 (8)
Cady[79]	1985	12	2 (16)
Morgan[80]	1985	16	2 (12)
Pakhomova[81]	1985	11	2 (18)
Samama[82]	1986	3	1 (33)
Halevy[69]	1987	8	0 (0)
Feng[83]	1987	9	1 (11)
Wilson[84]	1989	18	2 (11)
Halevy[5]	1989	22	1 (5)
Stephenson[119]	1990	31	0 (0)
Arnaud[53]	1994	44	3 (7)

* Percentages in parentheses.

elective procedures (7 vs 5.3%), with cardiac morbidity being the most prevalent in both groups. Operative mortality was significantly reduced for curative surgery (2.1%) compared with for palliative procedures (25%), thus confirming a higher operative morbidity for patients with disseminated disease. Wound infection occurred in 15.7% of emergency cases (vs 10% of elective cases).

A high incidence of anastomotic breakdown in emergency right colectomy has been reported, averaging 9–10%,[72,86] and this complication seems to be linked to the high prevalence of patients with advanced disease undergoing a palliative procedure. It has also been suggested that an ileocolonic anastomosis, should be avoided, substituting an ileostomy and mucous fistula;[86] however, ileostomies have their own complications, especially when performed as an emergency.[87] In the presence of an incompetent ileocaecal valve and disseminated disease, the patient might be treated by bypassing the tumour, although this is not strongly recommended (Table 9.5).

ON-TABLE LAVAGE

When a left-sided CRC is to be treated as an emergency, the bowel cannot be adequately

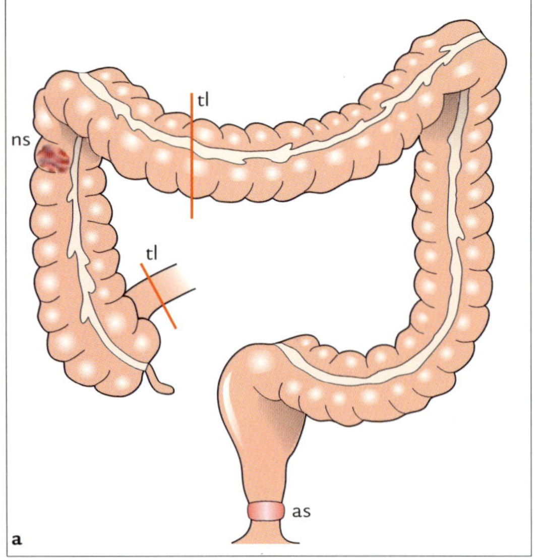

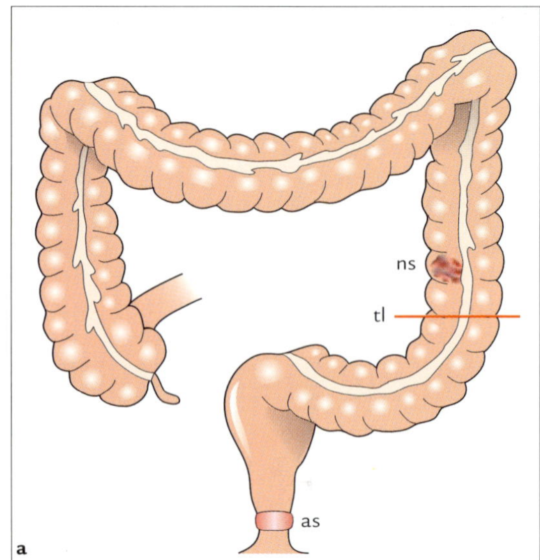

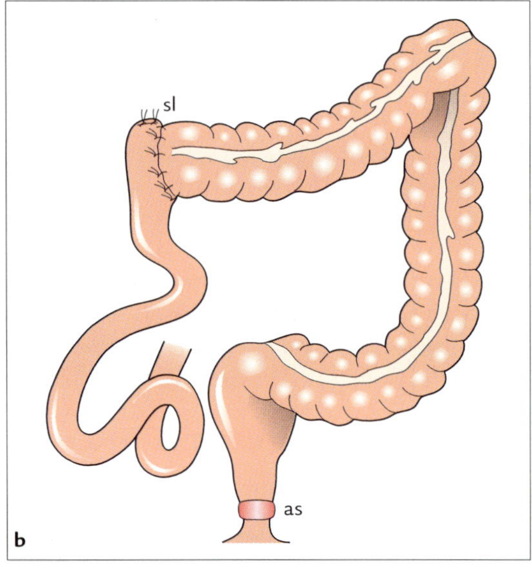

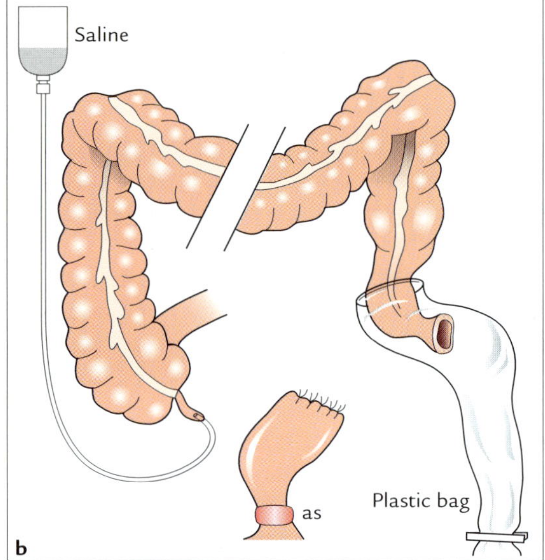

Figure 9.2: *Right hemicolectomy: the terminal ileal loop (a) is sutured to the transverse colon (b). as, anal sphincter; ns, neoplastic structure; sl, suture line; tl, transection line.*

Figure 9.3: *The washout technique (see text for explanation). ns, neoplastic structure; tl, transection line.*

prepared. The washout technique was introduced to reduce the bowel distension above the stricture, thus restoring the blood flow within the bowel wall. This favours the peristaltic movements and the synthetic processes at the anastomotic site. Finally, the washout significantly reduces the bacterial flora and decreases the prevalence of postoperative septic events.[90] Several authors take advantage of this procedure, which is relatively inexpensive and only moderately time consuming. From the practical point of view, the washout is performed as follows (Figure 9.3). Preoperative antibiotics are administered according to local practice (e.g. gentamicin 80 mg plus 600 mg clindamycin, or gentamicin 80 mg plus 500 mg metronidazole). The obstructed portion of the gut is prepared according to the standard technique (Figure

Table 9.5. *Right emergency hemicolectomy for obstructing/perforating CRC*

First author and ref. no.	Year	No. of patients	Operative deaths*
Hughes[67]	1970	17	0 (0)
Debas[86]	1973	43	10 (23)
Clark[41]	1975	23	8 (35)
Dutton[31]	1976	103	31 (30)
Valerio[68]	1978	22	2 (10)
Garrison[87]	1979	16	4 (25)
Fielding[88]	1979	54	10 (19)
Cohen[89]	1983	34	6 (18)
Smithers[72]	1986	57	4 (7)
Viale[42]	1991	11	2 (18)

* Percentages in parentheses.

9.3a). The prestenotic portion is also mobilized to allow adequate exteriorization out of the abdominal cavity, into a sterile plastic bag (Figure 9.3b). The gut is incised above the structure, to allow the outflow of fluids. Warm saline (3–30 litres) plus Betadine (povidone-iodine) or other solutions are freely introduced through a probe at the caecum. Some surgeons prefer to insert a Petzer drain at the caecum (through the abdominal wall, eventually left in site until postoperative day 10), whereas others prefer to insert a large Foley catheter 5 cm before the ileocaecal valve or into the appendix. It is essential to leave a clamp on the distal part of the small bowel while introducing the saline, to avoid inflation of this part of the gut and also of the stomach. A one-stage procedure is then performed according to standard technique.

It must be remembered that not every patient is suitable for this procedure, which should be undertaken only when the patient is a good surgical candidate. For the above-mentioned reasons, the washout procedure could safely be delivered to only one-third of the patients with a left colonic obstruction in a series reported by Peppas *et al.*[90] However, the postoperative dehiscence rate was still 19.5%, and the postoperative mortality rate 2.4%.[90] Conversely, a series from Japan, where a primary resection and anastomosis with intraoperative bowel irrigation was performed on 80% of subjects and compared with a staged resection offered to 20% of patients, showed no significant difference in the rates of curative resections, whereas postoperative infection, anastomotic dehiscence and postoperative mortality rates were reduced in the group of patients receiving a large bowel washout.[91] On-table colonic lavage and primary anastomosis is also currently conducted in the United Kingdom according to the Allen-Mersh report:[92] the results were comparable to those from a series of similar patients treated according to Hartmann's procedure, with no difference in perioperative mortality and morbidity.

HARTMANN'S PROCEDURE

In 1921 the results of a new surgical procedure were first presented by Terrier Henri Hartmann in Strasburg. This operation was specifically designed for obstructive lesions of the sigmoid colon, where patients receive a proximal colostomy while undergoing resection with closure of the rectal stump. This procedure was considered an option for those patients who were not amenable to abdominoperineal

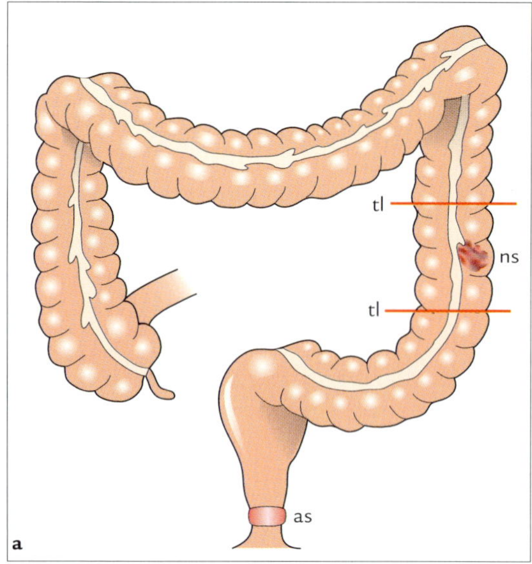

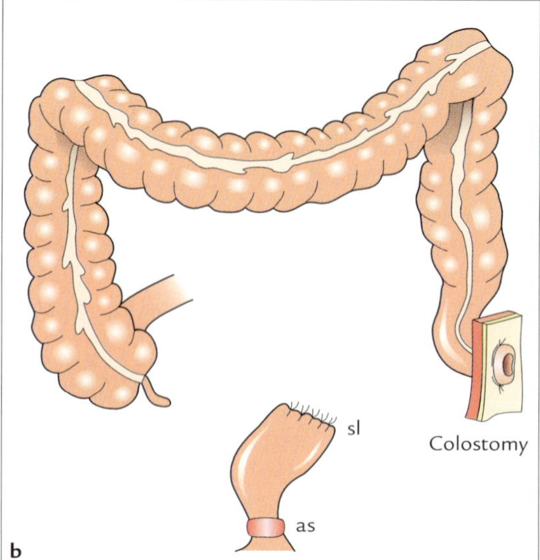

Figure 9.4: *The Hartmann's procedure: the rectal stump is transected and sutured on a purse-string (a). The distal colonic loop is sutured to the abdominal wall (b). as, anal sphincter; ns, neoplastic structure; sl, suture line; tl, transection line.*

resection. The original procedure included the transection of the rectum, which was closed at or below, the peritoneal reflection, where the bowel is supplied with blood by the inferior haemorrhoidal arteries (Figure 9.4).

The role of Hartmann's procedure has changed dramatically during the twentieth century: several authors, worldwide, have applauded this technique, which allows radical removal of the neoplasm and does not incur the risk of a problematic anastomosis in poor - risk patients with ill-prepared bowels. Technical advancements have been proposed such as avoidance of any mobilization/dissection of the sigmoid stump,[93] and the use of purse-string sutures[94]. A major pitfall with this operation is the low conversion rate, such that no more than one-half of the patients will have their bowel continuity successfully restored.[95,96] This is not specifically related to the emergency procedure: in a previous personal elective series, none of the 50 patients treated in this way had intestinal continuity re-established.[97] It is likely that these statistics will change significantly in the future, since the introduction of minimally invasive techniques allows a much easier anastomosis with minimal operative risk.

Hartmann's operation has also been performed and promoted as an elective procedure for rectal cancer, where an abdominoperineal excision is not needed and low anterior resection cannot guarantee acceptable continence;[98] however, operative mortality and morbidity can still be as high as 8–15% and 50–80% respectively, with one-third of the subjects developing pelvic or wound sepsis.[97–99] It was also claimed that the remaining rectal stump does not generate morbidity or discomfort, but the occurrence of carcinomas at the rectal pouch has been reported;[100] thus, a careful endoscopic follow-up of the rectal stump is required.

EMERGENCY ENDOSCOPY

Bowel decompression is the first goal in cases of acutely obstructing CRC. In certain cases, radical treatment is often beyond expectations, and a purely palliative approach can be considered in the respect of quality of life and health-economics evaluations, when long-term survival cannot be improved. The patients presenting with acute symptoms are often aged and at poor risk. On the basis of these considerations, a purely endoscopic approach has been introduced.[101] Palliative endoscopic management of inoperable CRC makes use of a variety of techniques: these include laser photocoagulation with neodymium–yttrium aluminium garnet

(Nd:YAG) source, mechanical or pneumatic dilatation, electrocoagulation, debulking with diathermal snare, liquid nitrogen cryotherapy, and their combined application.[102–107] Such emergency measures successfully restore bowel continuity while achieving decompression; they eventually represent a prelude to poor-risk elective surgery, waiting for improvements in the patient's general conditions.[101]

Arrigoni *et al.*[101] treated 17 patients in this way, who were unfit for surgery as a consequence of poor medical condition (electrolyte imbalance/dehydration, signs of heart failure, respiratory failure, decompensated diabetes, pneumonia). Emergency endoscopy was performed without preparation or premedication; antibiotics (piperacillin or ceftazidime) were given 1 hour before the procedure. A small volume of air was insufflated, and colonic gases were exchanged several times, by aspiration and CO_2 reinsufflation, before a diathermal snare or laser was used. As the endoscope could not be passed through the stricture, four different techniques were used: these included (1) pneumatic dilatation with Rigiflex TTS balloons (18 mm in diameter) 3–8 cm in length; (2) mechanical dilation with Savary dilators (12–18 mm in diameter) inserted through a guidewire previously positioned under fluoroscopic control; (3) Nd:YAG laser photocoagulation with a power rating of 60–70 W (the beam was moved forward to the lower pole of the neoplasm, at a dose of 8000–15,000 J for each session); (4) debulking with a diathermal snare cautery device, (the obstructing growth was removed with a combination of cutting and coagulating current).

A neoplastic stricture which was located at the rectosigmoid junction (four patients), sigmoid (four patients) and left colon (two patients). Patients were treated with a mean of one session (range 1–2 sessions), each session lasting 20–40 minutes. Patency was achieved in 11 cases (65%) in one single session, while five cases required two separate sessions; the procedure was unsuccessful in 1/17 cases. Pain was absent during laser treatment, and transient during balloon insufflation. No complications were noted.

The long-term results are also of interest: six patients died of cancer 2–9 months after the procedure. Recurrent stenosis was detected in two patients at 2 and 3 months from the procedure, respectively. The actuarial survival rates at 6 and 12 months were 63 and 23% respectively. This procedure should be considered in the management of the fragile patient, when surgery cannot be offered as a first step, if at all.

EXPANDABLE METAL STENT APPLICATION

A recent case report by Campbell *et al.*[108] confirms the feasibility of stenting obstructing colonic lesions, and expands the indications for stent application, even if the obstruction occurs at the right colon. This approach is indicated only when the patient is not a candidate for surgery, because of an excessively high operative risk. The authors describe the successful application of a metal stent in the right colon, allowing postponement of a particularly high-risk laparotomy.

MINIMALLY INVASIVE APPROACH

Patients with advanced malignancies often receive faecal diversion to relieve obstruction and other complications such as incontinence, perineal sepsis and fistulas. Laparoscopic faecal diversion does not require an abdominal incision (such as laparotomy) and does not limit intra-abdominal exploration. This procedure is technically simple, and can be performed easily with minimal equipment, even by inexperienced surgeons[109]. It allows the patient to recover without laparotomy, pain and related complications. Laparoscopic colostomy also decreases the complications rate of open colostomy, namely evisceration/incisional hernia and wound infection, which can affect 43% of the laparotomic group.[110] Bowel function returns more quickly after laparoscopy than laparotomy: furthermore, the small abdominal incision entails lower doses of narcotics because of less pain and a shorter procedure. A theoretical advantage is the reduced adhesion formation, while the surgeon is allowed to identify and mobilize the bowel segment accurately; however, in patients with a dilated colon or small bowel, visualization may not be enough to allow the surgeon to accomplish sufficient intestinal mobilization safely, and conversion to an open procedure may be required. No studies have compared open with laparoscopic colostomy, to confirm the theoretical advantages of the latter.[111]

STOMA COLOSTOMY

On the basis of the assumption that a primary anastomosis may be risky under emergency conditions, while supporting the resection of the primary CRC – if technically feasible – Lange *et al.*[112] proposed a new technique. This procedure, which they presented as the 'anastomotic stoma', consists of resection according to standard practice, followed by the configuration of a temporary stoma, when the loop is sufficiently mobilized: the distal and proximal loops are brought together, and they are anastomized on the posterior wall. The anterior wall is left open and fixed at the abdominal wall as a stoma. The anastomotic stoma protects the posterior wall from elevated pressure, while allowing control of the anastomosis (Figure 9.5).

Lange *et al.*[112] reported their results in 91 consecutive patients treated accordingly (73 as an emergency procedure), avoiding the disadvantage of a secondary laparotomy to restore bowel continuity. There was no operative death, however, one-quarter of the patients died as a consequence of the primary disease.

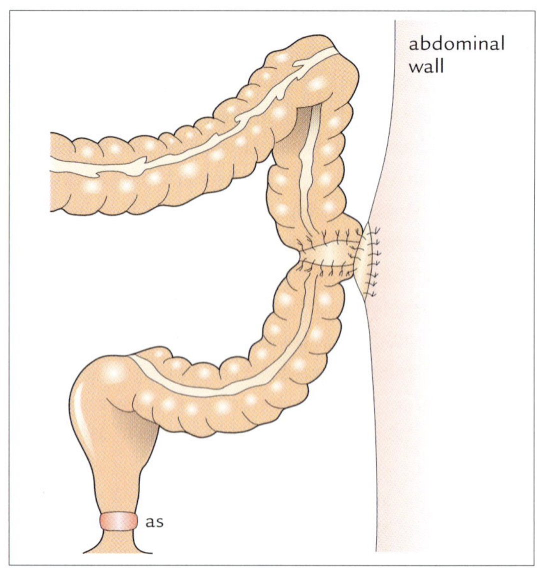

Figure 9.5: *Stoma colectomy: a primary colo-colonic anastomosis is hand sewn, while part of it is fixed at the abdominal wall and left open for regular checks*

CARCINOMATOSIS

Intraperitoneal seeding is frequent among subjects with recurrent CRC, although several cancer patients may present similar symptoms. Carcinomatosis and obstructive syndrome may result from other gastrointestinal primaries (gastric and pancreatic tumours), as well as breast and gynaecological tumours, or mesothelioma and other intra-abdominal sarcomas.

These patients have a poor prognosis, due to the advanced stage of disease. Unfortunately, most of these cases have minimal, if any, chance of being controlled by any sort of treatment. Their response rate to chemotherapy or radiation therapy is low, even when these are administered intraperitoneally. These subjects will present with bowel obstruction, vomiting and distended abdomen.

Combined cytoreductive surgery and intraperitoneal hyperthermic chemotherapy is being investigated as a treatment for peritoneal carcinomatosis from CRC. A few selected patients might benefit from this combined treatment modality, which appears to be less effective in patients with CRC than in those with other types of cancer.[94]

The role of enteral and parenteral nutrition requires critical supervision, and is best delivered by a specialized team, which should include a medical oncologist, pain-control specialist and oncological nurse. Risky, expensive and useless surgical procedures should be avoided.

Quality of life, the key issue here, should be a prime consideration. Any surgical procedure requires a conscious approach to the terminally ill cancer patient. Surgical oncologists should wisely address appropriate palliation, avoiding useless procedures such as the application of gastrostomy tubes or the implementation of an operative jejunostomy.[113]

Conclusions and recommendations

Colorectal emergencies represent a challenging proportion of the acute workload of general surgical units. Initial assessment and management should be directed towards the patient as a whole, taking into great consideration co-morbidities, risk factors, physical condition, and stage of disease.[114]

Emergency admission for CRC is to be considered a personal and resource disaster;[7] it is also highly expensive, as it has been shown that the median hospital stay is significantly longer than that for elective cases (16 vs 13 days; $P = 0.0001$).[7] Physical status is the principal determinant of outcome after emergency admission, given the poor general conditions of emergency patients.[3] Surgical strategies alone are probably only of marginal significance to the central problem determining poor outcome after emergency admission – the emergency patient is significantly more sick than the elective patient.[7]

Early diagnosis protocols and pre-symptomatic screening programmes are to be reinforced, with the aim of reducing the number of CRC patients presenting as a surgical emergency, particularly among high-risk groups (as is the case for elderly subjects). A more sensible dietary regimen might further decrease the incidence of this dramatic clinical presentation.[115]

Operative risk is increased overall, and the long-term results are hampered by a higher proportion of advanced stages (Dukes' 'D'). Other recognized risk factors are advanced age and membership of a low social class, where patients treated as an emergency are significantly less likely to have seen their primary care physician before admission.[7]

It is argued[64,115] that the non-specialized surgeon performing the procedure as an emergency has worst results, since the 5-year survival is poorer than that for elective surgery. However, it is likely that, disease-related variables (advanced stage),[8;116] or patient-related variables (patients age) may have a greater influence on ultimate survival than surgeon-related variables.[3,117]

Recently, a trend toward primary anastomosis had been established, but treatment is to be tailored according to the clinical presentation and the patient's general condition, as well as to the surgeon's preference and local facilities. The most favoured option for a single-stage procedure is segmental colectomy with on-table antegrade colonic irrigation and colo-colonic anastomosis.[118] Hartmann's procedure remains a popular choice, although one of three patients will never undergo reversal. Subtotal/total colectomy can be considered when several segments of the large bowel are obviously suffering ischaemia or perforation, or in the presence of multiple growths, where functional results are poorer than after segmental resection. New techniques, such as Nd:YAG laser photocoagulation and expandable metal stenting, may help to optimize patient selection for major curative procedures, while achieving satisfactory palliation.

References

1. Goligher JC, Smiddy FG. The treatment of acute obstruction for perforation and cancer of the colon and rectum. *Br J Surg* 1957; 45: 270–274

2. Waldron RP, Donovan IA, Drumm J *et al.* Emergency presentation and mortality from colorectal cancer in the elderly. *Br J Surg* 1986; 73: 214–216

3. Kingston RD, Jeacock J, Walsh SH. Physical status is the principal determinant of outcome after emergency admission of patients with colorectal cancer. *Ann R Coll Surg Engl* 1993; 75: 335–338

4. Runkel NS, Schlag PM, Schwarz V, Herfarth C. Outcome after emergency surgery for cancer of the large intestine. *Br J Surg* 1991; 78: 183–188

5. Halevy A, Levi J, Orda R. Emergency subtotal colectomy. *Ann Surg* 1989; 210: 220–223

6. Platell C. A community-based hospital experience with colorectal cancer. *Aust NZ J Surg* 1997; 67: 420–423

7. Scott NA, Jeacock J, Kingston RD. Risk factors in patients presenting as an emergency with colorectal cancer. *Br J Surg* 1995; 82: 321–323

8. Ponz de Leon M, Sassatelli R, Scalmati A *et al.* Descriptive epidemiology of colorectal cancer in Italy: the 6-year experience of a specialised registry. *Eur J Cancer* 1993; 29A(3): 367–371

9. Maghetti F, Fabiani P. Emergencies in cancer of the colorectum. *Ann Ital Chir* 1996; 67(2): 177–185

10. Myrvold HE. Surgical procedures in colorectal cancer emergencies. *Scand J Gastroenterol* 1988; 149: 120–124

11. McIntyre R, Reinbach D, Cuschieri A. Emergency abdominal surgery in the elderly. *J R Coll Surg Edinb* 1997; 42: 173–178

12. Uccheddu A, Cois A, Dessena M *et al.* Il cancro colorettale in etò geriatrica. *Minerva Chir* 1994; 49: 1215–1220

13. Audisio RA, Veronesi P, Ferrario L *et al.* Elective surgery for gastrointestinal tumours in the elderly. *Ann Oncol* 1997; 8: 317–326

14. Crucitti F, Sofo L, Doglietto GB *et al.* Prognostic factors in colorectal cancer: current status and new trends. *J Surg Oncol* 1991; 2(Suppl): 76–82

15. Hessman O, Bergkvist L, Strom S. Colorectal cancer in patients over 75 years of age – determinants of outcome. *Eur J Surg Oncol* 1997; 23: 13–19

16. Mulcahy HE, Patchett SE, Daly L, O'Donoghue DP. Prognosis of elderly patients with large bowel cancer. *Br J Surg* 1994; 81: 736–738

17. Koperna T, Kisser M, Schulz F. Emergency surgery for colon cancer in the aged. *Arch Surg* 1997; 132: 1032–1037

18. Wolters U, Isenberg J, Stutzer H. Colorectal carcinoma – aspects of surgery in the elderly. *Anticancer Res* 1997; 17: 1273–1276

19. Kemppainen M, Raiha I, Sourander L. Influence of age on colorectal cancer's 5-year survival. *Gerontology* 1995; 41: 145–151

20. Gatch W, Culbertson C. Circulatory disturbances caused by intestinal obstruction. *Ann Surg* 1935; 102: 619

21. Lopez-Kostner F, Hool GR, Lavery IC. Management and causes of acute large-bowel obstruction. *Surg Clin North Am* 1997; 77: 1265–1290

22. Coxon J, Dickson C, Taylor I. Changes in colonic motility during the development of chronic large bowel obstruction. *Br J Surg* 1985; 72: 690–693

23. Smith S, Connolly J, Gilmore O. The effect of faecal loading on colonic anastomotic healing. *Br J Surg* 1983; 70: 49–50

24. Sykes P, Boulter K, Schofield P. The microflora of the obstructed bowel. *Br J Surg* 1976; 63: 721–725

25. Sagar PM, MacFie J, Sedman P *et al.* Intestinal obstruction promotes gut translocation of bacteria. *Dis Colon Rectum* 1995; 38: 640–644

26. Bielecki K, Badi H, Kaminski P, Kubiak J. Postoperative wound infection in colorectal surgery. *Mater Med Pol* 1995; 27: 67–69

27. Greenlee HB. Proceedings: Acute large bowel obstruction. Comparison of county, Veterans Administration, and community hospital populations. *Arch Surg* 1974; 108: 470–476

28. Glenn F, McSherry CK. Obstruction and perforation in colorectal cancer. *Ann Surg* 1971; 173: 983–992

29. Peloquin AB. Factors influencing survival with complete obstruction and free perforation of colorectal cancers. *Dis Colon Rectum* 1975; 18: 11–21

30. Kronborg O, Backer O, Sprechler M. Acute obstruction in cancer of the colon and rectum. *Dis Colon Rectum* 1975; 18: 22–27

31. Dutton JW, Hreno A, Hampson LG. Mortality and prognosis of obstructing carcinoma of the large bowel. *Am J Surg* 1976; 131: 36–41

32. Irvin TT, Greaney MG. The treatment of colonic cancer presenting with intestinal obstruction. *Br J Surg* 1977; 64: 741–744

33. Annest L, Jolly P. The results of surgical treatment of bowel obstruction. *Am J Surg* 1979; 45: 718–721

34. Raftery TL, Samson N. Carcinoma of the colon: a clinical correlation between presenting symptoms and survival. *Am Surg* 1980; 46: 600–606

35. Kelley W Jr, Brown PW, Lawrence W Jr, Terz JJ. Penetrating, obstructing, and perforating carcinomas of the colon and rectum. *Arch Surg* 1981; 116: 381–384

36. Turunen MJ. Colorectal cancer obstruction: a challenge to improve prognosis. *Ann Chir Gynaecol* 1983; 72: 317–323

37. Umpleby HC, Williamson R. Survival in acute obstructing colorectal carcinoma. *Dis Colon Rectum* 1984; 27: 299–304

38. Hermaneck P Jr, Schweiger M, Gall FP. Colorectal carcinoma presenting in emergency situation. *Langenbecks Arch Chir* 1985; 366: 461–465

39. Phillips R, Hittinger R, Fry JS *et al*. Malignant large bowel obstruction. *Br J Surg* 1985; 72: 296–302

40. Waldron RP, Donovan IA. Mortality in patients with obstructing colorectal cancer. *Ann R Coll Surg Engl* 1986; 68: 219–221

41. Buechter KJ, Boustany C, Caillouette R, Cohn I. Surgical management of the acutely obstructed colon. *Am J Surg* 1988; 156: 163–168

42. Viale A, Ghisotti E, Ferraris C, Anselmetti GC. Le urgenze nella chirurgia delle neoplasie del colon. *Minerva Chir* 1991; 46: 25–30

43. Tobaruela E, Camunas J, Enriquez-Navascues JM *et al*. Medical factors in the morbidity and mortality associated with emergency colorectal cancer surgery. *Rev Esp Enferm Apar Dig* 1997; 89: 13–22

44. Michowitz M, Avnieli D, Lazarovici I, Solowiejczyk M. Perforation complicating carcinoma of colon. *J Surg Oncol* 1982; 19: 18–21

45. Edna TH, Bjerkeset T. Perioperative blood transfusions reduce long-term survival following surgery for colorectal cancer. *Dis Colon Rectum* 1998; 41: 451–459

46. Donohue JH, Williams S, Cha S, *et al*. Perioperative blood transfusion do not affect disease recurrence of patients undergoing curative resection of colorectal carcinoma. *J Clin Oncol* 1995; 13: 1671–1678

47. Darby CR, Berry AR, Mortense N. Management variability in surgery for colorectal emergencies. *Br J Surg* 1992; 79: 206–210

48. Clark Y, Hall AW, Mossa AR. Treatment of obstructing cancer of the colon and rectum. *Surg Gynecol Obstet* 1975; 141: 541–544

49. Fielding LP, Phillips R, Hittinger R. Factors influencing mortality after curative resection for large bowel cancer in elderly patients. *Lancet* 1989; 1: 595–597.

50. Aldridge MC, Phillips RK, Hittinger R *et al*. Influence of tumour site on presentation, management and subsequent outcome in large bowel cancer. *Br J Surg* 1986; 73: 663–670

51. Ohman U. Colorectal carcinoma – trends and results over a 30-year period. *Dis Colon Rectum* 1982; 25: 431–440

52. Irvin GL, Horsley S, Caruana JA. The morbidity and mortality of emergency operations for colorectal disease. *Ann Surg* 1998; 199: 598–603

53. Arnaud JP, Bergamaschi R. Emergency subtotal/total colectomy with anastomosis for acutely obstructed carcinoma of the left colon. *Dis Colon Rectum* 1994; 37: 685–688

54. Champault G, Adloff M, Arnaud JP *et al*. Colonic Occlusions. Retrospective cooperative study of 497 cases. *J Chir (Paris)* 1983; 120: 47–56

55. Mitchell W, Kovalick P, Gross G. Complications of colostomy closure. *Dis Colon Rectum* 1978; 21: 180

56. Mealy K, Salman A, Arthur G. Definitive one-stage emergency large bowel surgery. *Br J Surg* 1988; 75: 1216–1219

57. Hughes E, Cuthbertson A, Garden A. The surgical management of acute diverticulitis. *Med J Aust* 1963; 1: 780–782

58. Krukowski Z, Matheson N. Emergency surgery for diverticular disease complicated by generalised faecal peritonitis: a review. *Br J Surg* 1984; 71: 921–927

59. Ravo B, Mishrick A, Addei K. The treatment of perforated diverticulitis by one stage intracolonic by-pass procedure. *Surgery* 1987; 102: 771–776

60. Ryan P. The effect of surrounding infection upon leaking of colonic wounds: experimental studies and clinical experience. *Dis Colon Rectum* 1970; 13: 124–126

61. Pain J, Cahill J. Surgical options for left-sided large bowel emergencies. *Ann R Coll Surg Engl* 1991; 73: 394–396

62. Burgess AH. An address on acute intestinal obstruction. *Lancet* 1929; 1: 857

63. Wangesteen O. Cancer of the colon and rectum. *Wis Med J* 1949; 48: 591

64. Sjodahl R, Franzén T, Nystrom PO. Primary versus staged resection for acute obstructing colorectal carcinoma. *Br J Surg* 1992; 79: 685–688

65. Anderson JH, Hole D, McArdle CS. Elective versus emergency surgery for patients with colorectal cancer. *Br J Surg* 1992; 79: 706–709

66. Kronborg O. Acute obstruction from tumour in the left colon without spread – a randomized trial of emergency colostomy versus resection. *Int J Color Dis* 1995; 10: 1–5

67. Hughes ES. Subtotal colectomy for carcinoma of the colon. *J R Soc Med* 1970; 63: 41–42

68. Valerio D, Jones PJ. Immediate resection in the treatment of large bowel emergencies. *Br J Surg* 1978; 65: 712–716

69. Halevy A, Ponczek M, Orda R. Emergency subtotal colectomy for obstructing carcinoma of the left colon. *J Surg Oncol* 1987; 35: 256–258

70. Glass RL, Smith LE, Cochran RC. Subtotal colectomy for obstructing carcinoma of the left colon. *Am J Surg* 1983; 145: 335–336

71. Adloff M, Arnaud JP, Ollier JC. Emergency one-stage subtotal colectomy with anastomosis for obstructing carcinoma of the left colon. *Dig Surg* 1984; 1: 37–40

72. Smithers BM, Theile DE, Cohen JR *et al.* Emergency right hemicolectomy in colon carcinoma: a prospective study. *Aust NZ J Surg* 1986; 56: 749–752

73. Goligher JC. Treatment of carcinoma of the colon. In: Goligher JC (ed). *Surgery of the Anus, Rectum and Colon*. London: Bailliere Tindall, 1975, pp. 607–626

74. Klatt GR, Martin WH, Gillespie JT. Subtotal colectomy with primary anastomosis without diversion in the treatment of obstructing carcinoma of the left colon. *Am J Surg* 1981; 141: 577–578

75. Deutsch AA, Zelikovski A, Sternberg A, Reiss R. One-stage subtotal colectomy with anastomosis for obstructing carcinoma of the left colon. *Dis Colon Rectum* 1983; 26: 227–230

76. Terry BG, Beart R Jr. Emergency abdominal colectomy with primary anastomosis. *Dis Colon Rectum* 1981; 24: 1–4

77. Brief DK, Brener BJ, Goldenkranz R *et al.* An argument for increased use of subtotal colectomy in the management of carcinoma of the colon. *Am Surg* 1983; 49: 66–72

78. Weddel H, Banzhof G, Eissen M *et al.* Die notfallmassige colektomie mit primarer anastomose beim obturierenden linkseitigen colon carcinom. *Chirurg* 1983; 54: 582–588

79. Cady J, Godfroy J, Paclot R, Sibaud O. La colectomie sub-totale en un temps dans les occlusions intestinales aigues néoplastiques du colon gauche. *Ann Chir* 1985; 39: 377–380

80. Morgan WP, Jenkins N, Lewis P, Aubrey DA. Management of obstructing carcinoma of the left colon by extended right hemicolectomy. *Am J Surg* 1985; 149: 327–329

81. Pakhomova GV, Uteshev NS, Gurchumelidze TP. Subtotal colectomy in the treatment of intestinal obstruction in cancer of the left half of the colon. *Vestn Khir* 1985; 134: 58–62

82. Samama G, Brefort JL, Faaure A, Girard A. Cancers du colon gauche en occlusion. Traitment par colectomie sub-total avec anastomose iléosigmoidienne immédiate. *Presse Med* 1985; 25: 2070–2071

83. Feng Y-S, Hsu H, Chen S-S. One-stage operation for obstructing carcinomas of the left colon and rectum. *Dis Colon Rectum* 1987; 30: 29–32

84. Wilson RG, Gollock JM. Obstructive carcinoma of the left colon managed by subtotal colectomy. *J R Coll Surg Edinb* 1989; 34: 25–26

85. Substantial Colectomy vs On Table Irrigation and Anastomosis Study Group. Single-stage treatment for malignant left-sided colonic obstruction: a prospective randomized clinical trial comparing subtotal colectomy with segmantal resection following intraoperative irrigation. *Br J Surg* 1995; 82: 1622–1627

86. Debas HT, Thompson FB. Mortality in emergency right colectomy. *Can J Surg* 1973; 16: 399–402

87. Garrison RN, Shively EH, Baker C *et al.* Evaluation of management of the emergency right hemicolectomy. *J Trauma* 1979; 19: 734–739

88. Fielding LP. Large bowel obstruction caused by cancer: a prospective trial. *Br Med J* 1979; 2: 515–517

89. Cohen JR. Colorectal cancer at the Princess Alexandra Hospital: a prospective study of 719 cases. *Aust NZ J Surg* 1983; 53: 113–119

90. Peppas C, D'Ambrosio R, Rapicano G *et al.* Il wash-out nella chirurgia del colon in urgenza. *Minerva Chir* 1996; 51: 1029–1035

91. Mochizuki H, Nakamura E, Hase K, Tamakuma S. The advantage of primary resection and anastomosis with intraoperative bowel irrigation for obstructing left-sided colorectal carcinoma. *Surg Today* 1993; 23: 771–776

92. Allen-Mersh TG. Should primary anastomosis and on-table colonic lavage be standard treatment for left colon emergencies? *Ann R Coll Surg Engl* 1993; 75: 195–198

93. Sloan MS, Krebs HB, Wheelock JB. A simplified technique for intestinal reanastomosis after the Hartmann procedure. *Surg Gynecol Obstet* 1985; 161: 390–391

94. Rosenman LD. Hartmann's operation. *Am J Surg* 1994; 168: 283–284

95. Marien B. The Hartmann procedure. *Can J Surg* 1987; 30: 30–31

96. Keck JO, Collopy BT, Ryan PJ *et al.* Reversal of Hartmann's procedure: effect of timing and technique on ease and safety. *Dis Colon Rectum* 1994; 37: 243–248

97. Doci R, Audisio RA, Bozzetti F, Gennari L. Actual role of Hartmann's resection in elective surgical treatment for carcinoma of the rectum and sigmoid colon. *Surg Gynecol Obstet* 1986; 163: 1–5

98. Buhre LM, Plukker JT, Mehta DM *et al.* The extended Hartmann operation as an elective procedure for rectal cancer. A forgotten operation. *Eur J Surg Oncol* 1991; 17: 502–506

99. Block GE, Enker WE. Survival after operations for rectal carcinoma in patients over 70 years of age. *Am Surg* 1971; 174: 251–257

100. Lafreniere R, Ketcham AS. Hartmann's pouch carcinoma. *J Surg Oncol* 1985; 29: 26–27

101. Arrigoni A, Pennazio M, Spandre M, Rossini FP. Emergency endoscopy: recanalization of intestinal obstruction caused by colorectal cancer. *Gastrointest Endosc* 1994; 40: 576–580

102. Brunetaud LM, Maunoury V, Ducrotte P *et al.* Palliative treatment of rectosigmoid carcinoma by laser endoscopic photoablation. *Gastroenterology* 1987; 92: 663–668

103. Stone M, Bloom RJ. Transendoscopic balloon dilatation of complete colonic obstruction. *Dis Colon Rectum* 1989; 32: 429–431

104. Christiansen J, Kirkegaard P. A modified cutting loop for electroresection of rectal tumors. *Br J Surg* 1981; 68: 519

105. Heberer G, Denecke H, Demmel N, Wirshing R. Local procedures in the management of rectal cancer. *World J Surg* 1987; 11: 499–503

106. Mlasowsky B, Duben W, Jung D. Cryosurgery for palliation of rectal tumors. *J Exp Clin Cancer Res* 1985; 4: 81–83

107. Loizou LA, Grigg D, Boulos PB, Bown SG. Endoscopic Nd:YAG laser treatment of rectosigmoid cancer. *Gut* 1990; 31: 812–816

108. Campbell KL, Hussey JK, Eremin O. Expandable metal stent application in obstructing carcinoma of the proximal colon: report of a case. *Dis Colon Rectum* 1997; 40: 1391–1393

109. Hashizume M, Haraguchi Y, Ikeda Y. Laparoscopic-assisted colostomy. *Surg Laparosc Endosc* 1994; 4: 70–72

110. Castrati G, Scotti M, Fiorone E, Arrigoni G. Hartmann's operation in complicated lesions of the sigmoid and rectum. *Minerva Chir* 1989; 44: 1485–1488

111. Thompson DM, Tetik CA. Laparoscopic and other minimally invasive techniques in patients with advanced intraperitoneal malignant disease. In: Geraghty JG, Sackier JM, Young H, *et al.* (eds) *Minimal Access Surgery in Oncology. London:* Greenwich Medical Media, 1998. pp. 107–120

112. Lange R, Dominguez-Fernandez E, Friedrich J *et al.* The anastomotic stoma: a useful procedure in emergency bowel surgery. *Langenbecks Arch Chir* 1996; 381: 333–336

113. VanderMeer TJ, Callery MP, Meyers WC. The approach to the patient with single and multiple liver metastases, pulmonary metastases, and intra-abdominal metastases from colorectal carcinoma. *Hematol Oncol Clin North Am* 1997; 11: 759–777

114. DeFriend D, Hill J. A review of emergency colonic surgery. *Br J Hosp Med* 1996; 56: 326–329

115. Chester J, Britton D. Elective and emergency surgery for colorectal cancer in a district general hospital: impact of surgical training on patient survival. *Ann R Coll Surg Engl* 1989; 71: 370–374

116. Singh KK, Barry MK, Ralston P *et al.* Audit of colorectal cancer surgery by non-specialist surgeons. *Br J Surg* 1997; 84: 343–347

117. Isbister YM. Colorectal surgery in the elderly: an audit of surgery in octuagenarians. *Aust NZ J Surg* 1997; 67: 557–561

118. Koruth NM, Hunter DC, Krukowski ZH, Matheson NA. Immediate resection in emergency bowel surgery: a 7-year audit. *Br J Surg* 1985; 72: 703–707

119. Stephenson BM, Shandall AA, Farouk R, Griffith G. Malignant left-sided large bowel obstruction managed by subtotal/total colectomy. *Br J Surg* 1990; 77: 1098–1102

Chapter 10

RADIATION THERAPY FOR COLORECTAL CANCER

R.D. James

Introduction

Over the last ten years the use of cytotoxic chemotherapy (che0mo) and radiotherapy (XRT) in colorectal cancer has been increasing. In general, chemotherapy is most appropriate for colon cancer and XRT for rectal cancer. The treatment of intra-abdominal colon cancer by XRT cannot be routinely recommended outside a clinical trial.[1–3] *Research questions in colon cancer are different from those in rectal cancer and most collaborative research groups organize separate trials.*

This chapter is concerned only with rectal cancer. Most newly diagnosed patients with rectal cancer are referred to surgeons. If all comers are included, their crude tumour-free survival is probably as low as 40%, with around 40% dying with uncontrolled disease in the pelvis. The aim of perioperative pelvic XRT is to reduce local (pelvic) recurrence. Most prospective adjuvant trials that include a surgery-only arm have shown an improvement in local recurrence in favour of XRT (Table 10.1), but local recurrence rates, like survival rates, may be altered according to a definition of surgical procedure. Many series report local recurrence rates only after resections with curative intent. Patients with unresectable tumours may be considered as 'recurrent' from the first postoperative day or, alternatively, excluded from analysis. Other trials record local recurrences only if they occur with no evidence of distant metastases.[4] *Definitions of 'curative' surgery have varied from centre to centre and published local recurrence rates vary from 5 to 40%, depending on case selection. A more accurate way to define curative surgery is by a proper report on the lateral resection margins (LRM).*

A National Cancer Institute (NCI) Clinical Announcement advocated postoperative (postop) adjuvant combined XRT and chemo for patients with stage III rectal cancer.[5] *In Europe trials of preoperative (preop) XRT are more common. UK Guidelines recommend that preop XRT for patients with clinically operable rectal cancer should be considered.*[6] *Few XRT trials show improvements in mortality (Table 10.2), but a recent meta-analysis of the results of randomized studies of perioperative XRT vs no XRT*

Table 10.1. *Reported local recurrence rates in randomized trials of adjuvant radiotherapy for operable rectal cancer*

Radiotherapy	Trial (reference)	Dose (Gy)	No. patients randomized	Local recurrences		P value†	Endpoint
				Radiotherapy	Control		
Preoperative	MRC 1	5 or 20	824	255/549	112/275	NS	Local
	EORTC 2	34.5	466	6/152	21/166	**	Local only
	VASOG 2	31.5	361	37/180	40/181	NS	Residual or recurrent disease
	Stockholm	25	694	23/271	54/274	***	Pelvic recurrence
	MRC 2	40	261	41/129	50/132	NS	'Local recurrence'
	IRCF	25	478	'Significant difference'		*	'Local recurrence'
	North-west	20	284	26/143	58/141	***	'Local recurrence'
Postoperative	GITSG	40	202	15/96	27/106	NS	Local as the first sign of recurrence
	Denmark	50	494	18/244	20/250	NS	Local only
				38/244	44/250	NS	Local + distant
	NSABP	46.5	368	30/184	45/184	NS	Local ± distant
	MRC 3	40	369	14/180	42/189	***	'Local recurrence'

† NS, not conventionally significant; * $P < 0.05$; ** $P < 0.01$; *** $P < 0.001$.

Table 10.2. *Mortality in trials comparing adjuvant radiotherapy with no radiotherapy (including trials with identical chemotherapy for both treatment and control groups)*

Radiotherapy	Trial*	Dose (Gy)	Deaths/no. entered		O–E[†]	Variance	Odds ratio‡ comparing treatment with control mortality rates and (C.I.)
			Radiotherapy	Control			
Preoperative	VASOG-20	20	225/347	251/353	−11.0	38.1	
	Yale	40	9/15	11/16	−0.7	1.8	
	Toronto	5	46/60	52/65	−1.0	5.3	
	MRC 1	5/20	318/549	166/275	−4.5	44.5	
	EORTC-40761	34.5	55/201	61/209	−1.9	20.8	
	VASOG-28	31.5	121/180	114/181	3.8	20.6	
	Stockholm	25	147/351	140/343	1.8	42.1	
	North-west	25	83/143	84/141	−1.1	17.3	
	MRC-2	40	60/129	73/132	−5.7	16.4	
	Total preoperative		1064/1975	952/1715	−20.2	206.9	9% ± 7
Postoperative	Denmark	50	105/244	104/250	1.8	30.2	
	GITSG-7175	40	49/101	63/110	−4.6	13.2	
	NSABP R-01	46.5	113/184	116/184	−1.5	21.7	
	MRC 3	40	23/180	39/189	−7.2	12.9	
	Total postoperative		209/709	322/733	−11.6	78.0	14% ± 11
Total all trials			1354/2684	1274/2448	−31.8	284.9	11% ± 6

‡ For each trial the observed odds reduction in the figures is represented by a black square, with is 99% confidence interval (C.I.) as a horizontal line. A diamond shape represents the odds reduction and 95% C.I. for the overview of the individual trials.

* Data derived from ref. 91, except for MRC 1, 2 and 3 (ref. 92), Stockholm (ref. 47), North-west (ref. 31) and NSABP R-01 (ref. 75).

† O–E, observed–expected.

shows a reduction in cancer mortality of 14% for preop XRT compared with 7% for postop XRT (Gray 1997, pers. comm.).

Overviews focus on effectiveness measured by survival or local recurrence, but the way in which new treatments are adopted depends on the balance between effectiveness and side effects. Cost-effectiveness defines 'the intervention that results in the lowest cost for achieving a given outcome':[7] Improvements in effectiveness (efficacy) frequently involve an increase in cost and side effects.[8] The most reliable data on relative cost-effectiveness are from prospective, randomized clinical trials with a surgery-only arm. However, few of these report local recurrence, preservation of anal function, sexual effects, quality of life or degree of compliance with protocol drug and XRT doses.

The first section of this chapter ('Factors modifying the effectiveness and toxicity of perioperative pelvic XRT for rectal cancer') deals with cancer staging, an attempt to measure 'uncontrollable' variables that predict prognosis following conventional treatment, such as tumour size and fixity to surrounding pelvic structures, radio-sensitivity and imaging for local spread or metastases (Table 10.3). If these variables are not recorded prospectively, conclusions drawn from clinical trials of different treatments may be biased. In addition, clinical staging is an important guide to decisions taken before surgery about operability or surgical technique as well as the need for adjuvant XRT or chemotherapy. Clinicopathological staging (Dukes', Astler-Coller, LRM) determine appropriate treatment following surgery.

The second section ('Factors modifying the efectiveness and toxicity of perioperative pelvic XRT for operable rectal cancer controllable variables') deals with 'controllable' factors that determine the efficacy and side effects of XRT, such as XRT doses and field sizes as well as the timing of XRT and chemo relative to surgery. Other controllable factors affecting outcome include novel surgical and pathological techniques (Table 10.4).

The third section ('Recommendations: clinical trials') deals with recommendations on treatment and future clinical trials.

Table 10.3. *Staging in rectal cancer**

Preoperative	Tumour size/fixicity Tumour grade Distant metastases (radiology) Genetic markers of sensitivity to XRT/chemo
Postoperative	Degree of involvement of lateral resection margins Dukes' staging

* Factors determining local recurrence and metastases.
XRT, radiotherapy; chemo, chemotherapy.

Table 10.4. *Factors determining efficacy of treatment*

- Surgery: TME better than standard
- Pathology: LRM reporting better than Dukes' Astler Collier
- Radiotherapy: preop XRT better than postop XRT
- Chemotherapy: concomitant better than sequential

TME, total mesorectal excision; LRM, lateral resection margin; XRT, radiotherapy.

Factors modifying the effectiveness and toxicity of perioperative pelvic XRT for rectal cancer

SIZE, STAGE AND FIXITY OF TUMOUR

Large tumours are more likely than small tumours to be fixed to surrounding structures. Larger, more fixed tumours are less likely to be cured by XRT and surgery than small, mobile tumours. Modern radiological techniques such as computed tomography (CT), nuclear magnetic resonance (NMR) and endoluminal ultrasound (US) confirm the relationship between tumour size and operability associated with involvement of adjacent structures (see Chapter 2). York Mason[9] first documented the usefulness of digital examination in determining fixity. Experienced surgeons can probably achieve an accuracy of over 80%.[10, 11]

In the first Medical Research Council (MRC) trial of preop XRT (MRC I), surgeons were asked to record the degree of fixity before XRT was commenced. Patients with any degree of fixity had a probability of death from cancer twice that of those with mobile lesions, and a statistically significant reduction in the probability of having a 'curative' resection.[12]

A cure rate of at least 80% has been reported by most series for XRT alone for tumours of less than 5 cm in diameter,[13–19] however, in one series,[20] local control varied according to size and fixity from 97% (for superficial, exophytic tumours less than 3 cm in diameter) to 60% (for tethered tumours 3–5 cm in diameter). Gerard *et al.*[19] showed a similar reduction in local control from 93% for T1 to 60% for T2 tumours.

Brierley *et al.*[21] reported local control rates for XRT of 50, 30 and 9% for mobile, partially fixed and fixed tumours, respectively, in a retrospective analysis of 229 patients with rectal cancer who were unfit for or refused surgery. XRT for large, fixed, inoperable rectal cancer is even less effective: in one series of 29 such patients subjected to laparotomy 2 months after radical pelvic XRT, resection was impossible in 11; of the 18 tumours resected, only three showed complete clinical remission following XRT.[22] These results are confirmed in other publications.[22–25] Local control is only 15% for recurrent tumours, which often exceed 10 cm in size.[26]

Indirect evidence of the effect of tumour size/stage and fixity on XRT curability is seen from comparisons between trials of preop and postop XRT, which tend to include different patient groups. Two Medical Research Council (MRC) trials were launched simultaneously in order to test the relative effectiveness of preop and postop pelvic XRT in two different types of rectal cancer. MRC I included patients with advanced tethered or fixed tumours, whereas patients in MRC III were fit, postop and completely resected with a view to cure; XRT field sizes and doses were identical. Comparisons of efficacy between the two trials are inappropriate, as survival figures for patients allocated surgery alone in MRC II are significantly lower (23 vs 43%) than in the comparable arm in MRC III.[27, 28]

BIOLOGICAL ASSAYS

Clinicopathological staging is known to be inaccurate. Up to 40% of patients with Dukes' C cancer will be cured by surgery alone, so a policy of adjuvant treatment for all is wasteful. Laboratory-based research is dedicated to identifying tumour-tissue variables that refine predictability.[29,30] Assays of tumour sensitivity to XRT and chemo are an attempt to identify patients who need more intensive adjuvant treatment.[31] Cloned growth factors or genes might modify the interaction of chemo and XRT with surgery.

XRT side effects

The side effects of XRT are determined by organs and normal tissues surrounding the target tumour. The literature of XRT side effects in rectal cancer is dominated by those due to radiation small bowel disease (XRT enteritis). Preop XRT rarely causes XRT enteritis, but small bowel usually descends near the pelvic floor after radical rectal surgery and may be included in the XRT field (Fig 10.3–10.6). The incidence of XRT enteritis varies with uncontrollable factors such as hypertension, diabetes, vascular disease, diverticular disease, pelvic inflammatory disease, previous bowel surgery, physique and age. XRT enteritis may be acute or late.

When the gut is irradiated, an acute reaction, due to epithelial stem-cell death, appears approximately 2 weeks after XRT is started and continues for 2–3 weeks after its end. The epithelial lining of the gastrointestinal tract is depopulated by XRT because it sterilizes the self-renewal stem cells at the base of the intestinal crypts. Macroscopically, the villi shorten and shrink, giving rise to a syndrome similar to malabsorption. Acute XRT enteritis occurs during or shortly after treatment and is measured by diarrhoea, fatigue, weight loss and nausea. Following preop XRT, further complications of acute XRT enteritis may include anastomotic dehiscence; thus, the frequency of stomas may be a useful measure of any XRT enteritis.

The chronic or late XRT reaction appears months or years after the acute reaction has settled and is due to progressive endothelial changes. The serosal surface is thickened and several bowel loops may be matted together. Segments may show dilatation, variable lengths of stenosis and irregular defects of various sizes in the wall. Stenotic segments suggest features of late Crohn's or ischaemic bowel disease, with a cobblestone appearance to the mucosa. Microscopically, the lamina is fibrous and contains ectatic, thin-walled vessels, many of which are thrombosed. Capillaries exhibit intimal thickening and contain fibrin platelet thrombi associated with damaged endothelial cells.[32] Changes in small arterioles include medial necrosis due to ischaemia and medial hypertrophy, presumed to be secondary to the increased resistance to blood flow in the microvascular bed. Measurements of late XRT enteritis may require years of follow-up. Common symptoms include bowel disturbance and food intolerance; more serious are obstruction, bleeding and fistula formation. The most accurate measure is the frequency of late surgical interventions required for non-cancer causes. The true incidence of toxicity may have been underestimated because a number of trials have failed to report non-compliance with the trial protocol, due to dose reductions.

Although XRT enteritis is comparatively rare, surgeons may need to take these pathological changes into account when scheduling surgery following XRT. If radical surgery is scheduled within 3 weeks of the start of XRT, the acute reaction is unlikely to render the patient unfit for anaesthesia. However, when late XRT enteritis is established, there is serious danger of anastomotic breakdown if the full extent of affected bowel is not resected. Experienced surgeons may resect over 50 cm of small bowel to ensure that they are dealing with well-vascularized mucosa.[33]

PRACTICAL RESULTS OF PREOPERATIVE STAGING: A PREOPERATIVE TREATMENT PROGRAMME

On the basis of an assessment of tumour size/stage/fixity and appropriate radiology, patients can be divided into three groups preoperatively (Table 10.5). Information derived from surgery or from pathological examination of the operative specimen may be used postoperatively to modify the staging system. Indications for surgery, XRT and chemo in these groups is changing constantly with the results of research.[34, 35]

Small, mobile tumours in the lower rectum

Patients with fully mobile tumours should be assessed by a multi-disciplinary team. Most should be offered immediate surgery with no adjuvant XRT or chemo. Approximately 10% of these patients are suitable for some form of local surgical procedure. On digital examination the tumour should be mobile on deep structures and there should be no palpable mesenteric nodes. Intraluminal ultrasound may help to define those tumours that have not penetrated through the muscularis layer. In terms of effectiveness, there is little to choose between local excision, local XRT or diathermy. Conservative surgery for moderately small tumours is safer following preop XRT: of 34 patients with mobile or tethered tumours up to 6 cm treated by preop XRT followed 6–8 weeks later by a variety of conservative procedures (transanal, trans-sacral, anterior or local excision), 80% were alive at 2 years with only two colostomies.[36] Two similar series of 17 and 16

Table 10.5. *Rectal cancer treatment: clinical trials*

1. Small mobile tumours in the lower rectum (10%)
   Can XRT/chemo plus conservative surgery avoid APR?
2. Adjuvant treatment (80%)
   Is preop XRT better than selective postop XRT?
3. Inoperable/recurrent cancer (10%)
   What is the best combination of XRT/chemo/surgery?

XRT, radiotherapy; chemo, chemotherapy; APR, abdomino-perineal resection.

patients, respectively, reported local failure in only one patient each.[37, 38] In future, preop XRT may encourage more surgeons to perform sphincter-preserving surgery for selected tumours of the lower rectum.[39]

However, outside clinical trials, conservative radical XRT without surgery can be recommended only for well-differentiated tumours less than 3 cm in diameter. XRT requires little hospitalization but can be recommended only in centres with routine experience of intracavitary (contact) XRT. This specialized technique is becoming less widely available since the Phillips RT–50 machine is no longer being marketed. Contact XRT differs from conventional XRT in three important ways: first, it relies on the delivery of an extremely high (100–120 Gy) tumour surface dose which reduces to negligible intensity at a depth of 1.0 cm; secondly, the dose is given in three or four 5-minute treatments over at least 2 months in order to allow the tumour to shrink back between treatments; thirdly, the machine head is held in contact with the tumour during treatment, the patient being awake and in the knee–chest position. Because of the treatment position, considerable skill is required in treating tumours on the posterior rectal wall or those over 10 cm in diameter.

Operable rectal cancer

The second, largest group, comprising around 80% of patients, will be suitable for radical surgery with a view to cure. Advanced Dukes' B or C tumours are known to require extensive posterior dissection in order to reduce the risk of local recurrence;[40] less-careful dissection can be associated with permanent sexual or urinary problems.[41, 42] Details of adjuvant treatment for patients in this group are discussed below.

Fixed, inoperable, recurrent, rectal cancers

Most surgeons assess patients with rectal cancer for metastases and general fitness before surgery. Approximately 5% of patients have metastatic disease at presentation or are unsuitable for laparotomy on medical grounds; a further 10% have tumours so fixed to surrounding tissues as to discourage anything more adventurous than a defunctioning colostomy. These patients are suitable for combined XRT and chemo, with palliative surgery considered 6–8 weeks after XRT. The optimal XRT dose and chemo combination has yet to be determined. Low doses (30 Gy in 2 weeks up to 45 Gy in 3 weeks) and high doses (50–60 Gy over 5–6 weeks) are associated with similar resection rates of around 40%.[22–25, 43] Most oncologists would include patients with locally recurrent pelvic cancer following surgery in trials for fixed/inoperable tumours. Such trials help to determine safe doses of XRT and concomitant chemo for patients with operable rectal cancer.

POSTOP STAGING FOR OPERABLE RECTAL CANCER

The postop XRT trials detailed in Tables 10.1 and 10.2 selected patients for postop XRT using Astler-Coller/Dukes' staging, however the need for XRT is better determined by LRM positivity, and the need for adjuvant chemotherapy by lymph node positivity. Adam *et al.*[44] reported that 25% of specimens from patients thought to have undergone curative resection had a positive LRM; within 5 years, 78% of these had developed local recurrence, compared with 10% of those with clear margins. The relative figures from a Dutch series were 29 and 8%.[45] Clinical trials discussed below are designed to ask whether preop XRT is more cost-effective than selective postop XRT based on LRM examination.

Factors modifying the effectiveness and toxicity of perioperative pelvic XRT for operable rectal cancer controllable variables

XRT DOSE: HIGH-DOSE XRT IS BETTER THAN LOW-DOSE XRT (more effective, but more toxic)

Disappointing results of early XRT trials were due to inadequate overall biological XRT dose. Feigen *et al.*[46] reported local recurrence in 48 of 97 patients receiving 25 Gy postop in 2 weeks. However, a series of Swedish trials using 25 Gy preop in 1 week have shown improvements in local recurrence and survival compared with surgery alone.[47, 48]

A dose of 25 Gy over 1 week is clearly more effective than 25 Gy over 2 weeks, but may not be more effective than 50 Gy over 4–5 weeks.

The nominal standard dose (NSD)[49] is one method of estimating the biological effectiveness of XRT by taking into account radiation repair between separate daily fractions; it was not designed to compare tumour doses, but it gives an approximation of the cumulative effects of XRT on subcutaneous tissues. Data from non-randomized trials suggest a trend towards more effective local tumour control with higher XRT dose as measured by NSD.

Large doses per fraction allow radiotherapists to complete treatment more quickly, causing less delay before surgery, but may be associated with more serious late effects and they may be more difficult to combine safely with concomitant chemo. Two European trials of preop XRT (Figures 10.1, 10.2) launched in 1996 use daily fractions of 1.8 and 5 Gy.[50,51] The EORTC Trial protocol indicates that five fractions of 5 Gy given preop are considered equivalent to 28 fractions of 1.8 Gy given postop.

The planned XRT dose may be modified according to the presence or absence of adverse patient characteristics. Aleman *et al.*[52] retrospectively analysed the effectiveness of a variety of postop XRT doses dictated by the presence or absence of small bowel. A statistically significant ($P = 0.017$) trend for improved tumour control was noted with increased XRT dose in 206 patients with completely resected Dukes' B tumours. However, the relationship between dose and tumour volume is complex. Allee *et al.*[53] reported a positive correlation between postop XRT dose and effectiveness (local control) in patients with microscopic residual, but not for those with macroscopic, unresectable disease.

XRT FIELD SIZE AND SHAPE: SMALL XRT FIELDS ARE BETTER THAN LARGE XRT FIELDS (less toxic)

Optimal XRT planning uses small rather than large fields

The aim of both preop and postop pelvic XRT is to reduce the risk of regrowth at a positive LRM. Although the optimal pelvic XRT fields for rectal cancer have yet to be determined the least toxic are those of minimal size. Published trials have used a variety of field sizes and beam arrangements. Early studies conducted by the MRC, EORTC, ICRF and Stockholm Groups used large low-dose (34.5–40 Gy or equivalent) parallel opposed fields, sometimes extending into the abdomen. Large XRT fields increase acute XRT side effects such as diarrhoea[54] and postoperative non-cancer deaths.[55] Small bowel obstruction due to late XRT enteritis varies from 30% for extended abdominal fields to 9% for shaped pelvic fields.[56]

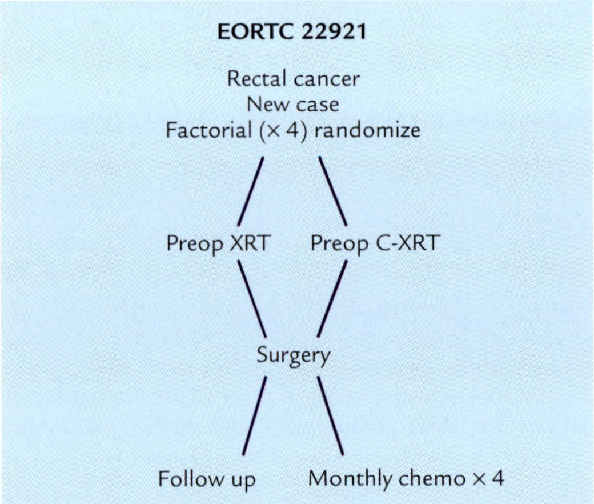

EORTC 22921

Rectal cancer
New case
Factorial (× 4) randomize

Preop XRT — Preop C-XRT

Surgery

Follow up — Monthly chemo × 4

Figure 10.1. *European Organization for Research and Treatment of Cancer (EORTC) trial of preoperative radiotherapy (XRT; 45 GY in 5 weeks) vs preoperative XRT with chemotherapy (C-XRT) with or without postoperative adjuvant chemotherapy (Mayo Clinic Regime (Fu/FA; 5-fluorouracil + folinic acid).*[51]

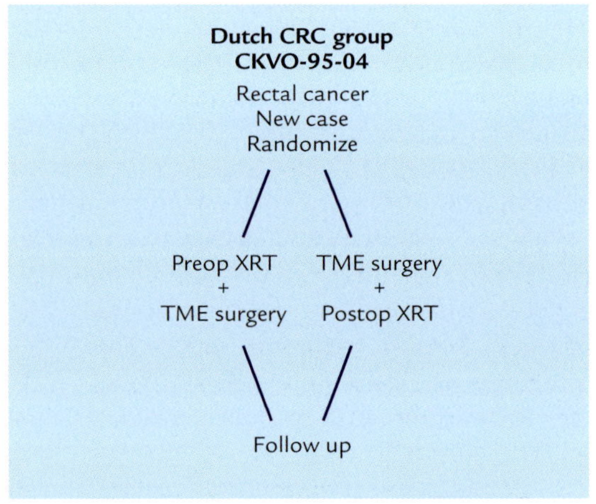

Figure 10.2. *Dutch Colorectal Cancer (CRC) Group trial of preoperative radiotherapy (Preop XRT; 25 Gy in 1 week) plus total mesorectal exusion (TME) vs TME plus postoperative XRT (Postop XRT; 50.4 Gy in 4 weeks), with no concomitant or sequential chemotherapy.*[50]

Mortality due to preop XRT has been due to large field sizes

In a subgroup analysis of the Stockholm–Malmo Trial,[47] postop non-cancer deaths were significantly higher in the XRT than the control arm (7 vs 2%: $P < 0.01$). Suggestions that this excess was due to an accelerated XRT dose schedule were discounted by a comparison with the Uppsala Trial,[57] which used a biologically higher dose (25 vs 25.5 Gy) and recorded no increase in mortality. Furthermore, a British Trial using a lower dose (15 Gy) also reported a significant increase in perioperative morbidity and mortality as well as in cardiovascular and thromboembolic complications in the XRT arm compared with surgery alone.[58]

It is now generally accepted that the excess of cardiovascular deaths in early trials was related to a preop XRT technique that irradiated an excess of small bowel. The XRT field size was much larger in the Stockholm than in the Uppsala trial (lower pelvis to L1–L2 interface, two fields vs lower pelvis to L3–L4 interface, three field, respectively). In a retrospective analysis of 1399 patients who received the same preop XRT dose and fractionation, postoperative mortality was significantly increased in patients irradiated with a two-field compared with a four-field technique.[59] The volume of small bowel in the high-dose XRT zone of a two field technique is more than twice that in a three- or four field technique.[55] Postoperative mortality in a subsequent Swedish trial using a four-field technique is identical (4 vs 3%) in the XRT and control arms.[48, 60]

Recent research has defined more accurately the areas most at risk. Local recurrence is usually a function of posterior or lateral spread of carcinoma into adjacent, unresected organs or the pelvic side wall. CT scanning of locally recurrent tumours confirms that the vast majority occur in the posterior pelvis.[61] Large XRT fields may not improve local control more than small fields. One trial of preop XRT (20 Gy in four fractions) which used standard field-sizes of 10 × 10 × 10 cm maintained a permanent CT scan record of the position of the field in the pelvis for each patient.[62] Of 16 patients with suspected local pelvic recurrence recalled for scanning, 10 had recurrence within the XRT field and six outside. The risk of recurrence following XRT within the field and outside the field was 7% and 4%, respectively. Whereas an increase in XRT dose (from 20 Gy in four fractions to 25 Gy in five fractions) might improve local control by up to 7%, an increase in field size (say, from 10 to 12 cm) might improve local control by only 4%.

Large tumours clearly require larger XRT fields than small tumours, but radiological and pathological studies suggest that it is most unusual for the longitudinal (luminal) or lateral dimension of a rectal tumour to exceed 10 cm. Regional (mesenteric) lymph nodes are removed by standard surgical resection, whereas side-wall (hypogastric, internal, external iliac) and inguinal nodes are rarely involved. It therefore seems illogical to attempt to include pelvic lymph nodes, the anterior pelvis or the perineum (for tumours of the middle or upper rectum) in the XRT field.

A margin of 2–3 cm beyond the CT or MR scan of a tumour includes malignant infiltration and takes into account the daily movement of the patient, organs and tumour. In addition, postoperatively there is uncertainty over the exact location of the tumour bed. An appropriate XRT field for rectal cancer is therefore a 'brick' or 'box' that encompasses the tumour bed involved within a margin of approximately 10 cm. During preop XRT planning the tumour is imaged by CT scanning and placed at the centre of the high-dose zone (Figures 10.3, 10.4).

There are practical reasons for treating patients in the prone rather than the supine position. The position of the centre of the high-dose 'brick' can be determined preoperatively by CT scanning or other imaging technology. Since the rectum lies in the curve of the sacrum, the depth of this 'brick' will vary, being most superficial (7–8 cm from the skin surface) in the mid-rectum and deepest (9–10 cm from the skin surface) in the upper or lower rectum. In the latter case, a tissue-equivalent 'bolus' may be needed to ensure that the perineum is uniformly irradiated.

For postop XRT, surgeons should be encouraged to leave clips in sites of residual disease. However, during postop XRT planning, the exact site of residual disease is often difficult to determine and, for this reason,

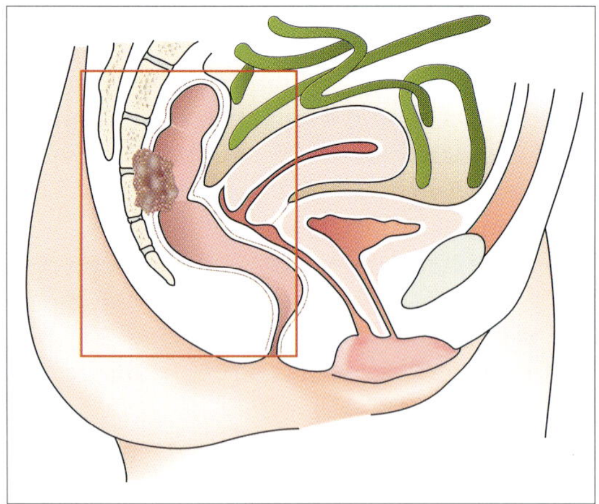

Figure 10.3. *Preoperative radiotherapy includes the tumour, but no small bowel within a posterior pelvic field.*

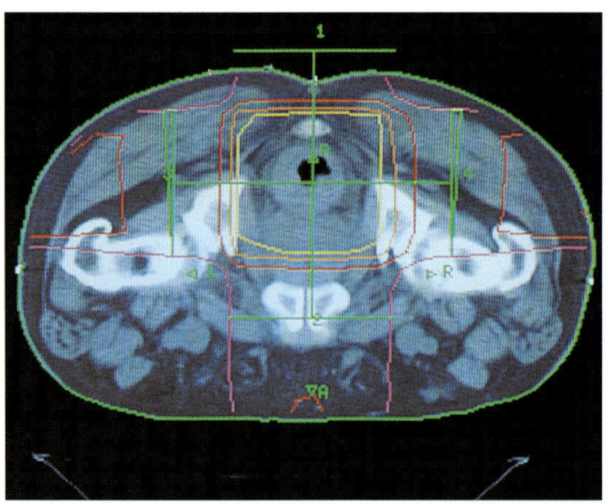

Figure 10.4. *Preoperative radiotherapy planning scan. Patient prone. Field centred 8 cm from skin of the natal cleft.*

postop XRT field sizes tend to be larger than those needed for preop XRT (Figures 10.5, 10.6). During XRT planning, Gastrografin (diatrizoic acid) contrast can be used to determine the proportion of the XRT field that contains small bowel, and field shaping may be used to exclude as much as possible.[63] In a retrospective series, the Houston group showed that mechanical devices that exclude small bowel from XRT fields can reduce late XRT enteritis from 9 to 3%.[56]

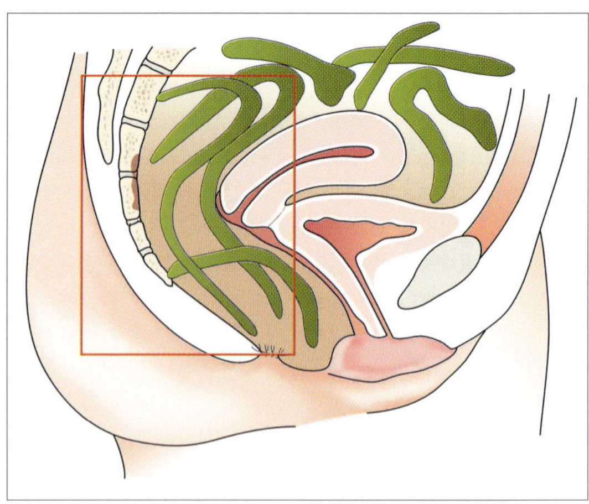

Figure 10.5. *Postoperative radiotherapy following AP resection. The lower pelvis usually contains small bowel and sites of residual disease are difficult to identify.*

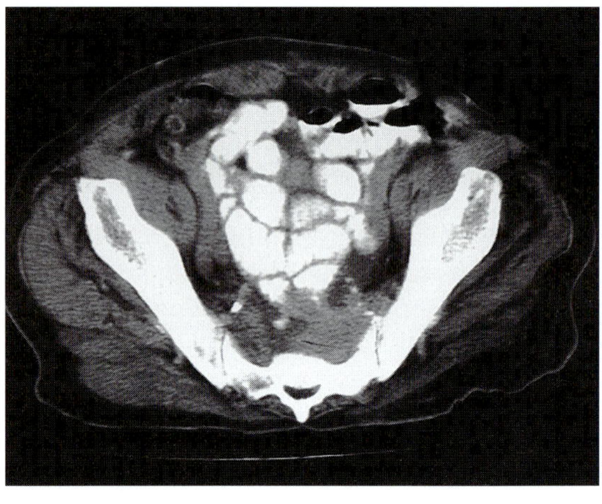

Figure 10.6. *Postoperative scan with small bowel contrast. Patient supine. Most of the imaged bowel would be included in the radiotherapy (XRT) field, causing acute and chronic XRT enteritis.*

TIMING OF XRT RELATIVE TO SURGERY – PREOP OR POST-OP? PREOP XRT IS BETTER THAN POSTOP XRT (more effective, less toxic)

Evidence is accumulating that pelvic XRT is more effective if given preop rather than postop for rectal cancer. A recent meta-analysis of published trials shows a reduction in local recurrence due to preop XRT of 43% compared with 32% for postop XRT (Gray, pers. comm.

1997). The reason for this difference remains obscure, but is probably multifactorial. Postop XRT is more toxic than equivalent doses of preop XRT and the reasons for this are more easy to define. However, preop XRT is more likely to give surgically curable patients unnecessary irradiation and delays surgery.

Delay in surgery: downstaging

Prolonged preop XRT schedules impose delays on surgery and are less likely to be acceptable to surgeons and patients. Short, sharp XRT schedules allow immediate surgery and are equally effective. This may be the reason why one UK preop trial (MRC II) recruited less rapidly (279 patients in 7 years) than did the UK postop trial launched simultaneously, MRC III (516 patients in 5 years).

Prolonged preop XRT alters the reliability of lymph node staging. Horn *et al.*[64] reported significant downstaging compared with controls in both lymph node invasion (18.4 vs 27.5%, $P < 0.05$) and tumour size ($P < 0.05$), as well as complete tumour regression in 4.4% of patients following 6 weeks' XRT. Following a similar biological dose, but with 93% of tumours resected within 2 weeks of the start of XRT, there were no detectable differences in tumour volume or Dukes' staging compared with controls.[31]

Uppsala trial

In the Uppsala trial,[65] 471 patients were randomly assigned to receive either preop or postop XRT through identical pelvic portals. The XRT doses were made as comparable as possible using the cumulative radiation effect (CRE) formula (preop CRE = 15.4; postop CRE = 17.0). Efficacy measured by survival was identical in the two arms; however, efficacy measured by local recurrence rates was significantly superior in the preop arm (13 vs 22%: $P = 0.02$).

National Swedish trials

The Stockholm Rectal Cancer Study Group[47] reported a significant reduction in local recurrence (25 vs 11%, $P<0.05$) in favour of preop XRT compared with surgery alone and an identical overall 5-year survival (XRT, 55%, control, 50%) for the two trial arms. A similarly designed national trial[48,60] on 1168 patients reported a highly significant reduction in local recurrence of approximately 65% (9 vs 24%, $P < 0.001$).

British trials

Measures of efficacy in two UK trials, MRC II (preop) and MRC III (postop), launched simultaneously, are interesting because the preop trial contained patients with more advanced disease.[27, 28] In MRC II there was a reduction in favour of the preop XRT arm compared with control of the following parameters: overall deaths ($P = 0.09$), cause-specific deaths ($P = 0.03$), metastases ($P = 0.02$). The corresponding figures for MRC III were less impressive ($P = 0.1$, 0.04 and 0.18, respectively). In contrast, although both trials showed a significant reduction in local recurrence in favour of XRT, the result was more impressive in the postop than the preop trial ($P = 0.001$ vs 0.04).

Non-randomized data

A multivariate analysis of 307 rectal cancer patients showed that preop XRT rather than postop XRT was the most important controllable variable predicting freedom from disease ($P = 0.001$). Of the patients receiving preop XRT, those given a 'short, sharp' schedule (20 Gy in five fractions) did as well as those receiving a more protracted, expensive schedule (40–50 Gy in 20–25 fractions) that caused 3 months' delay in surgery.[66]

Toxicity

Uppsala trial: side effects of XRT

In the Uppsala trial, in which patients were randomly allocated to receive either preop or postop XRT, there was a marked difference in direct and indirect costs between the two schedules.[57, 65, 67] First, the preop schedule was planned for 1 week, whereas the postop schedule was planned for 8 weeks. Second, in terms of compliance with planned treatment, postop XRT was significantly less likely to be delivered according to schedule: fewer than 50% of the patients allocated postop XRT were able to start XRT as planned (within 6 weeks of surgery), while only 60% completed XRT as planned (within 8 weeks). Third, more direct measures of toxicity seemed to favour preop XRT: all patients allocated to this arm experienced nil or minimal XRT-related morbidity and there was no measurable excess of postop mortality or anastomotic dehiscence, although significantly more patients in this arm experienced perineal wound sepsis.

In contrast, of those allocated to postop XRT, over 90% experienced XRT-related complications – 52% moderate or severe diarrhoea (5% requiring parenteral nutrition), 21% fatigue, 18% urinary disorders and 18% skin reactions. Furthermore, late small bowel obstruction due to XRT enteritis (defined radiologically or at laparotomy) was twice as likely in the postop as in the preop arm (11 vs 5%). Patients who live longer are clearly more at risk for developing late XRT enteritis than those who die early as a result of cancer recurrence, but this potential bias is not present in the Uppsala trial, since survival rates were identical.

MRC trial: side effects of XRT

MRC trials II and III confirm the impression that measures of cost, such as treatment compliance, favour preop over postop XRT. In MRC II, 90% of patients allocated preop XRT received it in the scheduled period; the corresponding figure for MRC III was 75%. Early XRT morbidity was also more common during postop than preop XRT: twice as many patients experienced nausea, abdominal pain and urinary symptoms. There was an excess of diarrhoea (46 vs 33%) and of obstruction and colovesical fistula (MRC, pers. comm.).

Non-randomized data

Because of concerns over small bowel irradiation, planned doses of XRT are less likely to be delivered on schedule if given postop rather than preop.[68] A study of quality control in one trial of postop XRT revealed that 8% of patients had major protocol deviations, 2% could not be evaluated and a further 2% had incomplete treatment because of disease progression or toxicity.[69]

An interim, non-randomized comparison of relative toxicity is available from the UK Adjuvant X-ray Infusion Study (AXIS). Patients randomly allocated to receive XRT were treated with a preop or postop schedule according to clinical preference. No serious morbidity was reported for any of the 69 patients who received preop XRT: one patient refused and another was not treated, in error. In contrast, of 124 postop XRT patients, two suffered severe diarrhoea requiring hospitalization and two suffered severe skin reactions requiring a break in treatment, while delayed starts were recorded in 16 patients (MRC, pers. comm.).

PRESENCE OR ABSENCE OF 5-FLUOROURACIL (5-FU) CONTAINING CHEMOTHERAPY

Introduction

Concomitant chemo enhances XRT damage in tumours or in small bowel because it is present when XRT-inflicted DNA damage is being repaired. Regimens using continuous ambulatory infusion (CAI) or 5-fluorouracil (5-FU) biomodulation prolong the biological half-life (*c.* 20 min) of bolus intravenous 5-FU. Controlled trials have shown them to be superior to bolus 5-FU regimes for metastatic colon cancer.[70–72] CAI and biomodulation are more likely to result in XRT enhancement than bolus 5-FU alone. CAI delivers 5-FU continuously 24 hours a day, 7 days a week at a dose level of around 300 mg/m2/day. Biomodulation of 5-FU uses folinic acid (FA, leucovorin) or methotrexate.

If chemo with 5-FU is not intended as a specific radiosensitizer, it may be given at another time: this technique is called sequential therapy. XRT might be given preop and chemo postop. Changes in local control rates due to pelvic XRT are less likely, than with concomitant but changes in survival may occur from changes in the pattern and timing of liver metastases.

Concomitant intravenous infusion of chemo plus XRT is more effective than sequential schedules but more toxic in terms of XRT enteritis. One method of overcoming this drawback is by spatial separation of schedules, using portal venous or arterial infusion.

Chemo plus XRT is more effective than perioperative XRT alone, but is also more toxic

Postop XRT plus chemo is more effective than postop XRT alone

USA postop trials GI-7175 and NCCTG 79-47-51 analysed by the National Cancer Institute (NCI) for the 1990 Consensus Statement showed a survival advantage for postop XRT plus chemo over, respectively, surgery alone and postop XRT.[73, 74] However, both used a combination of concomitant and sequential chemo. A three-armed trial conducted by the National Surgical Adjuvant Breast and Bowel Program (NSABP R-01) showed a survival advantage for adjuvant chemo but not for adjuvant postop XRT in a direct comparison with surgery.[75]

Postop chemo plus XRT is more toxic than postop XRT alone

However, GI-7175 reported severe acute non-haematological toxicity in 35% of those receiving combined-modality XRT–chemo, compared with 16% of those receiving postop XRT alone, while two cancer-free patients in the combined arm died of their complications. In NCCTTG 79-47-51 comparable figures were 20 vs 5%. Rominger and Gelber[76] reported severe late XRT enteritis (necrosis, stenosis and fistulas) more commonly in patients receiving postop XRT combined with concomitant and sequential chemo than in those receiving postop XRT alone (20 vs 14%); and 10 patients in the combined group developed life-threatening complications. A non-randomized pilot study of concomitant 5-FU with postop XRT reported severe late XRT enteritis in 35% of patients.[77]

NSABP C-03 combined postop XRT with bolus 5-FU 325 mg/m^2 modulated by low-dose FA. Only 15% of patients had normal bowel actions: 28% had more than seven bowel movements a day and 6% had an overall toxicity of at least grade 4.[78] Minsky *et al.*[79] attempted to deliver 12 postop cycles of chemo (bolus 5-FU plus FA 200 mg/m^2 daily for 5 days, repeated monthly) to patients receiving conventional postop XRT. They found that the maximum tolerated dose of 5-FU was significantly lower in the concomitant than in the sequential setting (250 vs 375 mg/m^2).

The same schedule of chemo plus XRT is more toxic if given postop than if given preop

Two studies[80,81] recorded significantly more cases of grade III–IV diarrhoea (50 vs 30% and 48 vs 13%) for postop chemo plus XRT compared with the same chemo schedule plus preop XRT. Both used conventional XRT fractionation. However, an interim report on the current NSABP R-03 trial showed no difference in treatment-induced toxicity between preop and postop XRT combined with two cycles of the 'Mayo' chemo regime.[82]

Preop chemo plus XRT is more toxic than preop XRT alone

An indirect comparison of toxicity due to preop XRT and concomitant chemo vs that due to preop XRT alone is available from two trials conducted by the European Organisation for Research on Treatment of Cancer (EORTC 40741 and 40761). Both used the same XRT dose, fractionation and field size, recruited patients of similar disease stage, and randomized between treatment and surgery alone; however, EORTC 40741 added concomitant chemo to preop XRT.

In Trial 40761 XRT was completed with no discernible toxicity in 162 of 166 patients and there was no reported increase in postop mortality compared with unirradiated controls.[83] However, in Trial 40741 which added chemo to XRT there was an increase, compared with surgical controls, in both postop (30-day) mortality (8.9 vs 5%) and in overall non-cancer intercurrent mortality (16 vs 5%), as well as a doubling of postop pulmonary complications (16 vs 8%). More patients experienced more severe acute XRT toxicity before surgery in the combined arm than in the XRT-only arm. This was particularly striking for weakness and pain (16 vs 5%, $P = 0.004$) and for severe diarrhoea (9 vs 1%, $P = 0.006$). Life-threatening XRT-related complications were not seen in the XRT-only arm, but occurred in 6% of patients in the combined arm.[84]

Infusional chemo is more effective and toxic than bolus 5-FU in combination with preop or postop XRT

A non-randomized study of concomitant 5-FU chemo and preop XRT in patients with primary unresectable cancer showed an improved resectability rate compared with historical controls.[43] A similar study of concomitant infusional 5-FU with preop XRT for 77 patients with advanced, operable (stage T3) rectal tumours achieved a local control rate of 99%, although median follow-up was short.[85]

However, a direct comparison of preop XRT and concomitant chemo vs preop XRT alone in resectable rectal cancer (EORTC 40741) showed no survival advantage.[86] An Eastern Co-operative

Oncology Group (ECOG) trial, which showed no survival advantage for postop XRT plus chemo, used a sequential technique.[87] A North Central Cancer Treatment Group Trial (NCCTG 86-47-51) compared the enhancement of postop XRT by concomitant 5-FU delivered by either bolus injection (500 mg/m^2 days 1–3 and 36–39) or continuous infusion (225 mg/m^2/day). Both groups received, in addition, postop sequential bolus chemo. With a median of 46 months follow-up, patients who received infusion had a significantly improved ($P = 0.01$) survival and time to relapse.[88] However, the incidence of severe/life-threatening diarrhoea was doubled (24 vs 14%) in the infusion compared with the bolus arm. Marsh *et al.*[89] reported that the maximum tolerated dose of continuous infusional 5-FU given with 5 weeks of preop XRT is 275 mg/m^2/day.

Leucovorin-modulated 5-FU is more toxic than non-modulated 5-FU in combination with preop XRT

A preop dose-escalation study of chemo plus XRT conducted by the EORTC reported a trebling of Grade III diarrhoea (from 7 to 20%) as a result of a 20% dose increment in bolus 5-FU.[90] The schedule adopted by EORTC Trial 22921[51] is 5-FU 350 mg/m^2 plus FA 20 mg/m^2 daily for 5 days every 4 weeks. Two courses of this are given during preop XRT (45 Gy in 5 weeks). A UK study confirmed acceptable toxicity with 5-FU 350 mg/m^2 plus FA 20 mg/m^2 during weeks 1 and 6 of preop XRT (Simpson and Glynne Jones 1996, pers. comm.). A similar schedule, adopted for NSABP R-03 has been reported to give acceptable interim toxicity.[82] However, a more intensive, weekly schedule (5-FU 400 mg/m^2 plus FA 80 mg/m^2), given for each of the 7 weeks of XRT produced an unacceptable 38% Grade III–IV cases of diarrhoea.[80]

Recommendations: clinical trials

XRT TECHNIQUE

Specific side effects of XRT and chemo should be explained and written, informed consent obtained. Pelvic XRT causes permanent sterility and sperm or ovum storage might be appropriate. Women of childbearing age should be asked about the risk of their being pregnant.

Meticulous planning of XRT is important. The volume at risk should be covered adequately, but small XRT fields are less toxic than large XRT fields. High-dose XRT is more effective than low-dose, but may be more toxic. Preop XRT is more effective and less toxic than postop XRT, but has the disadvantage of irradiating a number of patients needlessly.

Recommended doses for operable tumours are equivalent to 60 Gy in 30 fractions over 6 weeks, with dose reductions for small bowel tethering in the treatment volume, concomitant chemo, poor performance status and coincidental medical conditions such as diabetes and hypertension. A 4–6 week fractionation is recommended for postop XRT, but, for preop XRT, ‘short, sharp’ fractionation can be followed by immediate surgery with no change in lymph node status. Doses for fixed, inoperable or recurrent tumours are less critical: 30 Gy/2 weeks and 60 Gy/3 weeks give similar resection rates, probably because these are determined by general fitness for surgery and distant metastases rather than by volume reduction following XRT.

CHEMOTHERAPY PLUS XRT

Concomitant 5-FU containing chemo plus XRT is more effective than perioperative XRT alone, but also is more toxic. When the same schedule of concomitant chemo plus XRT is administered preop and postop, the latter is more toxic. The most effective and toxic 5-FU schedules in combination with XRT are those yielding longest serum half-lives (infusional or modulated).

CLINICAL STAGING: CLINICAL TRIALS

Close collaboration between surgeon and oncologist fosters patient selection. Preoperative evaluation using digital examination and radiology defines three broad stages for clinical trials (Figure 10.5). These monitor change in clinical practice over the duration of the trial, encourage the learning curve of new techniques, such as the benefits of LRM reporting. They provide the public with the best possible audit of treatment and clinicians with a framework of best current practice for patients treated off protocol.

Table 10.6. *Current trials of adjuvant XRT in operable rectal cancer*

Comparison	Trials	Arms
Preop XRT vs Postop XRT	Dutch CKV095-04	Preop XRT* vs Postop XRT
	NSABP R-03	Preop XRT† + chemo vs Postop XRT† + chemo
	UK-CR07	Preop XRT* + Postop chemo vs Postop XRT† + chemo
Preop XRT ± chemo	EORTC22921	Preop XRT† + Postop chemo vs Preop XRT† + chemo
Postop XRT ± chemo	USA Trials‡	Postop XRT‡ + chemo A vs Postop XRT‡ + chemo B

* Swedish' fractionation.

† Conventional fractionation.

‡ INT-0114, NCCTG-864751, NCIC C-04, NSABP -R02 (Stage B_2, C).

Small tumours in the lower rectum

Approximately 10% of rectal cancer patients are suitable for conservative (non-radical) surgery. For those with tumours in the lower rectum this means that they avoid a permanent colostomy. Preop external-beam XRT followed by conservative surgery (transanal, trans-sacral, anterior or local excision), appears to cure 80% of 5–6 cm tumours.

Fixed, inoperable, recurrent rectal cancer

Patients with fixed, inoperable, recurrent rectal cancer should be entered into phase I/II studies of combined XRT, chemo and surgery because the best way of controlling pelvic symptoms is by the judicious use of all three treatment modalities. Data from radio-sensitizing studies performed on 'inoperable' patients can be used to devise optimal XRT–chemo schedules for patients with operable rectal cancer using different XRT fractionation and new drugs such as raltitrexed, irinotecan and oxaliplatin.

Operable rectal cancer: USA and European approaches

Questions surrounding the 80% of patients with operable rectal cancer require large, adequately funded, collaborative studies. Trials conducted in the United States and in Europe, respectively, have defined what appear to be two equally effective policies for the optimal treatment of the majority of patients with operable rectal cancer; however, the relative costs of these two policies have yet to be determined. Surgeons could choose either approach with impunity. If they are uncertain of the best policy for individual patients, they should include them in a clinical trial. Not all questions can be answered in the same trial (Table 10.6)

The first approach consists of optimal total mesorectal exusion (TME) surgery with selective adjuvant postop XRT. In addition, node-positive patients and some node-negative patients (advanced Dukes' B or, where LRM data are available, node-negative LRM-positive) are most at risk of distant metastases and should be offered adjuvant chemo. If patients are not included in a trial, the optimal published schedule is probably a combination of bolus low-dose FA with 5-FU.

The second approach is a policy of preop XRT followed by surgery, chemo being given preop or postop. European preop XRT is by no means uniform. The so-called short 'Swedish' schedule of 1 week's XRT followed by immediate surgery is used in the current UK trial, CRO7. Prolonged preop XRT, used in the current EORTC Trial, 22921 (Figure 10.1), degrades lymph nodes and makes decisions regarding the need for postop chemo more difficult. A current Dutch Trial, CKVO-95-04, is evaluating the relative benefit of preop postop XRT. It differs from the UK Trial, CRO7 (Figure 10.7), in that all patients are expected to have TME surgery, but none get adjuvant chemo.

Acknowledgement

Tables 10.1 and 10.2 are reprinted, with permission, from the AXIS trial protocol.

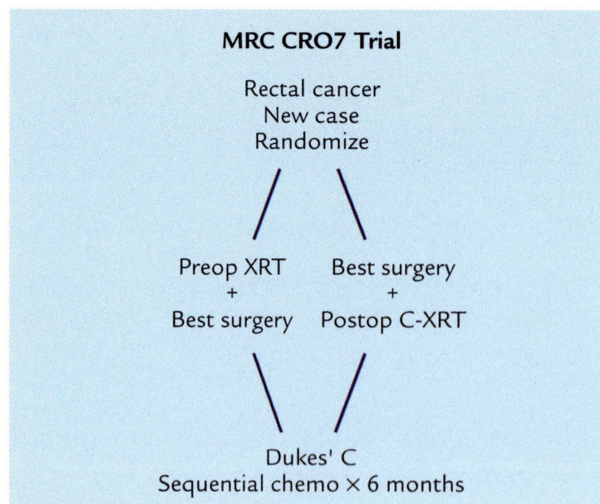

Figure 10.7. *MRC CRO7 trial of preoperative radiotherapy (Preop XRT; 1 week no surgical delay) vs selective postoperative radiotherapy plus concomitant chemotherapy.*

References

1. Meek AG, Lam CW, Order SE Carcinoma of the colon: irradiation by delayed split whole-abdominal technique. *Radiology* 1983; 148: 845–849

2. Fabian CJ, Reddy E, Jewell W *et al.* Phase I–II pilot of whole abdominal radiation and concomitant 5-FU as an adjuvant in colon cancer: a southwest oncology group study. *Int J Radiat Oncol Biol Phys* 1988; 15: 885–892

3. Minsky BD, Adjuvant radiation therapy for colon cancer. *Cancer Treat Rev* 1995; 21: 407–414

4. Marsh PJ, James RD, Schofield PF. Definitions of local recurrence after surgery for rectal carcinoma. *Br J Surg* 1995; 82: 465–468

5. National Cancer Institute 1989. Clinical announcement. Bethesda, MD: NCI

6. Royal College of Surgeons, Association of Coloproctology of Great Britain and Ireland, *Guidelines for the management of colorectal cancer.* 1996

7. Brown ML, Nayfield SG, Shibley LM. Adjuvant therapy for stage III colon cancer: economics returns to research and cost-effectiveness of treatment. *J Natl Cancer Inst* 1994; 86: 424–430

8. Gelber DG, Goldhirsch A, Cole BF *et al.* A quality-adjusted time without symptoms or toxicity (Q-TWiST) analysis of adjuvant radiation therapy and chemotherapy for resectable rectal cancer. *J Natl Cancer Inst* 1996; 88: 1039–1045

9. York Mason A. Rectal cancer: the spectrum of selective surgery. *Proc R Soc Med* 1976; 69: 30–36

10. Goligher JC. *Surgery of the Anus, Rectum and Colon*, 3rd edn, Springfield, Ill: Charles C. Thomas, 1977

11. Nichols RJ. The staging of rectal cancer. *Br J Surg* 1982; 69: 404–409

12. MRC Working Party. Second report. The evaluation of low dose preoperative X-ray therapy in the management of operable rectal cancer: results of a randomly controlled trial. *Br J Surg* 1984; 71: 21–25

13. Basrur VR, Knight PR. 'Intracavitary' radiation for rectal cancer. *J Can Assoc Radiol* 1983; 34: 42–46

14. Kovalic JJ 1988 Endocavitary irradiation for rectal cancer. *Int J Radiat Oncol Biol Phys* 1988; 14: 261–264

15. Lavery IC, Jones IT, Weakley FL *et al.* Definitive management of rectal cancer by contact (intracavitary) irradiation. *Dis Colon Rectum* 1987; 30: 835–838

16. Papillon J. Intracavitary irradiation of early rectal cancer for cure. *Cancer* 1975; 36: 696–701

17. Parturier Albot M, Albot G. Deux mille quarante cinq cas de cancer du rectum traités par radiotherapie de contact endocavitaire seule, ou preoperatoire, ou palliative. *Ann Gastroenterol Hepatol* (Paris) 1981; 17: 313–320

18. Sischy B, Hinson EJ, Wilkinson DR. Definitive radiation therapy for selected cancers of the rectum. *Br J Surg* 1988; 75: 901–903

19. Gerard JP, Ayzac L, Coquard R *et al.* Endocavitary irradiation for early rectal carcinomas T1 (T2). A series of 101 patients treated with the Papillon's technique. *Int J Radiat Oncol Biol Phys* 1996; 34: 775–783

20. Roth SL, Horiot JC, Calais G *et al.* Prognostic factors in limited rectal cancer treated with intracavitary irradiation. *Int J Radiat Oncol Biol Phys* 1989; 16: 1445–1451

21. Brierley JD, Cummings BJ, Shun Wong C *et al.* Adenocarcinoma of the rectum treated by radical external radiation therapy. *Int J Radiat Oncol Biol Phys* 1996; 31: 255–259

22. James RD, Schofield PF. Resection of 'inoperable' rectal cancer following radiotherapy. *Br J Surg* 1985; 72: 279–281

23. Dosoretz DE, Gunderson LL, Hedberg S *et al.* Preoperative irradiation for unresectable rectal and rectosigmoid carcinomas. *Cancer* 1983; 52: 814–818

24. Emami B, Pilepich M, Willett C *et al.* Effect of preoperative irradiation on resectability of colorectal carcinomas. *Int J Radiat Oncol Biol Phys* 1982; 8: 1295–1299

25. Glimelius B, Grafman S, Pahlman L *et al.* Preoperative irradiation with high dose fractionation in adenocarcinoma of the rectum and rectosigmoid. *Acta Radiol Oncol* 1982; 21: 373–379

26. James RD, Johnson RJ, Eddleston B *et al.* Prognostic factors in locally recurrent rectal carcinoma treated by radiotherapy. *Br J Surg* 1983; 70: 469–472

27. Oates GD, Stenning SP, Hardcastle JD *et al.* Randomised trial of surgery alone versus radiotherapy followed by surgery for potentially operable locally advanced rectal cancer. *Lancet* 1996; 348: 1605–1610

28. Arnott SJ, Stenning SP, Hardcastle JD *et al.* Randomised trial of surgery alone versus surgery followed by radiotherapy for mobile cancer of the rectum. *Lancet* 1996; 348: 1610–1614

29. Wilson MS West CML, Wilson GD *et al.* An assessment of the reliability and reproducibility of measurement of potential doubling times (T_{pot}) in human colorectal cancers. *Br J Cancer* 1993; 67: 754–759

30. Wilson MS, Anderson E, Bell JC *et al.* An evaluation of five different methods for estimating proliferation in human colorectal adenocarcinomas. *Surg Oncol* 1994; 3: 263–273

31. James RD, Haboubi N, Schofield PF *et al.* Prognostic factors in colorectal carcinoma treated by preoperative radiotherapy and immediate surgery. *Dis Colon Rectum* 1991; 34: 546–551

32. Carr ND, Pullen BR, Hasleton P *et al.* Microvascular studies in radiation bowel disease. *Gut* 1984; 25: 448–453

33. Schofield PF. Treatment of radiation pelvic disease. In: Schofield PF, Lupton EW (eds) *Causation and Management of Pelvic Radiation Disease*. London: Springer, 1989.

34. Buhre LMD, Mulder NH, Oldhoff J *et al.* The clinical staging of rectal cancer in patients treated by preoperative radiotherapy. *Clin Oncol* 1994; 6: 157–161

35. Fleshman JW, Kodner LJ *et al.* Adenocarcinoma of the rectum. *Dis Colon Rectum* 1985; 11: 810–816

36. Marks G, Mohiuddin M, Borenstein RD. Preoperative radiation therapy and sphincter preservation by the combined abdominosacral technique for selected cancers. *Dis Colon Rectum* 1985; 28: 565–571

37. Ramming KP, Juillard G, Parker R *et al.* Management of carcinoma of the rectum and anus without abdominoperineal excision. *Am J Surg* 1986; 152: 16–20

38. Rich TA, Weiss DR, Mies C *et al.* Sphincter preservation in patients treated with radiation therapy with or without local excision or fulguration. *Radiology* 1985; 156: 527–531

39. Billingham RP. Conservative treatment of rectal cancer. *Cancer* 1992; 70 (suppl): 1355–1363

40. Heald RJ, Husband EM, Ryall RDH. The mesorectum in rectal cancer surgery – the clue to pelvic recurrence. *Br J Surg* 1982; 69: 613–616

41. Enker WE. Potency, cure and local control in the operative treatment of rectal cancer. *Arch Sur* 1992; 127: 1396–1402

42. Williams NS, Johnston D. The quality of life after rectal excision for low rectal cancer. *Br J Sur* 1983; 70: 460–462

43. Frykholm GJ, Glimelius B, Pahlman L. Preoperative irradiation with and without chemotherapy (MFL) in the treatment of primarily non-resectable adenocarcinoma of the rectum. *Eur J Cancer Clin Oncol* 1989; 25: 1535–1541

44. Adam IJ, Mohamdee MO, Martin IG *et al.* Role of circumferential margin in involvement in the local recurrence of rectal cancer. *Lancet* 1994; 344: 707–711

45. Haas-Kock DFM, Baeten CGMI, Jager JJ *et al.* Prognostic significance of radial margins of clearance in rectal cancer. *Br J Surg* 1996; 83, 781–785

46. Feigen M, Cummings B, Hawkins N *et al.* Low dose postoperative adjuvant radiation therapy is ineffective. *Radiother Oncol* 1989; 1989 13: 181–186

47. Stockholm Rectal Cancer Study Group. Preoperative short term radiation therapy in operable rectal carcinoma. *Cancer* 1990; 66: 49–56

48. Swedish Rectal Cancer Trial. Initial report from a Swedish multicentre study examining the role of preoperative irradiation in the treatment of patients with resectable rectal carcinoma. *Br J Surg* 1993; 80: 1333–1336

49. Orton CG, Ellis F A. simplification of the use of the NSD concept in practical radiotherapy. *Br J Radiol* 1973; 46: 529–537

50. Dutch Colorectal Cancer Group. Total mesorectal excision (TME) with or without preoperative radiotherapy in the treatment of primary rectal cancer (CKVO 95-04). Trial protocol, 1996

51. European Organisation for Research and Treatment of Cancer. A four arm Phase III Clinical Trial for T3–T4 resectable rectal cancer comparing pre-operative pelvic irradiation to pre-operative irradiation combined with fluouracil and leucovorin with or without postoperative adjuvant chemotherapy, Study 22921. Trial protocol, 1996

52. Aleman BMP, Lebesque JV, Hart. Postoperative radiotherapy for rectal and rectosigmoid cancer: the impact of total dose on local control. *Radiother Oncol* 1992; 25: 203–206.

53. Allee PE, Tepper JE, Gunderson LL *et al.* Postoperative radiation therapy for incompletely resected colorectal carcinoma. Int *J Radiat Oncol Biol Phys* 1989; 17: 1171–1176

54. Letschert JGJ, Lrebesqu JV, Aleman BMP *et al.* The volume effect in radiation-related late small bowel complications: results of a clinical study of the EORTC Radiotherapy Cooperative Group in patients treated for rectal carcinoma. *Radiother Oncol* 1994; 32: 116–123

55. Frykholm GJ *et al.* Title. *Int J Radiat Oncol Biol Phys* 1996; 35: 1039–1048

56. Mak AC, Rich TA, Schultheiss TE *et al.* Late complications of postoperative radiation therapy for cancer of the rectum and rectosigmoid. *Int J Radiat Oncol Biol Phys* 1994; 28: 597–603

57. Pahlman L, Glimelius B, Graffman S. Pre versus postoperative radiotherapy in rectal carcinoma: an interim report from a randomised multicentre trial. *Br J Surg* 1985; 72: 961–966

58. Goldberg PA, Nicholls RJ, Grimsey JE *et al.* Low-dose preoperative radiotherapy for rectal cancer: a prospective randomized trial. Rectal Cancer Group (Imperial Cancer Research Fund). *Br J Surg* 1993; 80(Suppl): 21

59. Holm T, Rutqvist LE, Johansson H *et al.* Postoperative mortality in rectal cancer treated with or without preoperative radiotherapy: causes and risk factors. *Br J Surg* 1996; 83: 964–968

60. Pahlman L, Glimelius B, Cedermark B et al. Local recurrence rate in a multicentre trial of preoperative radiotherapy compared with operation alone in resectable rectal carcinoma. *Eur J Surg Acta Chir* 1996; 162: 397–402

61. Zheng G, Eddleston B, Schofield PF *et al.* Computed tomographic scanning in rectal carcinoma. *J R Soc Med* 1984; 77: 915–920

62. Marsh PJ, James RD, Schofield PF. Adjuvant preoperative radiotherapy for locally advanced rectal carcinoma: results of a prospective, randomised trial. *Dis Colon Rectum* 1994; 37: 1205–1214

63. Gallagher MJ, Brereton HD, Rostock RA *et al.* A prospective study of treatment techniques to minimise the volume of pelvic small bowel with reduction of acute and late effects associated with pelvic irradiation. *Inter J Radiat Oncol Biol Phys* 1986; 12: 1565–1573

64. Horn A, Morild I, Dahl O. Tumour shrinkage and down staging after preoperative radiation of rectal adenocarcinomas. *Radiother Oncol* 1990; 18: 19–28

65. Pahlman L, Glimelius B. Pre- or post-operative radiotherapy in rectal and rectosigmoid carcinoma. *Ann Surg* 1990; 211: 187–189

66. Myerson RJ, Michalski JM, King MD Adjuvant Radiation Therapy for Rectal Carcinoma: Predictors of Outcome. *Int J Radiat Oncol Biol Phys* 1995; 32: 41–50

67. Frykholm GJ, Glimelius B, Pahlman L. Preoperative or postoperative irradiation in adenocarcinoma of the rectum: final treatment results of a randomised trial and an evaluation of secondary effects. *Dis Colon Rectum* 1993; 36: 564–572

68. Brierley JD, Cummings BJ, Wong CS *et al.* Variation of small bowel volume within the pelvis before and during adjuvant radiation for rectal cancer. *Radiother Oncol* 1994; 31: 110–116

69. Martenson JA, Urias R, Smalley SR *et al.* Radiation therapy quality control in a clinical trial of adjuvant postoperative treatment for rectal cancer. *Int J Radia Oncol Biol Phys* 1995; 32: 51–55

70. Siefert P, Baker LH, Reed ML *et al.* Comparison of continuously infused 5-fluouracil with bolus injection in treatment of patients with colorectal adenocarcinoma. *Cancer* 1975; 36: 123–128

71. Lokich JJ, Ahlgren JD, Gullo JJ *et al.* A prospective randomised comparison of continuous infusion fluouracil with a conventional bolus schedule in metastatic colorectal carcinoma: a Mid-Atlantic Oncology Program Study. *J Clin Oncol* 1989; 7: 425–432

72. Weinerman B, Shah A, Fields A *et al.* Systemic infusion versus bolus chemotherapy with 5-fluouracil in measurable metastatic colorectal cancer. *Am J Clin Oncol* 1992; 15: 518–523

73. Gastrointestinal Tumor Study Group. Radiation and fluorouracil with or without semustine for the treatment of patients with surgical adjuvant adenocarcinoma of the rectum. *J Clin Oncol* 1992; 10: 549–557

74. Krook JE, Moertel CG, Gunderson LL *et al.* Effective surgical adjuvant therapy for high risk rectal carcinoma. *N Engl J Med* 1991; 324: 709–715

75. Fisher B, Wolmark N, Rockette H *et al.* Postoperative adjuvant chemotherapy or radiation therapy for rectal cancer: results from NSABP protocol R-01. *J Natl Cancer Inst* 1988; 80: 21–29.

76. Rominger JC, Gelber RD. Radiation therapy alone or in combination with chemotherapy in the treatment of residual or inoperable carcinoma of the rectum and rectosigmoid or pelvic recurrence following colorectal surgery. Radiat Therapy Oncology Group study (76-16). *Am J Clin Oncol* 1985; 8: 118–127

77. Danjoux CE, Catton GE Delayed complications in colorectal carcinoma treated by combination radiotherapy and 5-fluorouracil – Eastern Cooperative Oncology Group (ECOG) Pilot Study. *Int J Radia, Oncol Biol Phys* 1979; 5: 311–315

78. Wolmark N, Rockette H, Fisher B *et al.* The benefit of leucovorin modulated fluouracil as post-operative adjuvant therapy for primary colon cancer: results from National Surgical Adjuvant Breast and Bowel Project Protocol C–03. J Clin Oncol 1993; 11: 1879–1887

79. Minsky BD, Cohen AM, Enker WE *et al.* Phase I Trial of postoperative 5-FU, radiation therapy and high dose leucovorin for resectable rectal cancer. *Int J Radiat Oncol Biol Phys* 1991; 22: 139–145

80. Cooper SG, Bonaventurs A, Ackland SP *et al.* Pelvic Radiotherapy with concurrent 5-fluouracil modulated by leucovorin for rectal cancer: a phase II study. *Clin Oncol* 1993; 5: 169–173

81. Minsky BD, Cohen AM, Kennedy N *et al.* Combined modality therapy of rectal cancer: decreased acute toxicity with the pre-operative approach. *J Clin Oncol* 1992; 10: 1218–1244

82. Hyams DM, Mamounas EP, Petrelli N *et al.* A clinical trial to evaluate the worth of preoperative multimodality therapy in patients with operable carcinoma of the rectum: a progress report of National Surgical Adjuvant Breast and Bowel Project Protocol R–03. *Dis Colon Rectum* 1997; 40: 131–139

83. Gerard A, Buyse M, Nordlinger B *et al.* Preoperative radiotherapy as adjuvant treatment in rectal cancer. *Ann Surg* 1988; 208: 606–614

84. Gerard A, Loygue J, Liegois P *et al.* Controlled clinical trial for the treatment of rectal cancer using surgery, radiotherapy and chemotherapy-post-operative and delayed complications. In: Gerard A (ed) *Progress and Perspectives in the Treatment of Gastrointestinal Tumours*, pp. 76. Oxford: Pergamon Press, 1980

85. Rich TA, Skibber JM, Ajani JA *et al.* Preoperative infusional chemoradiation therapy for stage T3 rectal cancer. *Int J Radiat Oncol Biol Phys* 1995; 32: 1025–1029

86. Boulis-Wassif S, Gerard A, Loygue J *et al.* Final results of a randomised trial on the treatment of rectal cancer with preop radiotherapy alone or in combination with 5-fluorouracil, followed by radical surgery. *Cancer* 1984; 53: 1181–1818

87. Mansour EG, Letkopoulou M, Johnson R *et al.* A comparison of postoperative adjuvant chemotherapy, radiotherapy or combination therapy in potentially curable resectable rectal carcinoma (abstract). *Proc Am Soc of Clin Oncol* 1991; 10: 154

88. O'Connell, Martenson JA, Wieand HS *et al.* Improving adjuvant therapy for rectal cancer by combining protracted infusion fluouracil with radiation therapy after curative surgery. *N Engl J Med* 1994; 331: 502–507

89. Marsh R deW, Chu NM, Vauthey JN *et al.* Preoperative treatment of locally advanced unresectable rectal adenocarcinoma utilising continuous chronobiologically shaped 5-fluouracil infusion and radiation therapy. *Cancer* 1994; 78: 217–225

90. Bosset JF, Pavy JJ, Hamers BP *et al.* Determination of the optimal dose of 5-fluouracil when combined with low dose D,L-leucovorin and irradiation in rectal cancer: results of three consecutive studies. *Eur J Cancer* 1993; 29A: 1406–1410

Chapter 11

SYSTEMIC THERAPY OF COLORECTAL CANCER

R.S. Midgley, A.M. Young, D.R. Ferry and D.J. Kerr

Introduction

For many years, the chemotherapy of colorectal cancer (CRC) has been the subject of nihilism and ennui, apart from a few distinct and notable voices in the erstwhile wilderness.[1] There is a dual academic response to poor therapeutic results: optimize the use of conventional agents or search for mechanistically novel drugs; much recent laboratory and clinical research has been directed towards the former. Biomodulation of 5-fluorouracil (5-FU), most notably by folinic acid, and rescheduling of 5-FU by prolonged systemic infusion, have resulted in moderate but significant advances in the treatment of CRC. The benefits of improved response rates and prolongation of survival are offset, to an extent, by a rather different spectrum of toxicity, relative to single-agent bolus 5-FU. This chapter reviews the evidence describing the relative utility of chemotherapy and focuses on the search for novel anticancer agents and other therapeutic interventions, such as immunotherapy and gene therapy, that might be useful in treating CRC.

Chemotherapy for advanced colorectal cancer

The function of chemotherapy in advanced CRC is palliative, the goal being to improve the quality and, if possible, the duration of life rather than to offer cure. It is the acceptance of these limitations of treatment that has exacerbated the pessimism surrounding chemotherapy in this setting. However, five randomized trials of 5-FU-based chemotherapy have shown that, compared with best supportive care alone, early active treatment before symptoms occur results in a consistent pattern of improved survival (by 3–6 months) with at least as good, if not better, quality of life. Indeed, the overall benefits of chemotherapy are probably underestimated because of the high crossover to chemotherapy from the control arms when symptoms occur (60% in the Nordic study group).[2]

5-FLUOROURACIL

5-FU has been the mainstay of chemotherapy for CRC for 40 years. It is a prodrug which is converted intracellularly to various metabolites (5-fluorodeoxyuridine triphosphate [5-FdUTP] and 5-fluoruridine triphosphate [5-FUTP]) that inhibit the synthesis of thymidine, DNA and RNA; partly via inhibition of thymidylate synthase (TS), and partly by direct incorporation into the RNA and DNA molecules (Figure 11.1). Because of its action on TS, 5-FU is largely S-phase specific – cells are mainly susceptible to its effects when undergoing DNA replication. The early regimens of single-agent 5-FU – daily for 5 days every 4 weeks, or weekly bolus schedules – produced response rates of 10–15%, with an associated median survival of 8–10 months. Toxicity included nausea and vomiting, oral mucositis, diarrhoea and myelosuppression.

Biomodulation of 5-fluorouracil

Once it was established that 5-FU did have modest activity against CRC cells, this prompted a flurry of trials to find an appropriate biomodulator to augment this cytotoxicity. Levamisole (LEV) – an antihelminthic drug – was an early contender. However, the 5-FU/LEV combination was not found to produce any improvement, in terms of response rate or overall survival, compared with 5-FU alone, and no convincing mechanism of biological synergy between the two became apparent.

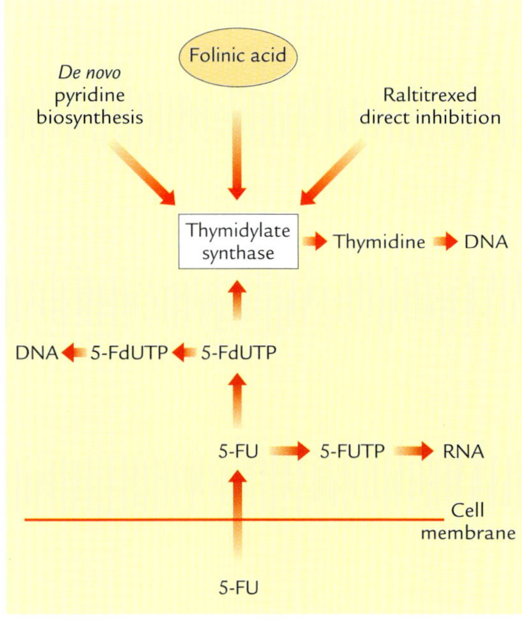

Figure 11.1 *The molecular pharmacology of 5-fluorouracil (5-FU) and the site of action of its modulators: FdUMP, 5-fluorodeoxyuridine monophosphate; FdUTP, 5-fluorodeoxyuridine triphosphate; FUTP, 5-fluorouridine triphosphate.*

Folinic acid

In contrast, folinic acid (FA; 5,10–methyltetrahydrofolate; leucovorin) has a described synergy with 5-FU and the effects of this have been borne out in randomized clinical trials. It has been shown that FA can stabilize the ternary complex of 5-fluorodeoxyuridine monophosphate (5-FdUMP) and TS, thus increasing the degree of thymidine depletion and augmenting the cytotoxicity of 5-FU. A recent meta-analysis of randomized studies comparing single-agent 5-FU with 5-FU/FA combinations, showed a highly significant increase in tumour response rates (11% vs 23%, respectively; $P < 10^{-7}$), and a trend towards improved overall survival, although this did not reach statistical significance. The pattern of toxicity alters with the addition of FA, cumulative diarrhoea being the most serious side effect.

Methotrexate

Methotrexate (MTX) is an inhibitor of dihydrofolate reductase, a key enzyme in folate metabolism. Synergistic antitumour activity after sequential administration of 5-FU and MTX was first seen in experimental rodent tumours, and cellular pharmacological studies have suggested that there is increased formation of FUTP. This increases incorporation of FUTP into RNA, reducing maturation rates and enhancing cytotoxicity in a synergistic manner. The sequence and interval of administration of each drug seems to be critical in obtaining optimal therapeutic effectiveness of the combination. In a clinical setting, a direct comparison between two schedules of 5-FU and MTX was performed in a randomized trial in which patients received MTX, 200 mg/m^2, followed by 5-FU, 600 mg/m^2, either 1 hour or 24 hours later. The 24-hour interval was associated with improved response rate and median survival compared with the 1-hour interval. A meta-analysis of a total of 1178 patients from eight randomized studies assessed the clinical benefit, objectively and quantitatively, of 5-FU/MTX combination compared with 5-FU alone.[3] Compared with 5-FU alone, the 5-FU/MTX combination provided a statistically significant advantage in response rate (10% vs 19.5%; $P < 0.0001$) and a small but significant advantage in median survival (9.1 vs 10.7 months; $P = 0.024$).

Infusional 5-fluorouracil

5-FU has a short plasma half-life (8–14 minutes) and is differentially cytotoxic to cells in the S-phase. A logical prediction might therefore be that continuous infusion (CI) of 5-FU could increase the proportion of susceptible cells and augment cytotoxicity. A meta-analysis of six randomized trials comparing CI with bolus 5-FU demonstrated a higher response rate (22% vs 14%) and a small improvement in overall survival (12.1 vs 11.3 months; $P = 0.04$) with CI. The pattern of toxicity was also significantly different, with decreased rates of mucositis, neutropenia and diarrhoea with CI 5-FU, but a significantly increased risk of hand–foot syndrome.[4]

In addition to infusional scheduling of 5-FU, it may be critical to maintain dose intensity, and biomodulation may also be appropriate. A high dose intensity with biomodulation is achieved with the de Gramont regimen, which comprises FA and bolus 5-FU, followed by a 48-hour infusion of 5-FU. A multicentre trial in France compared this schedule with the standard Mayo 5-FU regimen (bolus daily for 5 days every 4 weeks).[5] This trial was the first to demonstrate the superiority of modulated infusional 5-FU over the Mayo regimen in terms of both response rate (33% vs 14%; $P < 0.01$) and time to progression (6.2 vs 5.0 months; $P < 0.01$). The difference in overall survival just failed to reach statistical significance (15.5 vs 14.3 months; $P = 0.067$) but may have been masked by high crossover rates from the bolus regimen to the infusional regimen on progression. The de Gramont regimen was associated with a significantly lower incidence of severe (grade 3 or 4) toxicity than the bolus regimen.[5]

Modulation of infusional 5-FU by MTX has also been tested. The European Organization for Research and Treatment of Cancer (EORTC) compared high-dose infusional 5-FU (60 mg/kg) as a weekly 48-hour infusion alone or in combination with MTX (40 mg/m^2).[6] A significantly higher response rate for the combination treatment (23% vs 11%; $P = 0.025$) was associated with a non-significant trend towards improved survival (12.5 vs 9.3 months, $P = 0.123$).[6]

In summary, infusional regimens, continuous or intermittent, do appear to produce advantages, in terms of improved response rates and decreased toxicity, compared with bolus 5-FU. Attention is now focusing on improving overall survival by modulation with other drugs. It is important to bear in mind that infusional regimens incur extra costs because of the need for the insertion of Hickman lines or peripherally inserted central catheters, and pumps for the administration of treatment on an outpatient basis. Training of medical and nursing staff and patients is also required to avoid the risk of infection and thrombosis.

Oral fluoropyrimidines

To improve patients' quality of life and to reduce the cost of human resources in the administration of chemotherapy, there has been a trend towards developing oral fluoropyrimidines to replace conventional intravenous 5-FU. Work in this area was initially hampered by the erratic oral bioavailability of 5-FU (ranging from 0 to 80%); however, interest has been rekindled by results from randomized trials comparing oral uracil and tegafur (UFT) plus FA and the 5-FU-prodrug, capecitabine, with the standard Mayo 5-FU regimen.[7–10] A total of approximately 2400 patients were randomized in these four trials, and equivalence between the Mayo regimen and the oral agents was demonstrated in terms of response rate and overall survival. Toxicity was different with the two regimens, the oral agents being associated with decreased mucositis and decreased hospitalization rates but increased hand–foot syndrome. This pattern of toxicity is similar to that seen for infusional 5-FU regimens. It will be interesting to compare the oral agents directly with infusional 5-FU in terms of response and survival rates. If equivalence were observed, there would be much to gain from the oral agents in terms of health service resources and patient acceptability.

Regional 5-fluorouracil delivery

Regional chemotherapy relies on the premises that most cytotoxic agents have steep dose–response curves and that high drug concentrations can be generated within a target organ (e.g. the liver) because of differential drug clearance. Up to 20% of patients who relapse after apparently being cured of CRC by resection present with disease confined to the liver; this suggests that hepatic arterial chemotherapy could be a useful treatment for these patients. 5-FU and a derivative, fluorodeoxyuridine (FUdR), have high clearance rates and undergo significant arterial extraction, which makes them ideal drugs for hepatic arterial chemotherapy. Six major trials have compared hepatic arterial infusional (HAI) therapy with best supportive care or systemic therapy in patients with hepatic metastatic colorectal cancer. A meta-analysis of these trials showed a statistically significant improvement in response rate with HAI treatment (41% overall: complete response, 3%; partial response, 38%) compared with systemic treatment (14% overall: complete response, 2%; partial response, 12%) (overall $P < 10^{-10}$).[11] However, the difference in median duration of response was less impressive: 38 weeks for HAI therapy and 32 weeks for systemic therapy. The design of these trials has been criticized because of a reduced capacity to detect true differences in overall survival. The criticisms include the crossover from systemic to locoregional therapy on progression, the large proportions of patients deemed ineligible for treatment after randomization, and the variability in the systemic chemotherapy control patients.

A series of phase-I and -II trials allowed determination of an HAI 5-FU/FA regimen that mimics the de Gramont intravenous regimen in terms of schedule and steady-state systemic concentration. This HAI regimen is now being compared with the de Gramont systemic regimen in the Medical Research Council/EORTC/Cancer Research Campaign randomized phase-III CRO5 trial of patients with metastatic CRC confined to the liver. Conclusions from this trial will be a major determinant of HAI practice in this setting. If HAI is found to be superior to systemic chemotherapy, combinations of this regimen with other drugs, perhaps intrahepatic mitomycin C or intravenous irinotecan, are likely to be assessed.

Regional therapy via the hepatic artery is also being assessed in a quasi-adjuvant setting following resection of hepatic metastases. Recurrence after resection of hepatic metastases is unfortunately frequent, and is a solitary finding in 60% of patients (see Chapter 8). Two large trials have explored the administration of chemotherapy immediately after metastatectomy in an attempt to reduce recurrence rates. In a trial from Sloan-Kettering 156 patients were randomized to receive either HAI/FUdR/dexamethasone plus systemic 5-FU/FA or systemic 5-FU/FA alone as adjuvant treatment after resection. The total treatment period was 6 months. Compared with systemic 5-FU/FA alone, adjuvant treatment with HAI plus systemic 5-FU/FA significantly increased 2-year survival (85% vs 69%; $P = 0.023$) and hepatic-disease-free survival (89% vs 59%; $P = 0.00012$).[12] The Intergroup trial randomized patients preoperatively to either surgery alone (hepatic metastatectomy, $n = 56$) or surgery followed by continuous HAI of FUdR for four cycles plus systemic infusional 5-FU for twelve cycles ($n = 53$). Preliminary data from a mean follow-up time of 33 months indicate that the 3-year recurrence rate is significantly improved in patients receiving chemotherapy (34% vs 59%; $P = 0.039$). The liver was involved in 24 recurrences in patients receiving surgery alone and eight recurrences in those receiving chemotherapy ($P = 0.035$). There was also a trend towards an overall survival benefit in the chemotherapy-treated patients.[13]

NEW THYMIDYLATE SYNTHASE INHIBITORS

The success of 5-FU has encouraged the development of other compounds that directly bind and inhibit TS. Raltitrexed (Tomudex), the major competitor to 5-FU in this field, has undergone extensive phase-III evaluation in advanced CRC. More than 1000 patients have received raltitrexed in multicentre and international trials. These studies demonstrated equivalence of raltitrexed with the Mayo regimen and the Machover schedule in terms of response rates (15–20%). More recently, in the MRCO6 trial 905 patients with advanced CRC were randomized to receive raltitrexed (3 mg/m^2 three times a week), 48-hour infusional 5-FU fortnightly (de Gramont regimen), or continuous infusion 5-FU (Lokich regimen).

Response rates and overall survival (approximately 10 months) were identical for all three groups, but there was a significant advantage in progression-free survival for the de Gramont regimen compared with raltitrexed.[14] In addition, concern was raised over deaths associated with raltitrexed in this study, demonstrating that drug-induced diarrhoea and neutropenic sepsis need to be managed aggressively as they are often harbingers of serious morbidity and significant mortality rates. It is likely that raltitrexed will have a role as a single agent in selected groups of patients; it is also showing promise in combination with the novel agents described below.

Novel anti-cancer drugs for advanced colorectal cancer

It is increasingly apparent that biological and pharmacodynamic modulation of 5-FU and the use of other TS inhibitors is likely to produce only marginal improvement in survival for patients with CRC. Therefore novel chemotherapeutic agents that exploit different cellular mechanisms need to be developed. Two drugs are particularly noteworthy in this regard: irinotecan and oxaliplatin.

IRINOTECAN

Irinotecan (CPT-11) is a semi-synthetic camptothecin which works by inhibiting topoisomerase I. In early trials it showed modest activity as a single agent in previously untreated advanced CRC *and* did not show cross-resistance with 5-FU. Indeed, in phase-II trials of irinotecan in patients pretreated with 5-FU, the results appeared as good as those obtained in chemotherapy-naïve patients, with response rates of 13–18% and 19%, respectively. Subsequently, two phase-III studies compared irinotecan with best supportive care or with second-line infusional 5-FU for patients with 5-FU-resistant disease.[15,16] Both trials showed statistically significant benefits, with median improvements in survival of 2.9 and 2.3 months, respectively. The major toxicity of irinotecan is diarrhoea which is biphasic – an immediate acute cholinergic diarrhoea during treatment administration, which can be effectively counteracted and prevented by subcutaneous atropine, is followed by a delayed mucositic diarrhoea, with an onset 7–10 days after treatment. Because of this specific toxicity, oncologists were initially wary of using irinotecan in combination with 5-FU. However, two large randomized trials have now demonstrated that this hesitancy was largely unjustified.[17,18]

In a US trial, 683 patients were randomized to receive bolus 5-FU/FA alone, irinotecan alone, or a combination of 5-FU/FA and irinotecan. The toxicity of irinotecan plus 5-FU/FA was less than additive, perhaps even antagonistic, since it was no worse than with the same dose and schedule of irinotecan given as a single agent. However, whilst either 5-FU/FA or irinotecan gave almost identical progression-free-survival rates (median 4.4 vs 4.2 months) and response rates (22% vs 18%), the combination of 5-FU/FA and irinotecan significantly improved the progression-free-survival rate (6.9 months; $P < 0.005$) and response rate (40%; $P < 0.001$). This did not translate into improved survival but conclusions are hampered by significant salvage crossover from single agent to dual therapy.[17]

In a European trial, 387 patients were randomized to receive infusional 5-FU/FA with or without irinotecan. In this trial, toxicity was significantly increased with the addition of irinotecan but efficacy was also significantly augmented, with increased time to progression (median 6.7 vs 4.4 months; $P = 0.01$), improved response rate (41% vs 23%; $P < 0.001$) and improved overall survival (16.8 months vs 14.0 months; $P = 0.03$).[18]

OXALIPLATIN

Oxaliplatin, a third-generation platinum analogue which induces DNA cross-linking and apoptotic cell death, also showed promising early activity. From inception this drug has been used in combination with 5-FU for two reasons. First, *in vitro* experiments suggested 5-FU/oxaliplatin synergy and, secondly, the toxicity profiles of the two agents did not appear to overlap. In early phase-II trials, the response rate for single-agent oxaliplatin in 106 5-FU-resistant patients was 10%; the response rate in 46 patients pretreated with 5-FU who received an intensive 5-FU/FA/oxaliplatin schedule was 46%.[19] Because there are theoretical advantages to using combinations of non-cross-resistant cytotoxic combinations upfront (in terms of eradicating each cancer clone, particularly in the adjuvant setting) it is sensible to test drug combinations as first-line therapy. Hence, there have been recent trials of 5-FU/FA/oxaliplatin in patients with unpretreated metastatic colorectal cancer. Updated results from such a trial were reported at ASCO in 1999. Four hundred twenty patients were randomized to the de Gramont regimen with or without the addition of oxaliplatin. The addition of oxaliplatin increased toxicity but the combination was still extremely well tolerated.

The efficacy of the 5-FU/FA/oxaliplatin regimen was markedly better than 5-FU/FA alone, with an increase in progression-free survival (median 8.7 vs 6.1 months, $p = 0.0001$ and response rate (50% vs 22%, $p = 0.0001$). Although overall survival was not altered in a statistically significant fashion, this is partly accountable by imbalance in other variables between the two arms, since in multivariate analysis, allocation to 5-FU/FA/oxaliplatin arm predicted for survival ($p = 0.0001$).[20]

Both oxaliplatin and irinotecan are showing a great deal of promise both in terms of improved survival and tolerable toxicity. Each requires further work to define their optimal combinations and sequences of administration, but their translation from therapy for advanced disease into the adjuvant field appears likely in the future.

Chemotherapy for colorectal cancer in the adjuvant setting

Even though 80% of patients with CRC show complete macroscopic clearance of their disease by resection, 50% of these patients subsequently develop recurrence, presumably because of disseminated micrometastases present at the time of surgery, and eventually die of their disease. Adjuvant chemotherapy is administered with the intention of eradicating these circulating cancer cells before they become established and refractory to intervention. The Intergroup trial tested adjuvant chemotherapy after surgery in 318 patients with stage-B CRC, comparing surgery alone with surgery plus 5-FU/LEV. In addition, 929 patients with stage-C CRC received surgery alone, surgery plus LEV, or surgery plus 5-FU/LEV. In the patients with stage-C disease, there was a 33% decrease in the odds of death and a 41% decrease in the risk of recurrence amongst those who received 5-FU/LEV compared with those who received surgery alone.[21] More recently, three large prospective randomized trials have also shown increased disease-free survival and overall survival after adjuvant treatment with the combination 5-FU/FA regimens, usually for a total treatment period of 6 months (details reviewed elsewhere).[22] These results translate into a 25–30% reduction in the odds of dying from colon cancer or an improvement in absolute survival of 5–6% compared with control patients.

All prospective trials to date have largely concentrated on patients with Dukes' stage-C colon cancer and it is within this subgroup that the benefits of adjuvant chemotherapy are well established. There is continuing controversy surrounding the use of systemic adjuvant therapy in patients with rectal or Dukes' stage-B colon cancer. Current trials, in particular the uncertain arm of the QUASAR trial, will contribute useful information to this debate. It is likely that there will be a continuum of effect between stage-B and stage-C cancers, and there may be a particular subgroup of patients with Dukes' stage-B disease, perhaps with other poor prognostic markers, that will benefit as much as patients with Dukes' stage-C disease. However, on present evidence, the routine use of adjuvant chemotherapy in patients with Dukes' stage-B cancer is not justified. With respect to patients with rectal cancer, their pattern of relapse is different to that observed in colon cancer, with local recurrence usually the predominant feature. Local radiotherapy is therefore a much more useful tool in these patients; this is covered in detail in Chapter 10.

As in advanced CRC, infusional therapy has been tested in the adjuvant setting. This has largely been restricted to portal vein infusion (PVI), based on the observation that the liver is the most frequent site of metastatic relapse, and the belief that hepatic micrometastases less than 1–3 mm in size derive their blood supply from the portal vein rather than the hepatic artery. PVI adjuvant 5-FU has usually been administered as a single agent for 5–7 days immediately after surgery to remove the primary tumour. A meta-analysis of data from ten trials (including 4000 patients and 1557 deaths) of PVI compared with surgery alone showed that survival with and without PVI was similar for the first 2 years; however, at 5 years there was an absolute survival improvement of 4.7% with PVI ($P = 0.006$).[23] The early results of the AXIS trial, which randomized 4000 patients between PVI and observation, do not show any significant difference between the two treatments.[24]

With regard to the use of novel anticancer drugs in the adjuvant setting, this is of course the natural progression once they have been tested rigorously and found to be effective and safe in advanced disease. Oxaliplatin, irinotecan and the oral fluoropyrimidines are due to enter clinical trials in the adjuvant setting in the near future.

Innovative therapeutic interventions

Our evolving understanding of the biology of CRC and, in particular, recognition of genes that are switched on or off during carcinogenesis and of proteins that are preferentially expressed in CRC cells, is being translated into innovative immunotherapy and gene therapy techniques.

IMMUNOTHERAPY

Traditionally CRC has not been an obvious target for immunotherapy, especially bulky metastatic disease that is unlikely to respond to any immunological manipulation. The situation looks more promising in the adjuvant setting, where micrometastatic clusters of cells reside in mesenchymal tissues, surrounded by granulocytes, macrophages and killer cells, all effecting ready initiation of antibody-induced mechanisms of cytotoxicity and all potent inducers of apoptosis. In the early 1980s an anti-idiotypic anticolorectal cancer antibody was developed. It induced cellular cytotoxicity with human effector cells and prevented outgrowth of xenotransplanted human tumour cells in athymic mice. Toxicity studies in advanced CRC in 1991 suggested it was well tolerated. Riethmuller and colleagues did a randomized study of the antibody as adjuvant therapy in 189 patients with stage-C CRC compared with surgery alone.[25] Survival was significantly lengthened in the antibody-treated patients (5-year survival 51% vs 36%; $P = 0.025$), and the antibody is now being tested in combination with 5-FU/FA.

GENE THERAPY

Virus-directed enzyme prodrug therapy

The concept of virus-directed enzyme prodrug therapy (VDEPT) is to virally transduce the tumour cell with an enzyme (such as cytosine deaminase [CD]) capable of converting an inactive prodrug (5-fluorocytosine ([5-FC]) into an active cytotoxic species (5-FU). Tumour-cell specificity is created by splicing in the 5′ transcriptional regulatory sequences of the human carcinoembryonic antigen (CEA) gene (Figure 11.2). This promoter sequence effectively functions as an on–off switch, so that the downstream structural gene is transcribed only by cells that synthesize CEA, that is, CRC cells. Hence, tumour cells that express CD convert 5-FC to 5-FU, producing a high concentration of 5-FU which diffuses into and kills immediately neighbouring cells, the so-called bystander effect, leaving less proximate healthy cells intact. Clinical trials using this approach in patients with hepatic metastases are planned, with regional delivery of the viral vector with the CEA–CD construct, followed by oral administration of 5-FC.

Immunogenetic manipulation

Viral vectors can also be used to deliver immunomodulatory cytokines and co-stimulatory molecules to tumours, with a view to stimulating a host antitumour response. For example, the co-stimulatory molecule B7 (essential for optimal binding of a cytotoxic T cell to the target cell) can be transfected along with the stimulatory cytokine, granulocyte-macrophage colony-stimulating factor, into cancer cells, in an attempt to convert them into antigen-presenting cells. Transduction could be performed *in vitro* following *ex vivo* expansion of a tumour biopsy. The transduced cells would then be irradiated and transfused back into the patient as an autologous vaccine (Figure 11.3). Alternatively, viral vectors could be used *in vivo*, with tumour-specific promoters to ensure selective cancer expression and convert the tumour into an autologous vaccine *in situ*.

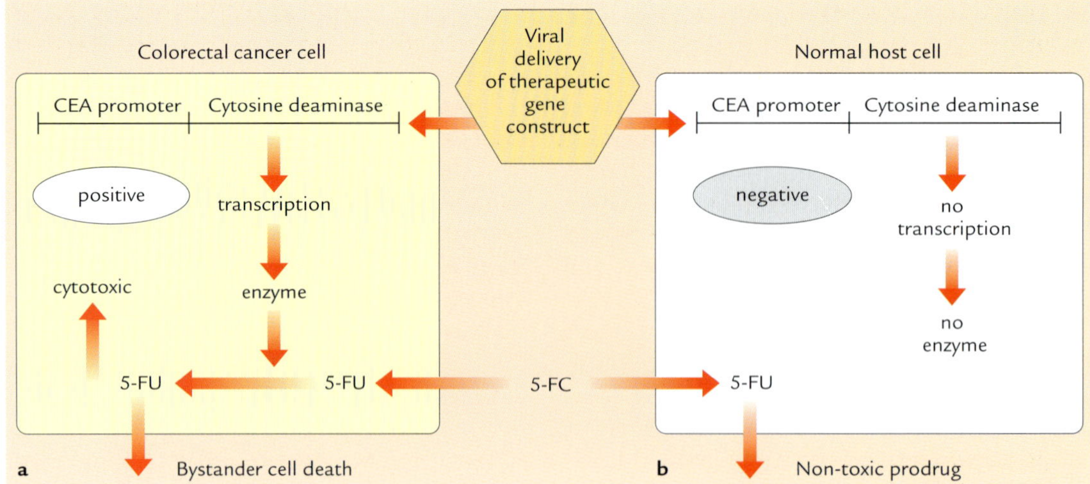

Figure 11.2 *(a) The application of virus-directed enzyme prodrug therapy (VDEPT) in colorectal cancer. (b) In the normal hepatocyte, the carcinoembryonic antigen (CEA) promoter will be transcriptionally silent and cytosine deaminase will not be expressed. 5-FU, 5-fluorouracil; 5-FC, 5-fluorocytosine.*

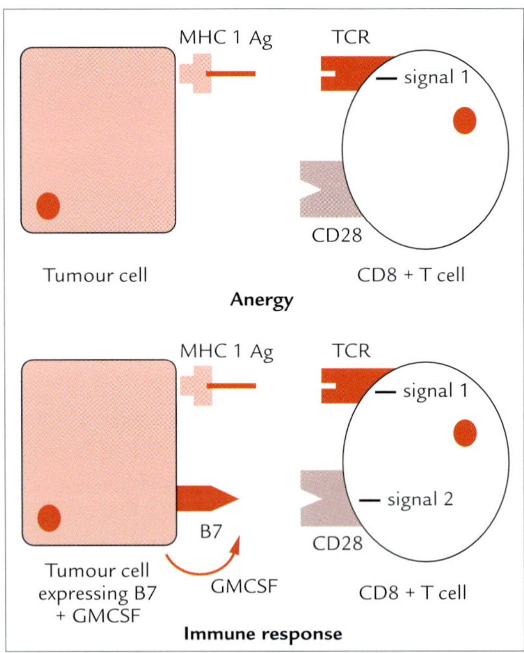

Figure 11.3 *Transfection with the co-immunostimulatory molecule B7 and GMCSF can convert the colorectal cancer cell into an antigen-presenting cell that is likely to be a promising target for a cytotoxic T-cell response. TCR, T-cell receptor; MHC I Ag, major histocompatibility class I antigen; CD, cell differentiation marker; GMCSF, granulocyte-macrophage colony-stimulating factor.*

References

1. Moertel CG. Chemotherapy for colorectal cancer. *N Engl J Med* 1994; 330: 1136–1142

2. Guidance on commissioning cancer services: improving outcomes in colorectal cancer. NHS Executive, London, 1997

3. The Advanced Colorectal Cancer Meta-analysis Project. Meta-analysis of randomised trials testing biochemical modulation of 5-fluorouracil by methotrexate in metastatic colorectal cancer. *J Clin Oncol* 1994; 12: 960–969

4. Meta-analysis Group in Cancer. Efficacy of intravenous continuous infusion of 5-fluorouracil compared with bolus administration in advanced colorectal cancer. *J Clin Oncol* 1998; 16: 301–308

5. de Gramont A, Bosset JF, Milan C *et al.* A randomised trial comparing monthly low-dose leucovorin/5-fluorouracil bolus with bimonthly high dose leucovorin/5-fluorouracil bolus plus continuous infusion for advanced colorectal cancer: A French Intergroup study. *Proc Am Soc Clin Oncol* 1997; 15: 808–815

6. Blijam G, Wagener T, Wils J *et al.* Modulation of high dose infusional fluorouracil by low dose

methotrexate in patients with advanced or metastatic colorectal cancer; final results of a randomised European Organization for Research and Treatment of Cancer study. *J Clin Oncol* 1996; 14: 2266–2273

7. Pazdur R, Douillard J-Y, Skillings JR *et al.* Multicentre phase III study of 5-fluourouracil (5-FU) or UFT™ in combination with leucovorin (LV) in patients with metastatic colorectal cancer (abstr). *Proc Am Soc Clin Oncol* 1999; 18: 1009

8. Twelves C, Harper P, Van Cutsem E. A phase III trial (SO14796) of Xeloda (capecitabine) in previously untreated advanced/metastatic colorectal cancer (abstr). *Proc Am Soc Clin Oncol* 1999; 18: 1010

9. Carmichael J, Popiela T, Radstone D *et al.* Randomised comparative study of ORZEL (oral uracil/tegafur) plus leucovorin (LV) versus parenteral 5-fluorouracil (5-FU) plus LV in patients with metastatic colorectal cancer (abstr). Proc Am Soc Clin Oncol 1999; 18: 1015

10. Cox JV, Pazdur R, Thibault A *et al.* A phase II trial of Xeloda™ (capecitabine) in previously untreated advanced/ metastatic colorectal cancer (abstr). *Proc Am Soc Clin Oncol* 1999; 18: 1016

11. Meta-analysis Group in Cancer. Re-appraisal of hepatic arterial infusion in the treatment of non-resectable liver metastases from colorectal cancer. *J Natl Cancer Inst* 1996; 88: 252–258

12. Kemeny N, Cohen A, Huang Y *et al.* Randomised study of hepatic arterial infusion (HAI) and systemic (SYS) versus SYS alone as adjuvant therapy after resection of hepatic metastases from colorectal cancer (abstr). *Proc Am Soc Clin Oncol* 1999; 18: 1011

13. Kemeny MM, Adak S, Gray B *et al.* Results of the Intergroup Eastern Co-operative Group (ECOG) and Southwest Oncology Group (SWOG) prospective randomised study of surgery alone versus continuous hepatic arterial infusion of FUdR and continuous infusion of 5-FU after hepatic resection for colorectal liver metastases (abstr). *Proc Am Soc Clin Oncol* 1999; 18: 1012

14. Maughan TS, James RD, Kerr D *et al.* on behalf of the British MRC Colorectal Cancer Working Party. Preliminary results of a multicentre randomised trial comparing three chemotherapy regimens (de Gramont, Lokich, and raltitraxed) in metastatic colorectal cancer (abstr). *Proc Am Soc Clin Oncol* 1999; 18: 1007

15. Cunningham D, Pyrhonen S, James RD *et al.* Randomised trial of irinotecan plus supportive care versus supportive care alone after fluorouracil failure for patients with metastatic colorectal cancer. *Lancet* 1998; 352: 1413–1418

16. Rougier P, van Cutsem E, Bajetta E *et al.* Randomised trial of irinotecan versus fluorouracil by continuous infusion after fluorouracil failure in patients with metastatic colorectal cancer. *Lancet* 1998; 352: 1407–1412

17. Saltz L, Locker P, Pirotta N *et al.* Weekly irinotecan, leucovorin and fluorouracilis superior to daily × 5 LV/FU in patients with previously untreated metastatic colorectal cancer (abstr). *Proc Am Soc Clin Oncol* 1999; 18: 898

18. Douillar J, Cunningham D, Roth A *et al.* A randomised phase III trial comparing irinotecan + 5-FU/FA to the same schedule of 5-FU/FA in patients with metastatic colorectal cancer as frontline chemotherapy (abstr). *Proc Am Soc Clin Oncol* 1999; 18: 899

19. de Gramont A, Vignoud J, Tournigant C *et al.* Oxaliplatin with high dose leucovorin and 5fluorouracil 48 hour continuous infusion in pre-treated metastatic colorectal cancer. *Eur J Cancer* 1997; 33: 214–219

20. Seymour M, Tabah-Fisch I, Hometin M *et al.* Quality of life in advanced colorectal cancer: a comparison of Q o L during bolus plus infusional 5-FU/leucororin with or without oxaliplatin. *Proz. Am. Soc. Ain. Oncol* 1999; 8: 901.

21. Moertal CG, Fleming TH, MacDonald JS *et al.* Levamisole and fluorouracil for adjuvant treatment of resected colon cancer. *N Engl J Med* 1990; 322: 352–358

22. Midgley RS, Kerr DJ. Adjuvant treatment of colorectal cancer. *Cancer Treat Rev* 1997; 23: 135–152

23. Liver Infusion Meta-analysis Group. Portal vein chemotherapy for colorectal cancer; a meta-analysis of 4000 patients in 10 studies. *J Natl Cancer Inst* 1997; 89: 497–505

24. James RD, AXIS Collaborators. Intraportal 5GU and perioperative radiotherapy (RT) in the adjuvant treatment of colorectal cancer – 3681 patients randomized in the UK Coordinating Committee on Cancer Research (UKCCCR) AXIS trial. *Proc Am Soc Clin Oncol* 1999; 18: 1013

25. Riethmuller G, Schneider-Gadicke E, Schmilok G. Randomised trial of monoclonal antibody for adjuvant treatment of resected Dukes C colorectal cancer. *Lancet* 1994; 343: 1177–1183

Chapter 12

OBSTRUCTING LARGE BOWEL CANCER

C.S. McArdle and J.H. Anderson

Introduction

Colorectal cancer is the second-commonest cause of death from malignancy in the United Kingdom: each year there are approximately 27,000 new cases and 19,000 deaths attributable to the disease.[1] Approximately 30% of patients present as emergencies with symptoms suggestive of obstruction, rectal bleeding or perforation. Outcome remains poor, largely as a result of the advanced stage of the disease at the time of initial presentation. Despite improvements in surgical technique, perioperative care and the use of antibiotic prophylaxis, population-based studies suggest that outcome has not altered substantially over the last three decades.[2]

Obstruction

Approximately 15% of all patients with colorectal cancer will present as emergencies with symptoms suggestive of incomplete or absolute obstruction. The risk is highest for lesions at the splenic flexure, nearly half of which present with obstruction. However, because of the high incidence of tumours in the distal colon, two-thirds of obstructing tumours lie at or distal to the splenic flexure. Obstructing rectal tumours are relatively uncommon: since symptoms, including tenesmus, occur early, few rectal tumours grow large enough to produce obstruction.

In the majority of patients, large bowel obstruction presents with lower abdominal pain, distension and constipation. Vomiting may also occur. Plain abdominal radiographs usually confirm the diagnosis, with gaseous distension of the large bowel proximal to the site of obstruction and a distal cut-off. Depending on whether the ileocaecal valve is competent, distension of small bowel may also be present. However, the clinical and radiological findings can be misleading. For this reason, urgent single-contrast enema studies should be undertaken to demonstrate the site of obstruction and to exclude other causes, including pseudo-obstruction, which occurs in approximately 10% of patients.

The timing of surgery is important. Patients with large bowel obstruction do not usually require emergency surgery unless the degree of abdominal tenderness suggests peritonitis, or abdominal radiography shows the caecum to be grossly distended, heralding impending perforation. Many of these patients will be dehydrated, oliguric and uraemic. Furthermore, many are elderly and are therefore more likely to have pre-existing cardiorespiratory insufficiency and consequently a higher risk of postoperative mortality. Careful resuscitation prior to surgery is essential and this might most appropriately be undertaken in the high-dependency or intensive therapy unit. Fluid losses should be replaced and a catheter inserted to monitor hourly urine output; it may also be prudent to insert a central venous line. In patients with an incompetent ileocaecal valve and small bowel distension, a nasogastric tube may be of value. The patient should be taken to theatre only when adequately resuscitated, with correction of fluid losses and electrolyte imbalance. Ideally, surgery should be performed during normal working hours by senior surgical and anaesthetic staff.[3] Prior to surgery, appropriate antibiotic prophylaxis and anti-thromboembolism measures should be initiated.

Surgical options

The aim of surgery should be the relief of the obstruction with minimal perioperative morbidity and mortality. Ideally, the tumour should be resected and a permanent colostomy avoided; this may involve more than one procedure. It is generally accepted that most obstructing colonic tumours at or proximal to the splenic flexure are suitable for primary resection and anastomosis. However, care is still required, since right-sided anastomoses may leak in up to 10% of cases and postoperative mortality may be as high as 17%.[4] In patients with an irresectable tumour, and in high-risk patients with extensive metastases, an internal bypass may be more appropriate.

In contrast, the optimal management of distal, obstructing colonic tumours remains controversial. Basically, three approaches are available – primary decompression followed by staged resection, primary resection with delayed anastomosis, or primary resection and anastomosis.

PRIMARY DECOMPRESSION FOLLOWED BY STAGED RESECTION

Traditionally, the most popular method of dealing with a large bowel obstruction has been to use a three-stage approach. First, a defunctioning colostomy was performed to relieve the obstruction; a secondary resection was then performed at a later date; ultimately, the patient was re-admitted for the closure of the colostomy. In theory, this provides a simple, life-saving operation which can be undertaken by relatively junior surgical trainees; however, it usually entails three separate admissions and delays potentially curative resection. Although the initial mortality is relatively low, cumulative mortality is around 20% when all patients with obstruction are included (Table 12.1). In studies where only the most poorly patients are treated in this way, operative mortality may be even higher. Furthermore, failure to remove the primary tumour in approximately one-third of patients often results in poor-quality palliation. Moreover, approximately one-half of those patients undergoing a staged resection fail to complete all three stages and are therefore left with a permanent stoma. More recently, intratumoral stents have been used to achieve primary decompression without the need to resort to laparotomy and stoma formation (see later).

RESECTION AND DELAYED ANASTOMOSIS

Concern that failure to remove the primary tumour at the time of initial surgery might compromise long-term survival led to the introduction of the Hartmann's procedure, where the tumour is resected with formation of an end colostomy and closure of the rectal stump or formation of a mucous fistula. This approach achieves the dual objectives of relieving the obstruction and resecting the tumour while avoiding the potential complications of an anastomosis performed under suboptimal conditions. Reversal of a Hartmann's procedure, however, is a major procedure with a not insubstantial complication rate. Morbidity occurs in about one third of patients and mortality is approximately 9% (Table 12.2). The major disadvantage of the strategy is that about 40% of patients may be unfit for (or refuse) further surgery, thereby ending up with a permanent colostomy.

Table 12.1. *Results of surgery for obstructing colorectal cancer (CRC): primary decompression followed by staged resection*

Reference	No. of patients	Pathology	Site	Percentage of total number of patients	No. of deaths*	Percentage resected	No. surviving all stages*	Median stay (days)
Hoffmann and Jensen 1984[18]	57	CRC	L	100	19 (33)	61	30 (53)	–
Phillips *et al.* 1985[4]	157	CRC	R/L	22	35 (22)	77	114 (73)	40
Buechter *et al.* 1988[19]	66	CRC	R/L	33	18 (28)	65	38 (58)	–
Ambrosetti *et al.* 1989[20]	26	CRC/benign	L	30	10 (38)	31	7 (27)	41
Gutman *et al.* 1989[21]	71	CRC	L	–	6 (9)	69	49 (69)	–
Kristiansen *et al.* 1990[22]	135	CRC	L	100	33 (24)	77	84 (62)	–
Runkel *et al.* 1991[23]	29	CRC	R/L	51	8 (28)	45	12 (41)	–
Gandrup *et al.* 1992[24]	53	CRC	L	41	1 (2)	100	46 (87)	30
Sjodahl *et al.* 1992[25]	48	CRC	R/L	42	7 (15)	83	36 (75)	45
Total	642	–	–	41	137 (21)	69	416 (65)	–

* Percentages in parentheses.

Table 12.2. *Results of surgery for obstructing colorectal cancer (CRC): primary resection and delayed anastomosis*

Reference	No. of patients	Pathology	Site	Percentage of total number of patients	No. of deaths*	No. surviving all stages*	Median stay (days)
Koruth *et al.* 1985[6]	29	CRC/benign obstruction/ peritonitis	L	31	1 (3)	17 (59)	26
Phillips *et al.* 1985[4]	141	CRC	R/L	20	–	–	–
Ambrosetti *et al.* 1989[20]	36	CRC/benign	L	41	4 (11)	17 (47)	21
Dixon and Holmes 1990[26]	32	CRC/obstruction/ perforation	L	32	3 (9	17 (53)	17
Allen-Mersh 1993[27]	35	CRC/benign obstruction/ infection	L	58	6 (17)	22 (63)	–
Total	273	–	–	25	14 (11)	73 (55)	–

* Percentages in parentheses.

PRIMARY RESECTION AND ANASTOMOSIS

More recently, primary resection with immediate anastomosis has been advocated. This approach achieves relief of the obstruction, removal of the tumour and restoration of intestinal continuity at one procedure. A potential disadvantage of this approach is that the bowel is unprepared. Some surgeons simply milk the solid faeces into the segment to be resected;[5] others employ on-table lavage to empty the large bowel proximal to the obstruction.[6] On-table lavage may be performed by inserting a Foley catheter into the caecum via an enterotomy or the base of the appendix and then irrigating the colon with warm Hartmann's solution; the effluent is collected via a closed drainage system. An alternative strategy is to perform a subtotal colectomy to encompass lesions as distal as the sigmoid colon, thus obviating the need to include distended, non-prepared colon in the anastomosis. This may be particularly appropriate in those patients with synchronous tumours or a non-viable caecum.

Clearly, avoidance of multiple operations and a stoma would be justified only if operative morbidity and mortality are no worse than that of primary resection with delayed anastomosis. This approach in selected patients is associated with an anastomotic leak rate of approximately 6% and an operative mortality of 9% (Table 12.3). However, immediate resection and anastomosis is technically more challenging than the alternative procedures and a primary anastomosis, particularly in the hands of an untrained surgeon, is fraught with potential danger: in the Large Bowel Cancer Project, the mortality rate of operations performed by trainees was almost twice that of operations managed by consultants.[4] As well as the seniority of the surgeon, their field of special interest is also of relevance: colorectal surgeons are more likely to perform primary resection and anastomosis than their non-colorectal colleagues.[7]

However, meticulous surgery alone will not guarantee anastomotic healing. Several studies have emphasized the importance of adequate tissue perfusion and oxygen delivery to the anastomosis.[8] There is a critical oxygen level below which anastomotic leakage is inevitable. Intra-operative fluid losses in these patients are often greater than realized; as a result, post-operative splanchnic perfusion is less than optimal. This may be compounded by significant hypoxaemia due to atelectasis or chest infection, to which elderly, frail patients are often prone. It is essential that adequate monitoring is continued into the postoperative period with prompt recognition and correction of adverse trends.

The above results, however, must be interpreted with caution. There is a real paucity of data. Few randomized, prospective comparisons of treatment for obstructing large bowel cancer have been undertaken. It is recognized that any individual surgeon's experience will be limited; therefore, the numbers required for such a study would entail either a long accrual time or a multicentre study, with its inherent intersurgeon variability.

None of the above studies was randomized: all but a few had small numbers and most were undertaken at least a decade ago. Many studies included either right-sided obstructing lesions or patients with benign disease. It is also often not clear whether all available patients were included in the analysis and, if not, what proportion were. Furthermore, the case mix within different studies is likely to vary widely. It is uncommon to provide a tight definition of 'obstruction' and 'emergency'. Some studies are based only on patients who were admitted with obstruction that failed to settle and underwent surgery during the acute phase, whereas others include patients in whom the obstruction settled following admission and subsequently underwent elective surgery, either during the same or at a later admission. There has also been a tendency to treat older, sicker patients by decompression only, and younger fitter patients by primary resection and anastomosis, so that direct comparisons of outcome following different procedures may be misleading.

There have been only two randomized trials. In the Danish study, Kronborg[9] compared three-stage surgery (transverse loop colostomy, then resection with anastomosis and, finally, reversal of loop colostomy) with two-stage surgery (resection with end colostomy and mucous fistula followed by secondary anastomosis) for obstructing large bowel cancer. There were no significant differences in cumulative operative mortality or survival between the two groups (Table 12.4).

Table 12.3. *Results of surgery for obstructing colorectal cancer (CRC): primary resection and immediate anastomosis*

Reference	No. of patients	Pathology	Site	Percentage of total number of patients	No. of deaths*	Anastomotic leak*	Median stay (days)
Amsterdam and Kuspin 1985[28]	25	CRC	L	17	3 (12)	1 (4)	15
Koruth *et al.* 1985[6]	47	CRC/benign	L	90	4 (9)	4 (9)	13
Phillips *et al.* 1985[4]	73	CRC	L	31	–	13 (18)	–
White and Macfie 1985[29]	35	CRC	L	100	3 (9)	4 (12)	18
Pollock *et al.* 1987[30]	41	CRC/benign	L	–	7 (17)	–	12
Naraÿnsingh and Ariyanayagan 1990[31]	30	CRC/benign	L	–	1 (3)	0 (0)	–
Stephenson *et al.* 1990[32]	31	CRC	L	57	1 (3)	3 (9)	17
Antal *et al.* 1991[33]	40	CRC	L	71	0 (0)	0 (0)	16
Murray 1991[34]	29	CRC/benign	L	–	0 (0)	–	–
Rosati *et al.* 1992[35]	29	CRC/benign	L	94	1 (3)	–	–
Stewart *et al.* 1993[36]	63	CRC/benign	L	86	4 (6)	4 (6)	15
Arnaud & Bergamaschi 1994[37]	44	CRC	L	37	3 (7)	2 (5)	–
SCOTIA Study Group 1995[12]	91	CRC	L	82	11 (12)	6 (7)	11
Biondo *et al.* 1997[38]	37	CRC/benign obstruction/ peritonitis	L	33	2 (5)	3 (8)	16
TOTAL	527	–	–	46	45 (9)	34 (6)	–

* Percentages in parentheses; –, information not available

Given the natural history of colorectal cancer, it is not surprising that primary decompression with delayed resection has little detrimental impact on survival when compared with resection at the initial operation. The poor prognosis for patients with colorectal cancer in general, and those presenting as emergencies in particular, is predominately related to the advanced stage of disease at the time of presentation. Even among those patients undergoing apparently curative resection, one-quarter will have occult disseminated disease at the time of surgery.[10] Studies have shown that this occult tumour has been present for several months prior to presentation;[11] the timing of resection is, therefore, unlikely to influence survival.

In the Scotia Study[12] subtotal colectomy was compared with segmental resection with on-table lavage: mortality was similar in both groups (Table 12.5); however, bowel function was less satisfactory in those undergoing subtotal colectomy. Diarrhoea and incontinence was often a problem in the early postoperative period and, although the frequency tended to settle with time, many patients, particularly the elderly, still had 2–5 motions a day.

In summary, therefore, although the results of primary resection and anastomosis can be excellent when undertaken by experienced surgeons, population-based audit has shown that, in less-practised hands, mortality remains high. In ideal circumstances, resection and primary anastomosis by an experienced colorectal surgeon may be appropriate in selected patients. However, when conditions are less favourable, there is still an important role for Hartmann's procedure.

Rectal cancer

Obstruction due to rectal cancer is relatively infrequent. Patients with high rectal tumours have been successfully treated by resection with or without immediate anastomosis. However, recent reports suggest that many patients may be better treated initially by decompression using a transtumoral stent or laser recanalization of the tumour.[13,14] Following relief of the obstruction, tumour resectability can be assessed, the bowel prepared and definitive surgery performed. In those patients with locally advanced lesions, preoperative radiotherapy can be utilized, thereby facilitating subsequent surgery. In patients who are medically unfit, or where there is evidence of metastatic disease, further surgery may not be required.

Table 12.4. *Results of surgery for obstructing colorectal cancer*

Type of surgery	No. of patients	No. of deaths*	No. resected*	No. surviving all stages*	Median stay (days)
Staged resection	28	3 (11)	17 (61)	16 (57)	38
Primary resection and delayed anastomosis	27	5 (19)	27 (100)	15 (56)	34

* Percentages in parentheses.
Adapted from ref. 9.

Table 12.5. *Results of surgery for obstructing colorectal cancer*

Type of surgery	No. of patients	No. of anastomotic leaks*	No. of deaths*	Median stay (days)
Subtotal colectomy	47	4 (9)	6 (13)	12
Segmental colectomy	44	2 (5)	5 (11)	11

* Percentages in parentheses.
Adapted from ref. 12.

Current practice

Pain and Cahill[15] recently reviewed current practice in the United Kingdom. Hartmann's procedure (44%) or sigmoid colectomy with primary anastomosis (40%) were considered to be the optimal choice for obstructing distal large bowel tumours. Alternative techniques, including on-table lavage, subtotal colectomy and 'protection' of an anastomosis with a proximal colostomy, were rarely employed.

Perforation

Approximately 5–10% of patients with colorectal cancer present with overt perforation. Perforation may be at the site of the tumour itself, owing to necrosis, or may occur more proximally, most commonly in the caecum, owing to distension and ischaemia.

Patients with overt perforation are usually extremely ill: features include dehydration, toxaemia, hypoxaemia, oligaemia and uraemia. Most patients also have an element of cardiac failure. Mortality is high. Such patients must be managed aggressively with adequate fluid replacement, correction of electrolyte and acid–base abnormalities, provision of adequate oxygenation including, if necessary, positive-pressure ventilation, and cardiac support. Monitoring should include central venous pressure measurements and hourly urine output. Invasive cardiovascular monitoring may be appropriate; the intensive therapists should be involved at an early stage.

Definitive surgery should consist of a primary resection with exteriorization of the proximal bowel. In the presence of established peritonitis, primary anastomosis is inadvisable, as the septic patient with incipient multiorgan failure is unlikely to achieve adequate perfusion of the anastomosis. In patients with a sigmoid perforation, a Hartmann's procedure should be performed; for more proximal lesions, an extended right hemicolectomy with formation of a mucous fistula may be appropriate.

Bleeding

Though many patients with colorectal cancer present with rectal bleeding, few require emergency surgery. Usually the bleeding is not catastrophic; most patients can be investigated and staged at leisure, secondary elective surgery being undertaken at a later date. Rarely, a colorectal cancer is found unexpectedly while operating for catastrophic colonic bleeding. In these patients the tumour should be resected; primary anastomosis should probably be avoided, especially if the patient has been shocked at any stage.

Outcome

There are a number of reasons why patients who present as emergencies have a poorer outlook than those who undergo elective surgery. These include the fact that patients who present as emergencies tend to be older, tend to present with more advanced disease than their elective counterparts and are less likely to have their tumour resected. Emergency patients also tend to have higher postoperative mortality rates and poor long-term survival.

For example, of 1128 patients presenting to Glasgow Royal Infirmary (GRI) with colorectal cancer between 1974 and 1984 (Table 12.6), 34% presented as emergencies.[16] Half those admitted for elective surgery had clinical evidence of local tumour fixity or disseminated disease at the time of presentation; 39% had a Dukes' A or B tumour; in contrast, two-thirds of those admitted as an emergency had clinical evidence of advanced disease at the time of initial presentation; only 27% had a Dukes' A or B tumour.

Resection rates were consistently lower in those presenting as emergencies; whereas the tumour was resected in 78% of those presenting electively, the tumour was resected in only 60% of patients presenting as emergencies (Table 12.7). Whether this difference reflects resectability *per se* is debatable. Whereas virtually all patients with no evidence of spread at the time of laparotomy underwent potentially curative resection, irrespective of whether they presented electively or as emergencies, the

Table 12.6. *Characteristics of patients undergoing surgery for colorectal cancer*

	Elective*	Emergency*
Total no. of patients	675	351
Age (years)		
< 55	114 (17)	57 (16)
55–64	176 (26)	72 (21)
65–74	242 (36)	112 (32)
> 75	140 (21)	111 (31)
Site of tumour		
Caecum Ascending colon Hepatic flexure Transverse colon	124 (18)	81 (23)
Splenic flexure Descending colon	70 (10)	96 (27)
Sigmoid colon	158 (23)	94 (27)
Rectum	298 (44)	70 (20)
Tumour spread		
None	329 (49)	127 (36)
Local	142 (21)	91 (26)
Distant	53 (8)	42 (12)
Local and distant	118 (17)	52 (15)
Dukes' classification		
A	39 (6)	5 (1)
B	225 (33)	91 (26)
C	167 (25)	78 (22)
Distand metastases	186 (28)	112 (32)

* Percentages in parentheses.

Table 12.7. *Relationship between extent of disease and treatment*

	Treatment*	
Extent	Elective	Emergency
No spread		
Curative resection	329 (100)	122 (100)
Local spread		
Curative resection	65 (46)	23 (25)
Palliative resection	33 (23)	25 (27)
Palliative diversion	43 (30)	40 (44)
Distant spread		
Palliative resection	40 (75)	22 (52)
Palliative diversion	10 (19)	13 (31)
Laparotomy only/no operation	3 (6)	7 (17)
Local and distant spread		
Palliative resection	58 (49)	19 (37)
Palliative diversion	47 (40)	21 (40)
Laparotomy only/no operation	13 (11)	12 (23)

* Percentages in parentheses.

curative resection rate in patients who presented as an emergency with evidence of local spread is only 25% compared with 46% of similar elective patients. Patients with evidence of distant spread were also less likely to have their tumours resected if they presented as emergencies (52 vs 75%). Furthermore, resection rates fell with age: for example, only 47% of those patients aged over 75 years presenting as emergencies underwent resection compared with 72% of those presenting electively. It appears, therefore, that resection rates may be influenced by the surgeon's perception of the extent of disease and a degree of pessimism about outlook.

Operative mortality was higher in the emergency group, particularly in elderly patients and those who underwent palliative diversion (Table 12.8): for example, 31% of emergency patients aged over 75 years died in the postoperative period compared with only 16% of those presenting electively; 41% of those undergoing emergency palliative diversion died compared with only 20% of those undergoing elective palliative diversion. Five-year survival was also poorer (Table 12.9): for example, only 26% of those patients presenting as emergencies and undergoing apparently curative resection survived 5 years compared with 45% of a similar group who presented electively.

These results are typical of population-based studies in the United Kingdom. In the Large Bowel Cancer Project, age-adjusted 5-year survival for emergency patients was only 25% compared with 45% for elective patients. Similarly, Serpell and his colleagues[17] showed that patients with obstructing colonic tumours had a significant reduction in 5-year cancer-specific survival compared with non-obstructed cases, even though there was no difference in the distribution of tumour stage between the groups.

Table 12.8. *Operative mortality*

Age (years)	Elective*	Emergency*
<55	4 (4)	9 (16)
55–64	18 (10)	12 (17)
65–74	18 (7)	22 (20)
> 75	23 (16)	34 (31)
Type of surgery		
Curative resection	22 (6)	11 (8)
Palliative resection	15 (11)	8 (12)
Palliative diversion	20 (20)	34 (41)
Total mortality	63 (9)	77 (22)

* Percentages in parentheses.

INTER-SURGEON VARIABILITY

Postoperative morbidity, postoperative mortality and ultimate survival also varied from surgeon to surgeon. In the GRI study, nine surgeons each supervised the management of more than 20 emergency patients (Table 12.10). Overall postoperative mortality of these patients varied among surgeons from 13 to 47%, and 5-year survival from 0 to 26%. The

Table 12.9. *Five-year survival (%) in patients undergoing surgery for colorectal cancer*

	Elective*	Emergency*
All cases: all-cause mortality (*n* = 675)	28	12
All cases: cancer-specific mortality (*n* = 675)	34	15
All resections: all-cause mortality (*n* = 529)	35	20
All resections: cancer-specific mortality (*n* = 529)	43	25
Curative resection: all-cause mortality (*n* = 398)	45	26
Curative resection: cancer-specific mortality (*n* = 398)	55	32
Palliative resection: cancer-specific mortality (*n* = 131)	6	8

Table 12.10. *Effect of the surgeon on 5-year survival following emergency admission*

All cases				Curative resections	
Surgeon	No. of cases	Postoperative mortality*	5-year survival (%)	No. of cases*	5-year survival (%)
A	48	14 (29)	5	25 (52)	9
B	30	6 (20)	10	13 (43)	23
C	27	10 (37)	7	6 (22)	17
D	19	6 (32)	0	5 (26)	0
E	25	8 (32)	4	8 (32)	12
F	23	3 (13)	26	13 (56)	46
G	17	8 (47)	12	5 (29)	40
H	24	5 (21)	21	14 (58)	36
I	20	6 (30)	10	5 (25)	40

* Percentages in parentheses

proportion undergoing curative resection varied from 22 to 58%; 5-year survival varied from 0 to 46%.

There is evidence to suggest that better results are achieved by senior anaesthetists and surgeons. In the authors' study, consultants performed the majority of the surgery on electively admitted patients. However, consultants were present at less than half of those emergency operations occurring within 48 hours of admission.

It might be argued that these are historical data and therefore bear little relation to the current situation. Preliminary analysis of current audit data from the West of Scotland shows that one-third of patients still present as emergencies. However, it is interesting to note that overall mortality has fallen from 22 to 10%, probably as a result of better preoperative preparation and postoperative support rather than of improvements in surgical technique.

Recommendations

In summary, patients who present as emergencies with large bowel cancer tend to be older and present with advanced disease. Especially in the elderly, resection rates tend to be lower, operative mortality higher and survival poorer. There is evidence to suggest that better preoperative preparation, appropriate surgery and improved postoperative care may reduce perioperative morbidity and mortality. Although the results of primary resection and anastomosis can be excellent when undertaken by experienced, individual surgeons, population-based audit has shown that in less-practised hands mortality remains high. In ideal circumstances, therefore, resection and primary anastomosis by an experienced colorectal surgeon may be appropriate in selected patients; however, when conditions are less favourable, there is still an important role for Hartmann's procedure.

References

1. Cancer Research Campaign. Cancer of the large bowel – UK Factsheet, London, 18.1.1993

2. Allum WH, Slaney G, McConkey CC, Powell J. Cancer of the colon and rectum in the West Midlands, 1957–1981. *Br J Surg* 1994; 81: 1060–1063

3. Campling EA, Devlin HB, Hoile RW *et al. The Report of the National Confidential Enquiry into Perioperative Deaths 1991/92*. London: Nuffield Provincial Hospitals Trust and Kings Fund for Hospitals, 1993.

4. Phillips RKS, Hittinger R, Fry JS, Fielding LP. Malignant large bowel obstruction. *Br J Surg* 1985; 72: 296–302

5. Mealy K, Salman A, Arthur G. Definitive one-stage emergency large bowel surgery. *Br J Surg* 1988; 75: 1216–1219

6. Koruth NM, Krukowski ZH, Youngson GG *et al.* Intra-operative colonic irrigation in the management of left-sided large bowel emergencies. *Br J Surg* 1985; 72: 708–711

7. Darby CR, Berry AR, Mortensen N. Management variability in surgery for colorectal emergencies. *Br J Surg* 1992; 79: 206–210

8. Anderson JH, McArdle CS. Obstructing large bowel cancer. *Curr Prac Surg* 1993; 5: 191–194

9. Kronborg O. The missing randomized trial of two surgical treatments for acute obstruction due to carcinoma of the left colon and rectum. *Int J Colorectal Dis* 1986; 1: 162–166

10. Finlay IG, McArdle CS. Occult hepatic metastases in colorectal carcinoma. *Br J Surg* 1986; 73: 732–735

11. Findlay IG, Meek D, Bruton F, McArdle CS. Growth rate of hepatic metastases in colorectal cancer. *Br J Surg* 1988; 75: 641–644

12. SCOTIA Study Group. Single-stage treatment for malignant left-sided colonic obstruction: a prospective randomized clinical trial comparing subtotal colectomy with segmental resection following intraoperative irrigation. *Br J Surg* 1995; 82: 1622–1627

13. Eckhauser ML, Imbembo AL, Mansour EG. The role of pre-resectional laser recanalization for obstructing carcinomas of the colon and rectum. *Surgery* 1989; 106: 710–717

14. Turegano-Fuentes F, Echenagusia-Belda A, Simo-Muerza G *et al.* Transanal self-expanding metal stents as an alternative to palliative colostomy in selected patients with malignant obstruction of the left colon. *Br J Surg* 1998; 85: 232–235

15. Pain J, Cahill J. Surgical options for left-sided large bowel emergencies. *Ann R Coll Surg Engl* 1981; 73: 394–397

16. McArdle CS, Wotherspoon H, Hole D, Murray GD. Colorectal cancer: a continuing problem. *GI Cancer* 1996; 1: 171–176

17. Serpell JW, McDermott FT, Katrivessis H, Hughes ESR. Obstructing carcinomas of the colon. *Br J Surg* 1989; 76: 965–969

18. Hoffmann J, Jensen HE. Tube cecostomy and staged resection for obstructing carcinoma of the left colon. *Dis Colon Rectum* 1984; 27: 24–32

19. Buechter KJ, Boustany C, Caillouette R, Cohn I. Survival management of the acutely obstructed colon. *Am J Surg* 1988; 156: 163–168

20. Ambrosetti P, Borst F, Robert J *et al.* L'exérèse-anastomose en un temps dans les occlusions coliques gauches operées en urgence. *Chirurgie* 1989; 115: 1–7

21. Gutman M, Kaplan O, Skornick Y *et al.* Proximal colostomy: still an effective emergency measure in obstructing carcinoma of the large bowel. *J Surg Oncol* 1989; 41: 210–212

22. Kristiansen VB, Sorensen C, Kjaergaard J, Jensen HE. Cecostomy can not be recommended as a routine method in the treatment of acute left-sided obstructive colon cancer. *Ugeskr Laeger* 1990; 152: 101–103

23. Runkel NS, Schlag P, Schwarz V, Herfarth C. Outcome after emergency surgery for cancer of the large intestine. *Br J Surg* 1991; 78: 183–188

24. Gandrup P, Lund L, Balslev I. Surgical treatment of acute malignant large bowel obstruction. *Eur J Surg* 1992; 158: 427–430

25. Sjodahl R, Franzen T, Nystrom P-O. Primary versus staged resection for acute obstructing colorectal carcinoma. *Br J Surg* 1992; 79: 685–688

26. Dixon AR, Holmes JT. Hartmann's procedure for carcinoma of rectum and distal sigmoid colon: 5-year audit. *J R Coll Surg Edinb* 1990; 35: 166–168

27. Allen-Mersh TG. Should primary anastomosis and on-table colonic lavage be standard treatment for left colon emergencies? *Ann R Coll Surg Engl* 1993; 75: 195–198

28. Amsterdam E, Krispin M. Primary resection with colocolostomy for obstructive carcinoma of the left side of the colon. *Am J Surg* 1985; 150: 558–560

29. White CM, Macfie J. Immediate colectomy and primary anastomosis for acute obstruction due to carcinoma of the left colon and rectum. *Dis Colon Rectum* 1985; 28: 155–157

30. Pollock AV, Playforth MJ, Evan M. Peroperative lavage of the obstructed left colon to allow safe primary anastomosis. *Dis Colon Rectum* 1987; 30: 171–173

31. Naraynsingh V, Ariyanayagam DC. Obstructive left colon: one-stage surgery in a developing country. *J R Coll Surg Edinb* 1990; 35: 360–361

32. Stephenson BM, Shadall AA, Farouk R, Griffith G. Malignant left-sided large bowel obstruction managed by subtotal/total colectomy. *Br J Surg* 1990; 77: 1092–1102

33. Antal SC, Kovacs ZG, Feigenbaum V, Engelberg M. Obstructing carcinoma of the left colon: treatment by extended right hemicolectomy. *Int Surg* 1991; 76: 161–163

34. Murray JJ. Nonelective colon resection. Alternatives to multistage resections. *Surg Clin North Am* 1991; 71: 1187–1194

35. Rosati C, Smith L, Deitel M *et al.* Primary colorectal anastomosis with the intracolonic bypass tube. *Surgery* 1992; 112: 618–622

36. Stewart J, Diament RH, Brennan TG. Management of obstructing lesions of the left colon by resection, on-table lavage, and primary anastomosis. *Surgery* 1993; 114: 502–505

37. Arnaud J-P, Bergamaschi R. Emergency subtotal/total colectomy with anastomosis for acutely obstructed carcinoma of the left colon. *Dis Colon Rectum* 1994; 37: 685–688

38. Biondo S, Jaurrieta E, Jorba R *et al.* Intraoperative colonic lavage and primary anastomosis in peritonitis and obstruction. *Br J Surg* 1997; 84: 222–225

INDEX

A

B

C

D

E

F

G

H

I

N

O

P

Q

R

S

T

U

V

W

X